The Clinical Nurse Specialist

Implementation and Impact

The Clinical Nurse Specialist

Implementation and Impact

Editors

Patricia S.A. Sparacino, M.S., R.N.
Clinical Nurse Specialist, Cardiovascular Surgery
Assistant Clinical Professor
The Medical Center at the University of California
San Francisco, California

Diane M. Cooper, Ph.D., R.N.
Robert Wood Johnson Clinical Nurse Scholar
School of Nursing
University of California, San Francisco

Formerly, Clinical Nurse Specialist
The Medical Center at the University of California
San Francisco, California

Pamela A. Minarik, M.S., R.N.
Psychiatric Liaison Clinical Nurse Specialist
Assistant Clinical Professor
The Medical Center at the University of California
San Francisco, California

APPLETON & LANGE
Norwalk, Connecticut

0-8385-1278-X

Copyright © 1990 by Appleton & Lange
A Publishing Division of Prentice Hall

90 91 92 93 94 / 10 9 8 7 6 5 4 3 2 1

Prentice-Hall International (UK) Limited, *London*
Prentice-Hall of Australia Pty. Limited, *Sydney*
Prentice-Hall of Canada Inc., *Toronto*
Prentice-Hall Hispanoamericana, S.A., *Mexico*
Prentice-Hall of India Private Limited, *New Delhi*
Prentice-Hall of Japan, Inc., *Tokyo*
Simon & Schuster Asia Pte. Ltd., *Singapore*
Editora Prentice-Hall do Brasil, Ltda., *Rio de Janeiro*
Prentice Hall, *Englewood Cliffs, New Jersey*

Library of Congress Cataloging-in-Publication Data

The clinical nurse specialist : implementation and impact / editors,
  Patricia S.A. Sparacino, Diane M. Cooper, Pamela A. Minarik.
  p.   cm.
  Bibliography: p.
  Includes index.
  ISBN 0-8385-1278-X
  1. Nurse practitioners.   I. Sparacino, Patricia S. A.
II. Cooper, Diane M.   III. Minarik, Pamela A.
  [DNLM: 1. Nurse Clinicians.   WY 128 C6385]
RT82.8.C56   1989
610.73'6—dc20
DNLM/DLC   89-6656
for Library of Congress   CIP

Acquisitions Editor: Janet Foltin
Production Editor: Lauren Manjoney
Designer: Janice Barsevich

PRINTED IN THE UNITED STATES OF AMERICA

Contributors

■ **Carrol A. Alvarez, M.S., R.N., C.S.**
Clinical Nurse Specialist, Psychiatry
Harborview Medical Center
Seattle, Washington

■ **Lora E. Burke, M.N., R.N.**
Cardiovascular Clinical Specialist
Collaborative Practice, Cardiology
Assistant Clinical Professor
University of California—Los Angeles School of Nursing
Los Angeles, California

■ **Margaret K. Chang, M.N., R.N, C., C.C.R.N.**
Clinical Nurse Specialist, Medicine and Gerontology
San Diego Veterans Administration Medical Center
San Diego, California

■ **Diane M. Cooper, Ph.D., R.N.**
Robert Wood Johnson Clinical Nurse Scholar
School of Nursing
University of California, San Francisco

Formerly, Clinical Nurse Specialist
The Medical Center at the University of California
San Francisco, California

■ **Lori Howell, M.S., R.N.**
Clinical Nurse Specialist, Pediatric Surgery
Assistant Clinical Professor
The Medical Center at the University of California
San Francisco, California

■ **Pamela A. Minarik, M.S., R.N.**
Psychiatric Liaison Clinical Nurse Specialist
Assistant Clinical Professor
The Medical Center at the University of California
San Francisco, California

■ **Diana L. Nikas, M.N., R.N., C.C.R.N., C.N.R.N.**
Clinical Nurse Specialist, Critical Care and Neuroscience Nursing
Director, Clinical-Professional Development and Research
Harbor–UCLA Medical Center
Torrance, California

■ **Patricia S.A. Sparacino, M.S., R.N.**
Clinical Nurse Specialist, Cardiovascular Surgery
Assistant Clinical Professor
The Medical Center at the University of California
San Francisco, California

■ **Margretta M. Styles, Ed.D., R.N., FAAN**
Professor and Livingston Chair in Nursing
School of Nursing
University of California, San Francisco
San Francisco, California

■ **Janet D'Agostino Taylor, M.S.N., R.N.**
Pulmonary Rehabilitation Clinical Specialist
St. Elizabeth's Hospital
Boston, Massachusetts

■ **Deborah Welch-McCaffrey, M.S.N., R.N., O.C.N.**
Oncology Clinical Nurse Specialist
Good Samaritan Cancer Center
Phoenix, Arizona

Reviewers

■ **Pamela F. Cipriano R.N., M.N.**
Director of Nursing Development
Medical University Hospital
Medical University of South Carolina
Charleston, South Carolina

■ **Sr. Rosemarie Donley, Ph.D., M.N.Ed., B.S.N., FAAN**
Executive Vice President and Associate Professor
Catholic University
Washington, D.C.

■ **Nancy Steiger, R.N., B.S., M.S.**
Vice President for Nursing
Santa Rosa Memorial Hospital
Santa Rosa, California

Contents

Preface

The time for passivity in nursing is over! Nursing exists in a dynamic present that is moving into an uncertain future (Sullivan et al., 1987). In the midst of this movement one group of nurses, clinical nurse specialists in particular, is caught in a controversy created by cost containment efforts and the nursing shortage.

Clinical nurse specialists have been labeled positively as "the salvation of nursing" and "catalysts for change." In contrast, others have referred to them as the "icing on the cake" and "high-priced luxuries." Situations continue to occur that demonstrate an ambiguous understanding of the role and the impact of clinical nurse specialists on care. In some settings hospital administrators and nurse executives question, on the basis of cost containment, the continuation or development of positions for clinical nurse specialists. Other clinical nurse specialists are forced to assume positions or function in roles that underutilize their capabilities and limit the scope of their effectiveness.

The clinical nurse specialist, however, is an identified role within the profession of nursing (Hoeffer & Murphy, 1984). Not only did the American Nurses' Association clearly define the clinical nurse specialist in 1980, but other specialty organizations and state nurses' associations have described formally the requisites and competencies of individuals who assume the title (American Association of Critical Care Nurses, 1987; California Nurses' Association, 1984). Further evidence of their acceptance came in 1982 when a separate Council of Clinical Nurse Specialists became a reality within the American Nurses' Association, and a study undertaken by the Council reported the existence of more than 19,000 registered nurses functioning as clinical nurse specialists within the United States (ANA, 1986). With increasing utilization of the role, the quarterly journal, *Clinical Nurse Specialist*, began publication. Born out of a recognized need for a forum where clinical nurse specialists could exchange ideas, this journal provides an avenue where strategies employed by specialists in role implementation and case management can be shared. Essential components of the clinical nurse specialist role are addressed and described through the organized presentation of articles on the clinical nurse specialist as researcher, consultant, educator, and executive.

In their book, *The Relationship of Theory and Research*, Fawcett and Downs (1986) define *theories* as "classified as descriptive, explanatory, or predictive" (p. 4). *Descriptive theories*, the most basic, "describe or classify specific dimensions or characteristics of individuals, groups, situations, or events by summarizing the commonalities found in discrete observations." Descriptive theories state "what is" (Fawcett & Downs, 1986, p. 5). As a means of ensuring that the nature of anything be understood, it must be well described. If circumstances change, new descriptions must follow. With the number of variables impacting the evolution of advanced practice in nursing, it will be some years before it can be said that specialists in nursing, the clinical nurse specialist in particular, have been over-described.

Definitions and competencies inherent in the role of the clinical nurse specialist are usually taught during formal education. Perhaps clinical nurse specialist students and practicing clinical nurse specialists are receiving adequate information on role theory and the strategies of role implementation. The effect of this input via peer discussions, journal articles, and regional clinical nurse specialist conferences might lead interested parties to the conclusion that the "is-ness" or "what-ness" of the clinical nurse specialist is known. Perhaps all that needs to be said about clinical nurse specialists appears to have been said. The contributors to this book, however, believe otherwise. This book has been written in response to the expressed need for a text that provides a picture of "how to" integrate effectively the components of the clinical nurse specialist role. It will be useful for clinical nurse specialist students in a graduate program and their faculty, for newly employed as well as experienced clinical nurse specialists, and for nursing administrators and other employers of clinical nurse specialists.

The book has been divided into three sections: Part One provides an overall framework, setting the stage for the chapters that follow. Issues addressed in Part One are the historical context from which the role evolved, the essential role components, the particulars of obtaining a position, moving into the role in the initial phase, role evaluation, and the assessment of the role through research.

Spurred on by the descriptive work done on the clinical nurse specialist role in the past, and realizing that there is yet much to be gleaned from analysis of successful clinical nurse specialists, the contributors to Part Two focus in some detail on the discrete aspects of individual clinical nurse specialist roles. This section chronicles the experiences of ten clinical nurse specialists, selected for their identified expertise. The section is introduced by a series of core questions that are central to the implementation of the role and assessment of impact. They are designed to encourage comparison of similarities and differences in the implementation of the role in varied specialties and practice settings. Through the medium of a self-selected case study, each clinical nurse specialist reveals a personal assessment and evaluation of the characteristics of clinical nursing specialization. To aid in comparison and analysis by the reader, each of the chapters contained in Part Two has been organized in the following manner. Initially a case study is presented. This is followed by the clinical nurse specialist's intervention, including method of patient selection and criteria used to determine the appropriate intervention; the method of communication used by the clinical nurse specialist with patients and other members of the health care team; and the clinical nurse specialist's assessment of the impact of the interventions on patient outcomes and cost/benefit ratios. Additionally, a description of the role within each of the practice settings is provided as well as how the clinical nurse specialist incorporates research in practice.

Each of these chapters concludes with specific questions that address particular aspects of the role described in each chapter. These questions have not been generated in an attempt to standardize the role or be critical of our peers. Rather, the questions are presented as basis for discussion and to elucidate the constant thread that is present in the definition of the role throughout existing differences in specialty, setting, and experience.

Finally, this being a time when some question the future of the role of the clinical nurse specialist, when others suggest that the differences between master's and baccalaureate expectations are becoming increasingly blurred, and when a growing number of writers suggest that the doctorate be established as the entry level to practice (Beecroft & Papenhausen, 1987; Christman, 1987), Part Three of this book discusses and challenges clinical nursing specialization in the future.

As in this book, the systematic logging of clinical practice by clinical nurse specialists can serve a number of significant functions, namely serving as anecdotes from which others can learn as well as providing data that can be used to build theory. Benner renewed our awareness of the power of a story in her book, *From Novice to Expert* (1984). Readers are privileged not only to read nurses' descriptions of positive "critical incidents" of their interactions with patients, but also are led through a process by which they are able to detect the fine gradations, the fine-tuning that distinguishes the expert nurse from the novice. As each nurse's story unfolds in Benner's book, the reader begins to identify the indications of the "mystery of expert nursing" (p.v). One reads what the nurses describe and one *sees* differences in levels of nursing skill. The invaluable contribution made by the nurses who were encouraged by Benner to tell their stories is that these significant interactions are logged, and therefore can act as graphic portrayals on which others can reflect. In order for clinical nurse specialists to identify and articulate their unique contribution to health care, they must be clear about the generic similarities in their role definitions as well as the gradations of skill in the implementation of the role. To insure this, the critical incidents in the clinical nurse specialist's practice must be told and systematically logged. The story-telling approach to descriptive research facilitates and accelerates the potential for the evolution of theory regarding the role of the clinical nurse specialist. At the same time, logging the critical incidents provides individual cases for ongoing analysis by clinical nurse specialists, nursing administrators, educators, and students.

In the past, clinical nurse specialists described their roles, particularly in hospitals, in some detail. Despite development of the role and the continued need for evolution in role descriptions, more recently due to changing economic trends in health care, clinical nurse specialists have focused on documenting their impact within various settings as a means of maintaining their positions. Although documentation of clinical nurse specialist activities certainly is necessary and should proceed with all haste, it is equally important not to move away too quickly from descriptions of the "is-ness" of the clinical nurse specialist in whatever practice setting.

This book, not unlike the report on *Magnet Hospitals* by the American Academy of Nursing in 1983, chooses among other things to focus on and "capture that which works" (Ferguson, 1983, p. vii) by including the personal role descriptions of clinical nurse specialists recognized for their expertise in the "is-ness" of clinical nursing specialization.

Unlike single journal articles or anecdotal accounts discussed between specialists or among students, it is the intent of the authors that this text, having gathered clinical nurse specialists' stories, surrounded them in historial context, and grounded them in role theory and futuristic thinking, will afford the reader a unique opportunity to focus deliberately and repeatedly on analysis of the essentials of clinical nursing specialization. In doing so, the text provides the reader a journey into the clinical nurse specialist's world as perceived through the eyes of individuals well-versed in the wealth of its realities and possibilities. The interested reader will be allowed to ponder in a more systematic manner the core or essence of the role, as well as the variations and gradations in skill in role implementation and impact.

Each of the contributors sincerely hopes that this book will offer a perspective different from the growing body of writings on the role of the clinical nurse specialist. To the clinical nurse specialist student, may the case studies help you determine the "is-ness" of what you strive for; to faculty, may first-hand, in-depth analyses of role components and role implementation serve as a basis for ongoing student discussion; and last, but certainly not least, to clinical nurse specialists, may the content of this book act as an ongoing reference, helping to rekindle and energize your efforts at excellence in practice through providing you with a series of alternative strategies in role performance. To all who read this book, may it be a reminder that there are specialists in the art and science of nursing practice "out there" who are firmly committed to the role of the clinical nurse specialist and to making and logging their significant and unique impact on patient care, and thus simultaneously on nursing practice.

BIBLIOGRAPHY

American Association of Critical Care Nurses. (1987). *AACN position statement: The critical care clinical nurse specialist: Role definition.* Newport Beach, CA: American Association of Critical Care Nurses.

American Academy of Nursing. (1983). *Magnet hospitals.* Kansas City, MO: American Nurses' Association.

American Nurses' Association (1986). *Clinical nurse specialists: Distribution and utilization.* Kansas City, MO: American Nurses' Association.

Beecroft, P., & Papenhausen, J. (1984). Editorial opinion. *Clinical Nurse Specialist* 1:53.

Benner P. (1984). *From novice to expert.* Menlo Park, CA: Addison-Wesley.

California Nurses' Association. (1984). *Position statement on specialization in nursing practice.* San Francisco, CA: California Nurses' Association.

Christman, L. (1987). The future of the nursing profession. *Nursing Administration Quarterly* 11:1–8.

Fawcett, J., & Downs, F. (1986). *The relationship of theory and research.* Norwalk, CT: Appleton & Lange.

Ferguson, V. (1983). Foreword. In *Magnet hospitals: Attraction and retention of professional nurses* p. VII. Kansas City, MO: American Nurses' Association.

Hoeffer, B. & Murphy, S. (1984). Specialization in nursing practice. In *Issues in professional nursing-practice.* p. 1–10. Kansas City, MO: American Nurses' Association.

Sullivan, T.J., Lee, J.L., & Warnick, M.L., et al. (1987). Nursing 2020: A study of nursing's future. *Nursing Outlook, 35,* 233–235.

Diane M. Cooper
May, 1989

Acknowledgments

To those with the vision to develop and expand the role.
To those with the conviction to support the role.
To those who have influenced each of us in our professional education, development, and growth.
To our patients for teaching us lessons in life and healing.
To the nursing staff with whom we have had the pleasure to work, for their clinical excellence and support.
To Cheyney Johansen, for her unfailing patience, editorial assistance, and willingness to type countless drafts.
To our families and friends for their endurance and humor in weathering our storms of creativity.
To each other—true colleagues!

part one

Framework for Practice

chapter one

A Historical Perspective on the Development of the Clinical Nurse Specialist Role

Patricia S. A. Sparacino

According to the American Nurses' Association (1980), specialization in nursing is currently well established and is indicative of the advancement of the nursing profession. Fiscal constraints in the current health care environment have led to questions about how well established the role actually is in some health care organizations. That does not negate the clarity in the profession about the clinical nurse specialist role, as illustrated in the following quotations.

> Specialization means a narrowed focus on a part of the whole field of nursing. It entails application of a broad range of theories to selected phenomena within the domain of nursing, in order to secure depth of understanding as a basis for advances in nursing practice (American Nurses' Association, 1980, p. 21).
>
> The specialist in nursing practice is a nurse who, through study and supervised clinical practice at the graduate level (master's or doctorate), has become expert in a defined area of knowledge and practice in a selected clinical area of nursing (ANA, 1980, p. 23).
>
> The clinical nurse specialist's role is multifaceted. The specialist is an expert in clinical practice, an educator, a consultant, a researcher, and may be an administrator.... The boundaries of the speciality are defined by the phenomena of interest to the clinical nurse specialist. These phenomena may change, reflecting the needs of society, and may therefore cause the boundaries to expand. (ANA, 1986a, pp. 2, 5)

To better understand how it is that the profession has arrived at this point, this chapter will present a historical perspective.

HISTORICAL DEVELOPMENT

The sequence of events that has guided the development of nursing specialization in general, and the role of the clinical nurse specialist in particular, can be attributed to a large increase in knowledge germane to specialization, new technology that requires intellectual competencies and complex skills, and a response to public need (Peplau, 1965). The first reference made in the nursing literature about specialities in nursing and its impact on the profession was DeWitt (1900), who attributed the development of nursing specialities to a response to "present civilization and modern science [which] demand a perfection along each line of work formerly unknown" (p. 1). While the nineteenth-century nurse was expected to perform household duties in addition to assisting the physician, DeWitt urged that "the new nurse is more useful, at least to the patient himself, and ultimately to the family and community. Her sphere is more limited, but her patient receives better care" (p. 1). She viewed speciality nursing as following the medical model, responding to a need for perfection within a limited domain, and generally limited to nursing certain types of patients or working for a speciality physician.

For most of the first half of the twentieth century, many nurses, particularly those employed in hospitals, worked for extended periods of time with specific populations of patients. In order to care for specific patient populations, these nurses established guidelines in an attempt to organize approaches to care. Within these general guidelines these nurses no doubt also established an "acuity" of symptoms which caused them to respond to the extremely ill in a manner different from the less acutely ill patient. Often these nurses became recognized and greatly respected for the wealth of information they possessed as well as their ability to appropriately intervene and provide direct care. Such nurses were often regarded as "specialists." Yet prior to World War II, most postgraduate courses beyond hospital training schools were functional courses aimed at preparing the nurse administrator or nurse educator. The few courses offered to provide advanced education in a clinical area were in response to social forces and were generally limited to public health nursing and its subspecialties (Hoeffer & Murphy, 1984).

In 1943 Frances Reiter promoted the idea of the "nurse-clinician". This concept embodied three aspects of clinical practice: (1) clinical competence in the dimensions of depth of understanding, range of function, and breadth of services; (2) clinical expertise for coordination of and responsibility for continuity of care; and (3) professional maturity in collaboration with the medical profession (Reiter, 1966). Also in 1943, the National League of Nursing Education (NLNE) began to address the basic principles that should determine advanced clinical nursing courses. Psychiatric nursing was chosen to illustrate the method. The NLNE's progress report recommended a plan to develop clinical nurse specialists, and the report urged qualified universities to undertake this experiment (Mayo, 1944).

During World War II, there was an acute nursing shortage, with insufficient numbers of generalists, let alone specialists.* In 1948 Esther Lucile Brown emphasized the necessity for specialists within clinical nursing as a basis for strengthening and developing the profession. As the NLNE made further recommendations, the emphasis was on shifting the focus from functional roles to developing competence and expertise in a clinical nursing area. The first program designed specifically to prepare clinical nurse specialists at the master's level began in 1954 when Rutgers University initiated a curriculum for psychiatric nurses. Subsequently, the National Working Conference on Graduate Education in Psychiatric Nursing developed curriculum recommendations to promote an in-depth knowledge base and expert skills (National League for Nursing, 1958).

During the 1960s there was a shortage of physicians, and this provided the milieu to expand nursing clinical specialization programs at the graduate level, with federal stipends available to prepare specialists in several clinical areas (Hoeffer & Murphy, 1984). Peplau (1965) raised the issues of whether nurse specialists should be categorized by area of practice, subspecialty of an organ or body system, age of the client, degree of illness, length of illness, nurse activity, field of knowledge, subrole of a staff nurse role, professional goal, or clinical services that would follow the medical model. She raised these issues to ensure that nursing would be defined in the situation of practice and that specifically clinical nurse specialists would be the ones to define standards of clinical practice.

By 1970 there were master's-level programs to prepare clinical nurse specialists and the role had been implemented in a variety of practice settings and specialty areas. Graduate education as entry level preparation, however, had not been mandated, and there was confusion about the multiple use of role titles such as nurse clinician, nursing specialist, expert clinician, clinical nurse scientist, and clinical nurse specialist. Lewis (1970) expressed the profession's concern by questioning the exact purpose, preparation, function, responsibility, and practice setting utilization of the clinical nurse specialist.

By 1980 the social policy statement of the American Nurses' Association defined specialization in nursing for its professional members and for society at large. The statement's greatest impact lies in the public

---

*A nurse generalist provides a comprehensive approach to health care and can meet diversified health concerns. Generalists in nursing provide the bulk of the care for most of the people served by nursing. A nurse specialist provides an expert approach to health focused on a refined body of knowledge and specialized practice competencies (American Nurses' Association, 1980, p. 19).

declaration of the criteria *required* to assume the title of clinical nurse specialist. Numerous bodies, including state nursing organizations and councils within the professional organization, have embraced the definition of the specialist in nursing as written and have supported the distinguishing characteristics in similar statements on specialization in nursing (American Association of Critical Care Nurses Position Statement, 1987; American Nurses' Association, 1986a; California Nurses' Association, 1984).

The support of the role by the professional association is demonstrated in the creation of the Council of Clinical Nurse Specialists. The first meeting of the executive committee of the American Nurses' Association Council of Clinical Nurse Specialists was held in February 1983. The council's creation evolved over a 3-year period during which the original idea of a council of advanced medical-surgical nurses changed to a council for master's-prepared clinical nurse specialists. Among its many functions, the council provides a forum for clinical nurse specialists and a central repository of documents and information about the role. The continued growth of the role and the council is evident in the publication of the clinical nurse specialist role statement (ANA, 1986a), a survey of clinical nurse specialist distribution and utilization (ANA, 1986b), and a collaborative research proposal to study the impact of the clinical nurse specialist on care outcomes of a specific patient population.

The clinical nurse specialist role has grown and developed from a vague concept at the beginning of the twentieth century to the clearly-defined and widely accepted role it is today. While clarity has been achieved in role definition, there remains a continuing lack of consistency in the core content of educational preparation.

EDUCATION FOR SPECIALIZATION

While the clinical nurse specialist role exists in a variety of settings and the boundaries of speciality practice may be determined by client need or specialist's interest, there is agreement that the entry level for clinical nurse specialist practice is the graduate level (master's or doctorate degree), with expertise in a selected area of clinical practice.

After the National League of Nursing Education made its many recommendations in the 1940s and graduate programs had been developed, further recommendations were made in 1969 by the National League for Nursing's Council of Baccalaureate and Higher Degree Programs to incorporate into the curriculum broad foundations in the theoretical sciences, specialized clinical practice, and research and teaching skills (National League for Nursing, 1969).

Out of this period of educational development, there have been a multiplicity of graduate programs, but with no consistency in preparation nor agreement about the balance between clinical specialist and other functional role preparation. There is also growing debate as to whether the master's degree should be the entry level for professional practice and the doctorate for speciality practice (Andreoli, 1986).

Graduate curricula for clinical nurse specialist preparation should have a framework (Diers, 1985; Feild, 1983; Hodges, Poteet, & Edlund, 1985; Oda, 1977) that addresses areas of common knowledge to all advanced-level health care providers so that there is a common basis on which providers can communicate. The clinical tracks offered in a program may be broad, may be divided into specific subspecialities, or may address an identified need such as gerontology. Whether broad or specific, the key components of preparation are theory content, clinical practice, and research (Feild, 1983).

Theory Content

The clinical nurse specialist's graduate program incorporates an extensive study of nursing theories and theories from related fields (American Nurses' Association, 1986a). This provides a scientific basis for advanced practice as well as a conceptual approach for utilization of the nursing process in complex situations and a basis for expert clinical judgment. Recommended content includes advanced level science courses, nursing theories, and related theories in role, role development, teaching-learning strategies, leadership, management, consultation, communication, change process, ethics, and legislative issues.

Clinical Practice Content

The range of human responses to actual or potential health problems and clinical nurse specialist decision making should be central to clinical practice. The clinical practice content cannot focus on the development of clinical expertise alone, but should be divided into two components: 1) a practicum focused on *skill development*, to increase clinical competence and to incorporate theory into practice, and 2) a residency focused on the development of the clinical nurse specialist *role*, with an emphasis on organizational skills and the integration of education, consultation, and leadership with the clinical practice component.

Research Content

While there is a lack of consensus about the level at which a master's-prepared clinical nurse specialist should be prepared in research skills (see Chapter 2), it is still expected that the clinical nurse specialist participates in research that explores the impact of nursing interventions on patient care outcomes and builds the scientific basis for nursing practice. Graduate research preparation at best stimulates scholarly inquiry, and at least provides the clinical nurse specialist with beginning research skills. Consensus about standardization of research preparation and competency at the master's level is still lacking.

Graduate study provides an opportunity to learn a scientific basis for practice, learn research methodology, and practice the integration of clinical judgment, management, education, and consultation skills in a clinical residency.

THE CLINICAL NURSE SPECIALIST TODAY

Where is the clinical nurse specialist role today? How have clinical nurse specialists established their practice? How is the role used? A survey conducted by the American Nurses' Association (1986b) provides information about the distribution and utilization of clinical nurse specialists. While the survey is limited by the representative sampling of association affiliates, the significant findings are: 98 percent are female, 96 percent are white, 98 percent are master's prepared, 64 percent are employed in a hospital setting, and 72 percent are in a staff position.

While in some organizations clinical nurse specialist positions are being considered for sacrifice in response to the need for cost containment in a prospective payment environment, that is not universally true. Many nurse executives and hospital administrators recognize the clinical nurse specialist role as a magnet to draw professional nurses committed to a high quality of care, limiting the impact of the nurse shortage. In these settings, positions are being maintained or new ones created. Additionally, settings such as home health care agencies have begun to utilize clinical nurse specialists.

Two related issues clinical nurse specialists currently face are coming together with master's-prepared nurse practitioners to wrestle with the definition of advanced practice and to discuss the similarities and differences in advanced practice. The definition of advanced practice is one currently being debated but about which there is no consensus. Suggested definitions have been, beyond the prerequisite of master's-degree preparation, "application of a broad range of theories" and "a broad set of post-graduate nursing skills" (California Nurses' Association, 1984), or "the deliberative diagnosis and treatment of a full range of human responses to actual or potential health problems" (Calkins, 1984, p. 27). Discussion of the similarities and differences in advanced nursing practice has focused on scope of practice, range of knowledge and skills, and domain of service. Presently the primary emphasis of the clinical nurse specialist is on client-centered practice, utilizing an in-depth knowledge base and emphasizing in-depth assessment, practiced within the domain of secondary and tertiary care settings. The nurse practitioner is responsible for providing a full range of primary health care services, utilizing a broad knowledge base, and practicing in multiple settings outside of secondary and tertiary care settings (Sparacino & Durand, 1986). While the realm of health care has proliferated in its subspecialities, and the scope of nursing knowledge, skills, and responsibility has expanded accordingly, nursing role titles and subtitles have also multiplied. Thus, it is time that the nursing profession examine those roles which provide specialized client care and come to agreement about singular definitions so that nursing services can be clearly specified, efficiently delivered, and accurately evaluated.

The future of clinical nurse specialists within the evolution of the nursing profession is addressed in Chapter 14 and Chapter 15. Clinical nurse specialists are in a pivotal position to turn current health care and professional challenges into exciting opportunities for tomorrow.

SUMMARY

The clinical nurse specialist role is clearly defined in respect to master's preparation and scope of practice. There is evolving clarity of core content of educational preparation and practice standards. While the role is widely accepted and is often considered to be a magnet to recruit and retain highly committed professional nurses, its popularity and use has weathered a stormy relationship in health care's cost-conscious environment. The role is experiencing a resurgence in interest because, in fact, clinical nurse specialists are measurably demonstrating a positive impact on patient care outcomes while reducing the cost of health care delivery.

REFERENCES

American Association of Critical Care Nurses. (1987). *The critical care clinical nurse specialist: Role definition.* Newport Beach, CA: American Association of Critical Care Nurses.

American Nurses' Association. (1980). *Nursing: A social policy statement.* Kansas City, MO: American Nurses' Association.

American Nurses' Association. (1986a). *The role of the clinical nurse specialist.* Kansas City, MO: American Nurses' Association.

American Nurses' Association. (1986b). *Clinical nurse specialists: Distribution and utilization.* Kansas City, MO: American Nurses' Association.

Andreoli, K.G. (1986). Specialization and the graduate curriculum: Where does it fit? In *Patterns in specialization: Challenge to the curriculum.* New York: National League for Nursing.

Brown, E.L. (1948). *Nursing for the future.* New York: Russell Sage Foundation.

California Nurses' Association. (1984). *Position statement on specialization in nursing practice.* San Francisco: California Nurses' Association.

Calkin, J.D. (1984). A model for advanced nursing practice. *Journal of Nursing Administration, 14* (1), 24–30.

DeWitt, K. (1900). Specialties in nursing. *American Journal of Nursing, 1* (1), 14–17.

Diers, D. (1985). Preparation of practitioners, clinical specialists, and clinicians. *Journal of Professional Nursing, 1* (1), 41–47.

Feild, L. (1983). Current trends in education and implications for the future. In A.B. Hamric & J. Spross (Eds.), *The clinical nurse specialist in theory and practice.* Orlando, FL: Grune & Stratton.

Hodges, L.C., Poteet, G.W., & Edlund, B.J. (1985). Teaching clinical nurse specialist to lead . . . and to succeed. *Nursing and Health Care, 6* (4), 193–196.

Hoeffer, B., & Murphy, S.A. (1984). *Specialization in nursing practice.* Kansas City, MO: American Nurses' Association.

Lewis, E.P. (1970). *The clinical nurse specialist.* New York: American Journal of Nursing, Educational Services Division.

Mayo, A.A. (1944). Advanced courses in clinical nursing. *American Journal of Nursing, 44* (6), 579–585.

National League for Nursing. (1958). *The educational preparation of the clinical nurse specialist in psychiatric nursing.* New York: National League for Nursing.

National League for Nursing. (1969). *A review of the preparation and roles of the clinical nurse specialist: Extending the boundaries of nursing education.* New York: National League for Nursing.

Oda, D. (1977). Specialized role development: A three-phase process. *Nursing Outlook, 25* (6), 374–377.

Peplau, H. (1965). Specialization in professional nursing. *Nursing Science, 3* (4), 268–287.

Reiter, F. (1966). The nurse-clinician. *American Journal of Nursing, 66* (2), 274–280.

Sparacino, P.S.A., & Durand, B.A. (1986). Editorial on specialization in advanced nursing practice. *Momentum, 4* (2), 1–4.

chapter two

The Role Components

Patricia S.A. Sparacino
Diane M. Cooper

Challenging and multifaceted, the role of the clinical nurse specialist incorporates the primary components of expert clinical practice, consultation, education, and research. Integration of these role dimensions is difficult, but a necessary requirement for successful implementation of the role. Maintaining some distinction between the role components clarifies both for the clinical nurse specialist and others the varying role responsibilities. Although agreement is widespread that these are the four primary components of the clinical nurse specialist role, some would also add change agent and role model to the list. Change agent and role model, however, are descriptive labels indicating processes used to accomplish particular aspects of the role, hence they cannot be considered role components per se.

In some settings, the clinical nurse specialist also may function as an administrator. This fifth possible role component is the most controversial, eliciting debate as to how much one can maintain a client-based practice and yet successfully manage administrative responsibilities. The authors of this chapter adhere to the premise that the clinical nurse specialist role has four primary components and may have a fifth. To fulfill the role, clinical nurse specialists must simultaneously perform the four primary components, always ensuring that the primary emphasis of all activities concerns client-based practice.

Direct and indirect care are terms applied to aspects of the clinical nurse specialist role. Direct care is part of the clinical practice component and refers to actual interaction with selected clients, families, or groups. Direct care includes assessment, diagnosis, planning, therapeutic intervention, and evaluation. Indirect care refers to services, such as education and consultation, which enhance patient care and are provided to the care providers actually involved with the patient.

Although integration of the four primary components is essential, this chapter will describe each separately in an attempt to clarify and distinguish between the clinical nurse specialist's varying responsibilities. The administrator component will also be described here and in Chapter 3. This chapter serves as a generic description of the dimensions of the clinical nurse specialist role. The dynamic nature of role implementation as influenced by setting, speciality, and experience is described by practicing clinical nurse specialists in the chapters in Part II of this book.

CLINICIAN

Despite some variation, the clinical nurse specialist position has been described most often as consisting of four role components: expert clinician, educator, consultant, and researcher (American Nurses' Association, 1980; Malone, 1986, Montemuro, 1987). Whether one ascribes to this definition or attaches additional functions to the role, the fact remains that the activities considered by most as essential to successful role implementation concern those surrounding the clinical nurse specialist's skill as an expert clinician (Topham, 1987; Walker, 1986; Werner, Bumann, & O'Brien, 1988).

Anecdotal reports from the past describing the clinical nurse specialist have focused heavily on the clinical aspects of the role, as well as on methods for gaining entry into the clinical environment (Jackson, 1973; McGann, 1975). Establishing oneself as an expert clinician has long been viewed as a crucial accomplishment if the clinical nurse specialist ultimately desires to fulfill the other role components and be successful. The chapters in part two of this book are purposely framed in a clinical situation (i.e., "critical incident") stemming from a significant interaction each clinical nurse specialist had with a patient precisely because of the clinical nurse specialist's contributions and impact as an expert clinician.

Although the majority of writers describing clinical nursing specialization agree that the clinical aspect of the role is pivotal, opinions vary regarding the optimal amount of time thought necessary to ensure its implementation (see Table 2–1). Even so, the clinician aspect of the clinical nurse specialist role is most often accorded the greatest percentage of time when each of the four role components is evaluated separately. In the past, allocations for each subrole within nursing specialization were proposed somewhat arbitrarily; more recently, studies have been undertaken logging the actual time clinical nurse specialists spend in accomplishing each of the role components (Baker, 1987; Beecroft & Papenhausen, 1985; Robichaud & Hamric, 1986). Additionally, investigators have interviewed clinical nurse specialists and nurse executives to ascertain their respective assessments of appropriate time allotments for each of the clinical nurse specialist subroles (Malone, 1986; Tarsitano, Brophy & Snyder, 1986; Walker, 1986). Interestingly, discrepancies exist between nursing executives and clinical nurse specialists in their assessments of the proportion of time that should be allotted to

TABLE 2–1. STUDIES EVALUATING PERCENTAGE OF CLINICAL NURSE SPECIALIST'S TIME IN CLINICIAN ROLE

Investigator(s)	Sample Size	Group Questioned	Percentage as Clinician
Baker (1987)	1	CNS	70–75% (first two years)
Beecroft & Papenhausen (1985)	262	CNS	>60%[b]
Donoghue & Spross (1985)	186	CNS	Primary focus practitioner and change agent
Malone (1986)	?	CNS & NA	50%[c]
Robichaud & Hamric (1986)	15	CNS	40%[b] (42%[c])
	9	NA	40%[b] (42.5%[c])
Tarsitano, Brophy, & Snyder (1986)	54	NA	32.40%[a]
	35	CNS	34.80%[a]
Walker (1986)	81	NA	34%[c]

[a]	=	"perceived importance"
[b]	=	actual
[c]	=	optimal
NA	=	Nursing Administrators
CNS	=	Clinical Nurse Specialists

each subrole including the role of clinician. Not only do variations exist between the nurse executives and the clinical nurse specialists but similiar differences exist between the time the clinical nurse specialists think should be spent performing certain role functions and that which they actually spend in practice (see Table 3–3).

Historical Background

In reviewing the history of the clinical nurse specialist role (see Chapter 1) it is easy to see why, despite changes in the health care system, clinical nurse specialists continue to be committed to focusing primary attention on the patient. Almost four decades ago a pattern emerged which revealed that in order to achieve status in nursing, qualified practitioners moved away from the bedside and into administrative positions (Kinsella, 1973). Cognizant of the potential deleterious effect this ongoing drain could have on the level of expertise of the nurse at the bedside, and aware of the increasing dissatisfaction of the American public with the abilities of those ministering to them when they were ill, Frances Reiter (1966) proposed a new position in nursing, the "nurse clinician". This individual, later referred to as the clinical nurse specialist, was to be a "master practitioner throughout all the dimensions of nursing practice", and was to be committed "to the provision of the highest quality of nursing care". Although the staff nurse, according to Reiter, was concerned with the *amount* of care. The nurse-clinician, by contrast, is concerned with the *kind* of care" (p. 278). So determined was Reiter with insuring this nurse's impact on the clinical practice of nursing that she stated: "No matter how skilled a nurse may be in the teaching arts, for instance, I would not consider her a nurse-clinician unless she couples her teaching activities with continuing clinical practice" (Reiter, 1966, p. 279).

The American Nurses' Association echoed Reiter's sentiments regarding the role when in 1976 they stated, "while the roles may change by circumstances for a certain period of time, this practitioner ceases to be recognized as a clinical nurse specialist when the patient-client-family ceases to be the basis of practice" (p. 5).

Over the past 20 years the need for and the understanding of clinical nursing specialization has evolved. In 1980 the American Nurses' Association defined the role and reemphasized the predominant role clinical expertise must play if an individual is to be defined as a *clinical nurse specialist*. Statements such as the following, excerpted from the section on "Specialization in Nursing Practice" in *Nursing: A Social Policy Statement* (1980) attest to that: "Unlike generalist nurses, who upon licensure and entry into practice are expected to be competent at least at a *minimum safe level*, specialists are expected to have *expert competence*" (p. 25). Or again, "Expert competence is an abstraction—the difference between a generalist and a specialist cannot be seen until it has been made concrete through practice, over time" (p. 25).

Today over 20,000 registered nurses can be counted among those nurses with graduate degrees who, responding to the mandate of Reiter and others, call themselves clinical nurse specialists (American Nurses' Association, 1986a). It is doubtful that there is an area of nursing practice in which some nurse with advanced educational preparation and clinical skills is not prepared. With increased technology and the changing needs of society with respect to health care, the demand continues to increase for the services of these highly skilled, creative, advanced clinical practitioners whose primary focus is on the patient (Fralic, 1988; Styles, 1987). Even with some insight into the evolution of the role, some still might ask what is accomplished when clinical nurse specialists excel as clinicians?

Significance of Demonstrating Clinical Expertise

In addition to improving the level of care received by those patients with whom the clinical nurse specialist interacts directly, the ultimate goal of any clinical nurse specialist is to improve, through role modeling, the overall quality of care delivered by nurses (Christman, 1965; Hamric, 1983). The impact of clinical nurse specialists' clinical expertise should be felt on the units and within the institution in which they work, as well as through their writings, continuing education offerings, and research programs. A prerequisite to effective and sustained impact on clinical practice is the clinical nurse specialist's ability to prove skills as a clinician. Although such efforts are paramount for the novice clinical nurse specialist, they are equally essential for the experienced clinical nurse specialist moving into a new organization or faced with new technology and ongoing need to integrate research with practice.

Proving one's skills as an expert clinician is the method by which the clinical nurse specialist establishes credibility with nurses and other members of the health-care team, as well as with patients and their families. It is the prime mechanism by which the clinical nurse specialist gains entry into patient situations and sustains that activity. If the clinical nurse specialist lacks technical skills, or is not the clinical expert purported, nursing staff will assess the individual as knowing less about bedside care than they do and, as Hamric (1983) so aptly put it, will be "understandably dismayed and even hostile" (p. 42). Or again, if nurses assess the clinical nurse specialist as possessing theoretical knowledge but lacking the experience and skill to realistically and comfortably translate that knowledge into directives for use in the practice setting, they will devalue the clinician's suggestions until such skills are demonstrated. Baker and Kramer (1970) captured the dissatisfaction experienced by staff nurses who, having been exposed to an unskilled clinical nurse specialist, made the following comments: "Her suggestions aren't always practical", or again, "What does she know about good patient care? All she's ever learned is from a book" (p. 50).

In addition to establishing one's credibility as a clinician and as an advanced practitioner, there are numerous other reasons supporting the importance of the clinical nurse specialist demonstrating skills as a clinical expert. Some of the more obvious reasons cited in the literature are: 1) that "direct care activities increase the visibility and accessibility of the clinical nurse specialist" (Felder, 1983, p. 59) and "that availability on the patient units is key to utilization of the CNS" (Gleason & Flynn [1987] [p. 131]); 2) increased contact with staff enhances the clinical nurse specialist's ability to serve as a staff advocate; 3) functioning in direct care situations increases the team's interdisciplinary effort, reinforcing other professionals' awareness of the significant impact the nurse has in patient care (Felder, 1983; Fralic, 1988); 4) clinical skill on the part of the clinical nurse specialist and involvement in patient care situations increase the collaborative and collegial relationship that the clinical nurse specialist creates with physicians (Barrett, 1972); 5) clinical nurse specialists with joint appointments who are clinically involved, or those who precept graduate students, can provide reality based examples for use in teaching both in their area of specialization, as well as in strategies for role implementation; 6) maintaining one's clinical skills can provide clinical nurse specialists opportunities for continued development of their own practice, allowing them to remain current; 7) provides the mechanism by which the clinical nurse specialist is better able to fulfill other aspects of the role, especially highlighting areas for continuing education programs, inservice topics, or questions that might form the basis of clinical nursing research (Felder, 1983); 8) affords multiple opportunities for incorporating research findings into the direct care of patients and thereby advances practice (Munro, 1987); 9) demonstrates accountability for the quality of nursing practice rendered (Kinsella, 1973). In a very real sense then the clinical aspects of the role of the clinical nurse specialist form the "glue" binding the other role components together, while at the same time acting as a catalyst energizing the clinical nurse specialist's work.

Perhaps there is no more basic reason for the importance of developing and maintaining one's skills as a clinical expert in the specialized area of nursing practice than the fine tuning and increased discrimination in patient care such activity affords (Kinsella, 1973). The clinical nurse specialist who has been involved directly in every phase of a disease state, has observed multiple patient responses, and has integrated these observations with theory and research, can function as a "well-spring" to other clinicians. Once acknowledged as an expert this clinical nurse specialist is able to provide staff with additional assessment skills, multiple and varied nursing interventions, research based rationale for carrying out patient-care activities, evaluation criteria by which to assess patient progress, and praise when theory-based, knowledgeable nursing practice has been rendered.

Due to limited numbers and wide variation in speciality areas, clinical nurse specialists once perceived each other as equally educated, equally qualified advanced practitioners. Now, as a result of increasing numbers and duplication among specialties, clinical nurse specialists are realizing that gradations in skill exist among them. Variations in level of expertise exist both within clinical nurse specialists' areas of expertise, as well as within their ability to implement the role. It is the depth of one's skill as a clinical expert, gained through repeated exposure, observation, and evaluation of patient care situations that distinguishes the refined expert from the developing one. A high level of expertise coupled with ongoing study and research are distinguishing trademarks of expert nursing specialization. As a greater number of clinical nurse specialists function in the role for longer periods of time, and as more clinical nurse specialists obtain doctoral degrees, these gradations in practice and skill among them will only become more obvious.

A statue standing outside Presbyterian-University of Pennsylvania Medical Center in Philadelphia captures the esteem true clinical expertise can hold for the peers of the expert. In life size proportions, this work entitled "Consultation," depicts five physicians engaged in discussion. The piece is noteworthy for the message it delivers. Even after only brief observation, one can determine the roles of the various characters: the intern, wearing a short coat, pockets stuffed with books, and necktie flying in the breeze appears late for rounds and engrossed in all that has befallen him; the young attending, prim and proper in his long, white, starched lab coat, is made to appear as if he is trying to look older and more scholarly than either his years or experience warrant. Most poignantly though, the passerby cannot but help noticing the older serious but pleasant, calm appearing attending physician. The observer assesses that individual in the grouping to be the attending physician because of the pivotal position he has been accorded by the others in the group. He is the individual towards whom the others have focused their attention. He is reflective, attentive, and wise in his appearance. It is not difficult to assess him as drawing in the list of symptoms being presented by each of the members of the group. He exudes the ability to ask crucial questions and to provide answers, not just one answer but another and another and another. The attending has been sculpted in such a way that he stands as a resource for the others; they appear to value his direction because they have witnessed his discriminating abilities. For them, he is the embodiment of the saying "he knows of what he speaks." This true to life individual, the focal point of the statue, is *attending* to all the aspects of the patients being discussed. He listens and hears differently from the others. The other physicians in the group value his expertise in a way difficult to put into words.

Daily in some hospitals this scenario is replicated both by expert attending physicians and "attending nurses." Someday a statue like the one outside "Presby" will exist elsewhere but the professionals being depicted will not be physicians, rather they will be nurses. The individual towards whom the nurses lean will be identified by all as the refined expert, the clinical nurse specialist—the "attending nurse" (Cooper, 1983). Whoever poses as the model for the latter statue will exude the confidence and skill that can only be gained as the result of years of direct clinical activity with patients.

Evolution of Clinical Expertise in the Clinical Nurse Specialist's Practice

Most articles written by and about clinical nurse specialists in the past described individuals whose experience in the role was limited (Hamric, 1983). In fact, numerous conferences attended by clinical nurse specialists during the 1970s and 1980s repeatedly addressed strategies for assisting the novice to successfully gain entrance into the role. More recently clinical nurse specialists with more extensive periods of time in the role have chronicled their activities at stages beyond that of entrance into the role and shared them with peers (see Table 2–2). One consequence of an increased number of experienced specialists logging their activities has been the elucidation of a series of time-phased activities considered to be crucial if success as a clinical nurse specialist is to be

TABLE 2–2. PROPOSED DEVELOPMENTAL ROLE MARKERS

	Year 1	Year 2	Year 3	Year 4	Year 5
GOAL:	*Establish role identity and visibility*	*Successfully Implement role*	*Expand education and research components* ***Maintain clinical expertise***		***Expand consultant component*** ***Refine and integrate role components***
Clinical Practice	Establish clinical specialty expertise Demonstrate high level of competency Develop own conceptual framework within specialty area	Identify subspecialty, dependent on client care needs	Plan, give, evaluate care within specialty area Define and circumscribe subspecialty	Re-examine subspecialty Test own conceptual framework within specialty area	Maintain clinical practice expertise Evaluate client care outcomes Combine theory, clinical research, and clinical expertise to change practice "Attending nurse" Serve as clinical consultant within specialty practice to external consumers Identify additional client-centered services or programs
Consultation	Develop informally Articulate own consultation style	Develop skill with own consultation style Assist staff with providing care within specialty area	Formalize consultation style Demonstrate flexibility in responding to priorities Serve as a resource to health professionals for clients in specialty area	Refine skill at discriminating consultation priorities	

18

Education	Focus on staff and client/family individually or in groups Role-model direct patient care	Establish and conduct interdisciplinary care conferences Establish relationship with associated school of nursing Develop patient education materials	Plan and teach clients/families within specialty area Publish clinical experiences/knowledge in professional journals Expand programs to community, state, and national levels Serve as preceptor to graduate students	Maintain and refine teaching skills Use own conceptual framework within specialty area as a basis for teaching	Develop and facilitate formal programs Teach at the national level Consider doctoral education
Research	Use research findings in specialty practice Identify researchable problems	Plan collaborative projects Establish contacts in specialty area	Conduct small collaborative research studies on clinical nursing problems	Communicate research results to colleagues Demonstrate research continuity within specialty area of practice	Develop larger collaborative clinical research studies Seek external funding Publish

Adapted from Baker (1987), Cooper (1983), Holt (1987), University of California, San Francisco (1986).

insured. Obviously if these trajectories were analyzed separately variations in the tasks could be noted (Baker, 1987; Cooper, 1983; Holt, 1987; University of California at San Francisco, 1986). Synthesis of the four as presented in Table 2–2, however, demonstrates many similarities.

After brief review, it is apparent that early on the clinical nurse specialist's energy must be focused on establishing a specialty and demonstrating clinical competency. Initially direct care activities can be carried out, either by assigning oneself to patient care on selected days, by working along side nurses as they implement care, or by working in the role of a staff nurse for a period of time prior to assuming the other aspects of the role. Whichever method is selected, clinical nurse specialists must assess whether or not the activities undertaken with patients advance their own clinical skills and serve to demonstrate to staff a different level of expertise. At the same time the clinical nurse specialist must take pains to insure that such direct patient care activities are not viewed by staff as invasive, condescending, or disruptive. Once clinical nurse specialists' skill in direct patient care is proven, then they will be sought out as knowledgeable resources for years to come. Maintaining and honing direct patient care activities over time will increase the likelihood that the clinical nurse specialist eventually will be viewed as an expert, if not a refined expert.

As clinical nurse specialists progress in the role, it is obvious that the effect of their clinical expertise is directed towards larger groups of patients and professionals. Additionally, the clinical nurse specialist focuses on measuring the effects of interventions on outcomes as well as clinical research that adds to the knowledge base for nursing practice. Yet, maintaining clinical practice expertise remains such an inherent aspect of clinical nursing specialization that some direct care activities must *always* form a percentage of the clinical nurse specialist's time. The experienced clinical nurse specialist might find that the amount of actual time spent in direct care activities decreases as tenure in the position increases. The goal, however, is not to become "advanced" to the degree that direct care activity is seen as unnecessary or "too time consuming". Only through ongoing direct involvement with the patient, client, or family can the clinical nurse specialist justifiably, professionally, and ethically continue to assume the title.

The clinical nurse specialist has been labeled as the "most expensive nurse" (Beecroft & Papenhausen, 1987, p. 149). With increasing demands being placed on health care professionals to deliver efficient, quality, cost effective care, it is important that multiple issues be considered when the clinical nurse specialist chooses to be involved in direct patient care activities. Cognizance of economic factors, the importance of visibility if effective utilization is to occur, and the need to influence broadly the quality of patient care, are just a few of these issues. The

TABLE 2–3. ASSESSMENT QUESTIONS FOR CLINICAL NURSE SPECIALIST INVOLVEMENT IN DIRECT PATIENT CARE ACTIVITIES

1. In terms of your area of specialization, do you deliver the same or different care than the clinical nurses (i.e., staff nurses) do?
2. Have you determined ways by which to assess the difference in the level of care you administer to patients versus that delivered by the clinical nurses?
3. As regards the clinician aspect of your role where do you fit on the "Developmental Role Markers" (See Table 2–2)?
4. How have your direct care activities changed over time?
5. Can you distinguish between direct care activities and indirect care activities in your work?
6. Have you defined "appropriate" direct care activities in which you should be involved?
7. Would you be able to articulate the specific reason you have chosen to be involved with this (these) patients?
8. Are staff, including the head nurse and your supervisor, aware of your direct care involvement? Do they understand the rationale for it?
9. Are your clinical skills advancing? Which ones?
10. Are your advanced skills becoming more refined and more readily discernable to others as a result of your involvement in direct patient care situations?
11. Could you complete the total care on an extremely complex patient within your specialty? Do you think you should be able to?
12. If you were required to bill for your services as a clinician, do you have an idea of the level(s) of care you provide and what that would cost?
13. Is there any discrepancy between the percentage of time you think you should be involved in direct care activities and that which you actually do? If the percentages vary, can you identify the reason?
14. If you are employed in a tertiary care center, could you comfortably operate all the "machinery" used in the care of patients in your area of specialization?
15. When reading nurses' notes, or discussing patient care, can you assess that the nursing care plans you initiate are being followed? If not, are you able to exclude the possibility that they make unrealistic demands on the staff?
16. Have you considered requesting a fellow clinical nurse specialist in your area of specialty (either within or outside of your setting) to critique your suggestions regarding direct care activities with patients for their relevancy and basis in theory?
17. Have you requested a clinical nurse specialist skilled in role implementation to provide you with feedback regarding the time and strategies you use to carry out your direct care activities?
18. Do you believe that a decline in the quality of care, or an increase in the length of stay of the patients with whom you interact, would occur if your position was deleted from the organization?

questions in Table 2–3 are proposed to assist the clinical nurse specialist who is determining the degree and appropriateness of involvement in direct patient care. The clinical nurse specialist new to the role or the organization, or experienced clinical nurse specialists deliberating the appropriateness of their involvement in direct patient care will be assisted by reflecting on their answers to these questions.

The Clinical Component and the Future

The debate continues over the essential components of the clinical nurse specialist role. Noll (1987) proposed that as with other professions, so too nursing specialization will find that the "main action" of the advanced practitioner will be consultation. In this way clinical nurse specialists "can incorporate the 'subroles' of practice, education, and research as 'methods' for solving problems and effecting change" (p. 50). Montemuro (1987) stated:

> "The emphasis seems to have changed of late from direct caregiver to a more integrated broader approach of consultant, teacher, and researcher. This changing emphasis has resulted as nurses have begun to examine how the agency in which they work can attain maximum utilization of a person prepared at the master's level and have begun to appreciate the full scope of professional practice" (p. 108).

Certainly the words of both these authors make sense and deserve serious discussion by clinical nurse specialists. Besides challenging our thinking, these perspectives on the future of the role bring the serious clinical nurse specialist directly into the process of shaping this evolving role.

Clinical nurse specialists, skilled as clinicians, will continue the struggle to frame their practice. In all of this though, it is important to recall that although no clinical nurse specialist can succeed merely as a result of clinical expertise (Stevens, 1976), those skills, and the discrimination one brings to the bedside, form the bedrock that gives meaning or brings merit to all else the clinical nurse specialist does.

The future will bear testimony to the value that society and health care professionals reassign to clinical expertise. Werner, Bumann, and O'Brien (1988) pointed out "The demand for nurses with advanced clinical knowledge and expertise is as urgent today as it was when the CNS role was initially developed" (p. 15). Furthermore, after undertaking an extensive review of the literature for the purpose of organizing an annotated bibliography on the role of the clinical nurse specialist, they were left with several impressions, one of which was:

> "Clinical expertise remains the cornerstone of CNS practice. The value of the CNS lies in the theoretical and clinical knowledge that makes the CNS a clinical expert able to function as an influential leader, educator, and role model. Expertise in clinical decision making and an understanding of functioning within the health care system enable the CNS to assure quality nursing care for clients" (p. 15).

The clinical nurse specialist who continues to excel as a clinician will stand in good stead for years to come. In discussing the future of the profession of nursing, Christman (1987) pointed out, "The possessors of . . . expert knowledge will become the prime participants in the provision of care" (p. 3).

CONSULTANT

Definition and Framework

Hamric (1983) summarized the essential components of consultation; it is "a process in which an individual with recognized expertise is invited by another to assist in resolving a problem" (p. 41). Classically, consultation has been divided into three types or subcategories, each of which is accomplished in a different manner. The key types of consultation are 1) expert, 2) resource, and 3) process. The expert consultant is assessed by the consultee as possessing unique skills and is called upon to prescribe approaches or solutions for specific problems in specific situations. The resource consultant, on the other hand, provides relevant information to enable the consultee to make decisions based on the widest range of alternatives. Finally, the process consultant brings about changes in a situation that enables the consultee to make a decision in the particular instance and in future situations (Kohnke, 1978).

Using a different framework, Caplan (1970) proposed four models for consultation: client-centered case consultation, consultee-centered case consultation, program-centered administrative consultation, and consultee-centered administrative approach. Each of the models proposed by Caplan differs from the others based on the individual or system with which the consultant interacts.

Regardless of the framework used, it is important that early on the consultant identify the type of consultation being requested by the consultee. Such identification will assist the consultant in evaluating the appropriateness of the strategies employed both during and after the consultation.

Obviously no one utilizes the same approach to consultation at all times. Selection of the most appropriate type of consultation is determined by numerous factors, among them the type of request from the consultee, time constraints and, in the case of patient care, the acuity of the patient situation.

Components of the Consultative Process

Regardless of the particular approach utilized, all forms of consultation possess identifiable components:

- It is initiated by the consultee.
- The relationship between the consultant and the consultee is temporary.

- The role is advisory.
- The consultant has no responsibility for implementation.

Ideally the consultant also has no administrative relationship to the consultee (Kohnke, 1978). This last issue, namely the consultee's relationship to the consultant, brings up another method by which consultations can be classified: internal or external.

Traditionally in nursing the majority of consultations that have occurred did so in hospitals. There, staff nurses, having recognized another's expertise, sought that individual out in relation to some aspect of patient care. This form of consultation, "a verbal agreement to work on a problem with a colleague", is termed informal (or internal) consultation. External consultation, on the other hand, more often "follows specific steps and involves negotiating a contract." Frequently the outside consultant "works from an expert framework to solve system-wide problems" and is hired from outside of the institution, thus the term external, or outside (Edlund, Hodges, & Poteet, 1987, p. 88). There are advantages and disadvantages inherent in each of these approaches to consultation.

The discussion that follows will focus primarily on internal consultation. It should be kept in mind, though, that requests for clinical nurse specialists to undertake external consultations are on the rise. Astute preparation for such undertakings can be facilitated by reviewing the literature on the "essentials" of external consultation (Beare, 1988; Edlund, Hodges, & Poteet, 1987; Poteet, 1987).

In spite of whether one chooses to function as an internal or external consultant, there is increasing clarity regarding the behaviors and atmosphere surrounding the clinical nurse specialist that are more likely to ensure one's success as a consultant. Similarly, circumstances that have the potential to impact the consultative process negatively are being logged.

Perhaps one of the most threatening deterrents to success in the role as a nursing consultant is lack of support from nursing administration. Certainly such an attitude can threaten the very existence of the role of the clinical nurse specialist within an institution. Without administrative support, requests for clinical nurse specialist consultations will be sparse, if they occur at all. Edlund, Hodges, and Poteet (1987) pointed out, "Positive sanction conveys power. Therefore, the most critical element of all is administrative support for the consultant role. Administration must establish that consultation is a norm and expect the staff to seek out consultants" (p. 88).

Another deterrent to use of a nurse consultant, although decreasing some as of late, has been an attitude among nurses that they should be capable of meeting *all* the patients' needs; to indicate otherwise would demonstrate serious inadequacies on their part. When confronted with difficult patient situations, staff nurses often turn to physicians for assistance with problem solving, even when clinical nurse specialists are available and the patient care problem is amenable to nursing intervention.

The increased emphasis on utilization of resources during a nursing student's preparation, coupled with the increased presence of nurses with advanced preparation in multiple settings are causing a decrease in the need for individuals to strive to be "supernurses." The result of such an attitude change is recognition that nurses can depend on one another and work together for the good of the patient. In such an atmosphere, requests for consultations by clinical nurse specialists increase and become the norm.

It is very important that clinical nurse specialists who desire success in the role of the consultant not lose sight of the possible vulnerability of the nurse who initiates the consultation. Thus awareness of interpersonal dynamics during the consultative process is necessary. Clinical nurse specialist utilization trends, collected over time by the clinical nurse specialist, should reveal one's ability to "market" one's skills as a consultant. Frequently, underutilization of the clinical nurse specialist finds its roots in unpolished interpersonal skills. More specifically, within the confines of patient safety, the clinical nurse specialist should avoid judgmental behavior if the care plan is not carried out exactly as directed. Barron (1983) pointed out that "the consultant is not a supervisor" nor there to prescribe the " 'perfect' approach . . . the emphasis in consultation is on effective, practical problem solving" (pp. 104–105).

If the clinical nurse specialist is overextended in the job and projects a negative or hurried manner, or is not prompt in responding to requests for services, these behaviors, too, will influence the number and quality of the consultations initiated by staff. Confusion about the clinical nurse specialist role also can act as a deterrent, as well as lack of specialized knowledge or experience in the consultative process.

Gleason and Flynn (1987) identified clinical nurse specialist behaviors that increase the potential for requests for consultations. Their research described circumstances surrounding the consultations requested of a surgical clinical nurse specialist in a tertiary setting. The clinical nurse specialist involved assessed the consultations carried out in relation to the way the process was initiated: what the nature of the request was, who initiated the consultation, and what clinical problems were identified. Of interest was the finding that "requests for consultation occurred when the clinical nurse specialist was visible on the patient care unit" (p. 131), and that the majority of the requests (60 percent) were initiated informally. The linkage between visibility, availability, and consultations is supported by several other writers (Barron, 1983; Edlund, Hodges, & Poteet, 1987). Gleason and Flynn (1987) also noted that "consultation in the surgical intensive care unit . . . whether direct or indirect care activities, revolved around use of high technology equipment in patient care" (p. 130). This latter finding speaks again to the importance of in-depth knowledge and skill in the care of those patients for whom one purports to be a clinical nurse specialist. If deficiencies are identified, the clinical nurse specialist should schedule some direct care patient days, perhaps with a nurse recognized for expertise in the clinical nurse specialist's area of weakness. Although many clinical nurse specialists avoid exposing their deficiencies to staff, those who are willing to work at building new skills by working with staff reap rewards.

In all successful consultative relationships, the clinical nurse specialist must focus initially on the problem as perceived by the consultee. This is paramount, as it respectfully acknowledges the validity of the nurse's identification of the problem. Frequently other problems can be identified as one moves along in the discussion and diagnosis of the issues involved. Except in rare cases, unless the nurse's identification of the problem is acknowledged and addressed, little else of what the clinical nurse specialist says will find its way into practice.

This mandate of accepting the statement of the problem as the consultee defines it can be seen as particularly important when acting as a consultant to other members of the health-care team. In order to broaden the use of the clinical nurse specialist across the team, as well as to increase the other members' awareness of nursing's unique contribution to patient care, it is particularly critical in dealing with nonnurses that the specialist begin by perceiving the problem through the eyes of the consultee. Often the success of the clinical nurse specialist in initial interactions will lead to repeated requests for consultative input. Although a request for a consultation from a physician should be viewed objectively and not seen as superior to any other request for consultation, it would be naive to ignore the potential for affecting patient care in a positive manner over time as a result of the physician's acknowledgment of the clinical nurse specialist's contributions to patient care.

Other qualifications that have the potential for ensuring the clinical nurse specialist's success as a consultant are: "common sense, analytical ability, sense of organizational climate, productive imagination, reasoning power, sense of humor, high frustration point, and a sense of timing" (Noll, 1987, p. 49).

Perhaps the apex of nursing consultation occurs when more than one or several clinical nurse specialists come together and, with the input of the staff nurses involved, formulate a plan for the patient that is theoretically-based and cohesive. In such a situation, clinical nurse specialists provide a richness of practice that can only benefit the patient (see Chapter 12). Furthermore, such interactions stimulate the clinical nurse specialists involved and provide evidence for peer review, role development, etc. Most of all, though, these interactions where multiple clinical nurse specialists consult on a patient's care role-model to the "bedside" nurse clinical practice at its best for, here, the nurse:

1) Learns from the sharing of in-depth content
2) Observes nursing as a valuable resource to both the patient and other nurses
3) Learns from expert clinicians deferring to one another, questioning one another, and collaborating for the benefit of the patient
4) Observes the acceptability of questioning or not having to "know it all"
5) Feels the pride and respect that comes from observing the clinical nurse specialist seek one's input as vital while at the same time learning new areas of observation or understanding

Numerous clinical nurse specialists consulting over one patient have an obligation to conduct these sessions well, acknowledging all input as valuable, for they are being critically assessed by staff members. Clearly, the goal must be the formulation of a plan that is clear, prioritized, and manageable for the nurses carrying it out. Most often this situation is facilitated if one clinical nurse specialist agrees to assume primary responsibility for the synthesis of the nursing care, with clinical nurse specialist colleagues being available as situations pertaining to their specialities arise.

In some instances clinical nurse specialists find themselves alone in an institution or with few peers. Creative individuals in these situations have initiated contact with major health-care centers and have utilized clinical nurse specialists there for input regarding patient care situations in their settings. These consultations can be extremely satisfying to both clinical nurse specialists and lead to effective networking for subsequent patient transfers. The possibility of developing common research interests is also a benefit that can arise from such exchange.

Stages/Steps of the Consultative Process

Wherever and with whomever the consultation takes place, it evolves through a series of steps. Some have suggested that the steps in the consultative process are the same as those used to define the nursing process: identifying the problem, assessing, planning, intervening, and evaluating (Barron, 1983; Blake, 1977). Laureau (1985), on the other hand, proposed six steps: gaining entrance into the system, negotiating with the consultee, identifying the problem, developing interventions, intervening, and evaluating. One can see how easily Laureau's steps could be incorporated into the nursing process.

Blake (1977) proposed four steps to the process of consultation: entry, diagnosis, response, and closure. Although these terms could be easily renamed to fit within the nursing process, their clarity regarding the activities engaged in by the consultant give them an added dimension. Whatever the terms used to describe the stages, it is important during the consultation process for the consultant to be aware of the current stage. As Barron (1983) noted, "while the boundaries between phases can be somewhat fluid, keeping the outline and sequences of the stages clearly in mind can give structure and direction and help to establish the objectives and the limits of the consultation process" (p. 96).

Consultation: The Foundation or a Subrole?

Consultation has long been noted as one of the essential functions of the clinical nurse specialist. Many writers have described it as a subrole of clinical nurse specialist practice (Blake, 1977; Fife & Lemler, 1983; Gresham, 1983). Noll (1987) made the case for consultation being not a subrole of the clinical nurse specialist role, but rather the foundation from which the roles of educator, researcher, and clinician spring. Noll referred to Kohnke (1978), who stated, "All professions have members who are prepared beyond the general professional practice area. These people are generally called consultants and have additional knowledge in specific areas of the practice. It is the consultant's role that is prescribed for the master's degree nurse in the clinical area" (p. 55). Noll went on to urge that if clinical nurse specialists using internal consultation employed the framework suggested by Kohnke, where consultation is the basis for practice, they could "incorporate the subroles of practice, education, and research as methods of solving problems and effecting change" (p. 50). As clinical nurse specialists continue to discuss the roots of their practice, it may be useful to consider the statements of Kohnke, Noll, and others as regards the key role consultation plays in advanced practice.

Place for Consultation in Clinical Nurse Specialist Role Development

As the clinical nurse specialist develops in the role, behaviors change. In several of the "role marker" trajectories cited in Table 2–2, it is significant to note that the longer one is in the position of clinical nurse specialist, the greater the emphasis on time spent in consultation. Although by definition the clinical nurse specialist always participates in direct patient care, the percentage of time in this activity gradually reduces as time progresses, with the percentage in consultation increasing. Observing that the consultant role is "often one clinical specialists wish to develop first," Gresham (1983) went on to say, "a sound consultative practice is often the last aspect of one's role to evolve. It is worth waiting and working for. To be sought out as a consultant . . . implies an earned reputation for expertise" (p. 136). Again, "consultation," stated Barron (1983), "is a complex and highly professional aspect of the role of the clinical nurse specialist that challenges the practitioner to blend science with art, theory with practice, and the real with the ideal" (p. 113). Perhaps more discussion and writing on the realities of role implementation, particularly as concerns the novice clinical nurse specialist, will reduce some of the pressures to "be all things to all people" immediately.

The Future of Consulting

Poteet, the editor of the section on consultation in the quarterly journal *Clinical Nurse Specialist*, forecasts that the consultative role of the clinical nurse specialist will increase in the future. She stated, "a more visible and influential role awaits the clinical nurse specialist in the area of consultation" (Poteet, 1987, p. 85). Among the areas of influence listed are: "promoting collaboration with other professionals and health care agencies, identifying strategies to deliver more cost efficient and effective patient care, establishing standards and definitions of nursing care, and identifying mechanisms of change within sociopolitical, economic, and legislative arenas as well as the system of health care delivery itself" (Poteet, 1987, p. 85).

Nurses in the role of consultant have been described as "catalysts for change" (Hendrix & La Godna, 1982). In addition to promoting change, they are to be leaders, role models, teachers, skilled communicators, expert practitioners, reviewers of the literature, researchers—to name a few of the descriptors. Lange (1979) poignantly reminded us that "the primary function of any consultant is to facilitate human potential, in other words, to develop the capacity for self-renewal within individuals, groups, and the total system" (p. 30).

Describing the relationship that occurs between the consultant and the consultee, Barron (1983) stated,

> The relationship that develops . . . is limited in duration and focus yet can be profoundly influential. Applying the process . . . is arduous at times. Yet it is the process that creates the opportunity for mutual creative problem solving . . . that is so necessary for the ongoing development of nursing practice (p. 113).

In closing, if we take Noll's (1987) premise to its logical conclusion, perhaps it can be said that the clinical nurse specialist is never more a professional than when interacting in a consultative manner to improve care. In giving away what is known to others, and in listening for the strategies of nurse colleagues, a new atmosphere is created that can only bring healing to the patient and renewed vigor to the consultee.

EDUCATOR

The educator role is one of the most commonly described components of the indirect practice aspect of the clinical nurse specialist role. The clinical nurse specialist teaches clients, families, groups, communities, undergraduate and graduate nursing students, colleagues, peers, and other health care providers. Unique as an educator, the clinical nurse specialist is in a position to integrate theory and advanced nursing practice in the practice setting (Sills, 1983).

The clinical nurse specialist as educator and role model is in a pivotal position to influence client, family, and health care team member behaviors. A theoretical knowledge base and expertise in a defined area of clinical practice is brought by the clinical nurse specialist to a teaching-learning situation, but it is not only what one says but what one does that creates an impact, and this is the basis for role modeling. An impression cannot be created merely by listening; the learner must react verbally as well as functionally in order to incorporate the impression into behaviors and into conceptual ideologies. That impression may be more successfully made when the instruction is objective, experimental, and anecdotal, associating the new with the old. If an impression does not modify the learner's behavior, then it is useless, as the impression has not produced the desired effect nor does it create an acquired capacity (James, 1958).

A method of effective role modeling in the practice setting is the practice of prescheduled clinical days, in which the clinical nurse specialist takes a patient assignment on a preplanned basis. This practice provides an opportunity to work side by side with a new nurse who may need further instruction in assessments or interventions. It provides an opportunity to role model, to incorporate research-based innovations into the nursing plan of care, and to demonstrate a comprehensive client approach.

Client and Family

The clinical nurse specialist's influence on client and family learning goes beyond that which the nurse generalist is able to provide. The clinical nurse specialist, by assessing a client's unique physical condition, emotional state, or other particular need, and by applying teaching-learning theories and the wisdom of clinical experience, is able to individualize the content for the learner and tailor the content for the setting. This instruction can incorporate theoretical principles into practical approaches and associate new approaches with that which is familiar and comfortable, thus creating the desired impression or motivation. An illustrative situation would be the following difference in approach to a client-teaching situation. Instead of the more traditional approach of "I've come to tell you what you will need to know about your surgery tomorrow", the clinical nurse specialist incorporates the adult learning theories of Redman (1980) and Johnson and colleagues (1978) to approach the same situation with the introductory question of "What questions may I answer for you regarding your surgery tomorrow?" The clinical nurse specialist's educational as well as experiential preparation provide the basis on which the impression, or motivation, is modified to change the learner's behavior and introduce a new learner capacity.

Nursing Staff

The nurse generalist also learns from the clinical nurse specialist. The clinical nurse specialist's own case load may provide a way of sharing patient-specific instruction. Instructing staff while caring for the client (role modeling) will stimulate others to increase their clinical competencies (Armacost, 1973; Dirschel, 1976; Everson, 1981; Smith, 1974). More formal educational intervention may be made by coordinating, facilitating, or leading interdisciplinary conferences and learning situations that are related to the clinical nurse specialist's area of expertise. Necessity may require assisting the nurse generalist to learn a concept or procedure quickly, and so the clinical nurse specialist's expertise facilitates the process of simplifying the problem at hand, identifying quickly attainable learning goals, compiling information from the literature, and providing the essential inservice instruction. By assisting other nurses to learn the theoretical concepts that apply to the clinical question, to incorporate those concepts into the resolution of a client care problem, and to learn new approaches to old problems, the clinical nurse specialist employs the instructional mode which is one of objectivity, experimentation, and associating new information with old practices. Hence, presumably, an impression is made and the impact will modify the nurses' behaviors (James, 1958).

Other Health Care Providers and Consumer Groups

Educational intervention with professional colleagues should not be limited to the nurse generalist but should extend to the interdisciplinary members of the health care team, client groups such as those that are organized around a shared life experience, and the general public. By knowing how and when to tailor the instructional method to the learning needs of the situation at hand, the clinical nurse specialist not only contributes to the attainment of a client care or health goal but, by virtue of that contribution, demonstrates the clinical nurse specialist's impact on client outcomes.

Formal Educational Programs

The clinical nurse specialist as educator of client and family, nurse generalist, and members of the health care team is a well-accepted and widely used component of the role. Although the clinical nurse specialist may also be selectively involved in basic nursing programs, it is more imperative that the clinical nurse specialist be actively engaged in graduate nursing programs. By serving as a role model and preceptor, the practicing clinical nurse specialist can demonstrate to the graduate nursing student 1) integration of theoretical principles and clinical expertise,

2) combined technical and humanistic expertise in the provision of innovative client care, 3) dissemination of expert knowledge and resources, 4) effective health care team collaboration in achieving exemplary client care, and 5) the spirit of inquiry that generates practice-based research. Only by observing and working collaboratively with such a role model in a clinical residency setting will the graduate nursing student comprehend the individualized role responsibilities of the clinical nurse specialist and be able to more easily and effectively actualize the role upon employment.

The clinical nurse specialist's involvement with graduate nursing programs should also extend to the contribution of critical clinical expertise to the design of new curricula, the evaluation and update of current curricula, formal lectures and presentations on speciality content, and leadership of clinical residency or role development seminars. For this type of collaboration between clinical nurse specialist and graduate educator to be productive and credible, the clinical nurse specialist needs to seek an appointment, whether salaried or nonsalaried, in the school of nursing. The nonsalaried faculty appointment generally requires a minimum number of hours yearly that the clinical nurse specialist contributes in the way of lectures, preceptorships or residencies, consultations, or thesis committee participation. A nonsalaried appointment permits the clinical nurse specialist to incorporate the contributions into daily client-related activities, maximizing time utilization and role efficiency.

A salaried joint appointment may be the preferable alternative for personal or professional reasons. While a salaried joint appointment may allow the clinical nurse specialist to work toward seniority in the academic ranks, the main disadvantage of such an arrangement is that rarely does a part-time appointment remain part-time. The time spent in responding to client needs competes with academic requirements, and the clinical nurse specialist with salaried joint appointments will find that either two part-time positions have developed two full-time needs or that a sense of dissatisfaction pervades due to doing neither job well.

The following partial description of the educator component from *The Role of the Clinical Nurse Specialist* (ANA, 1986b) is an excellent summary of the important aspects of this component.

> The clinical nurse specialist provides information when there is a knowledge deficit and when new information is needed to resolve a health problem or improve the quality of care. The clinical nurse specialist functions as a role model and preceptor for nurse generalists and faculty and students in a variety of clinical arenas. The clinical nurse specialist may also provide input and critique for curriculum design and development, may be responsible for teaching specific content in basic nursing programs and teaching specialty content in mas-

ter's nursing programs, and may update nurses' knowledge in continuing education programs (p. 3).

RESEARCHER

The function of the clinical nurse specialist as researcher is, perhaps, the least exercised of the four role components (ANA, 1986c; Oda, Sparacino, & Boyd, 1988). Numerous reasons have been proposed for the least amount of time being spent on the research component: 1) insufficient preparation at the master's degree level (Hodgman, 1983), 2) incongruity in role expectations between administrators and clinical nurse specialists (Holt, 1984; Tarsitano, Brophy, & Snyder, 1986), 3) immaturity in the role with research assuming a lower priority for the novice than for the experienced clinical nurse specialist, 4) the institutional value placed on clinical research including the amount of time the clinical nurse specialist is expected to be involved in research activities (Robichaud & Hamric, 1986), and 5) the clinical nurse specialist's competency to use research findings to improve clinical practice or to participate in research projects (Fenton, 1985; Wyers, Grove, & Pastorino, 1985). The research component is, however, one of the most essential aspects of the role, as only in this way will the scientific basis for nursing practice be expanded (Jacox, 1974).

Master's-level preparation in research methodology varies from program to program for the clinical nurse specialist. While there is debate as to whether the clinical nurse specialist should be a consumer of research or a researcher, it is at least agreed that master's-level graduate students need more and consistently uniform research preparation. Regardless of the extent of educational preparation, the clinical nurse specialist can and must be involved in nursing research at some level, whether as initiator or collaborator, so that the scientific basis for nursing knowledge and practice can be tested and the quality of client care improved (Dirschel, 1976; Peplau, 1965).

The clinical nurse specialist, whether novice or experienced, should evaluate whether research is a realistic performance goal at a given time in a particular setting. Is the organization ready for nursing research? Is the individual clinical nurse specialist ready?

Nursing research in the practice setting has a better chance of succeeding if the nursing administration actively supports it, both philosophically and practically. Examples of commitment are inclusion of research in the organization's as well as the department of nursing's philosophy or goals, a department of nursing research committee that both actively supports nursing research and reviews all proposals that affect nurses or nursing care, nursing representation on the institution's committee on human research, commitment of organizational resources, and an atmosphere of scientific inquiry among nursing staff and nursing managers (Cronenwett, 1986a).

As important as organizational readiness is the readiness and commitment of the clinical nurse specialist to conduct research. Readiness is determined by assessing the clinical nurse specialist's graduate research preparation, experience with previous research projects as a research assistant or co-investigator, evidence of strong writing skills, and success in publication. When the clinical nurse specialist is ready, the nursing administrator can be of assistance by collaborating on reasonable and appropriate expectations (Cronenwett, 1986a).

When the clinical nurse specialists value research and realize that research outcomes can have a significant impact on practice, then conviction is present. With conviction comes commitment and the challenge. "The clinical nurse specialist promotes scientific inquiry in clinical practice, using the research process to improve that practice" (ANA, 1986b, p. 3). The clinical nurse specialist is expected to be knowledgeable about nursing and medical research related to the area of speciality practice and may contribute to research in numerous ways (ANA, 1986b; Cronenwett, 1986b; Munro, 1987; Pollock, 1987; Sneed, 1987). Many of these are listed below:

- Documenting problems to establish priorities for problem solving
- Generating and refining research questions
- Analyzing, evaluating, and applying research findings to change clinical practice when appropriate
- Educating other nurses about research findings
- Replicating or participating in the conduct of research based in the speciality area
- Conducting clinical trials of new innovations in practice
- Collaborating in the design and conduct of research
- Communicating research findings through publication
- Acting as a research preceptor for students or staff

The clinical nurse specialist's success in research can be enhanced by participating in collaborative research between the specialist and the academic researcher. The need for collaborative research is supported by the proposal that the improvement of nursing care, the reduction of health care costs, and the testing of a scientific basis for nursing knowledge need to take a greater priority than the previous emphasis on theory and heuristics (Barnard, 1980; Gortner, 1980; King, Barnard, & Hoehn, 1981). Collaborative research utilizes the unique but separate roles of the clinician and the researcher. The clinical nurse specialist can advise which clinical problems are current and can identify relevant researchable questions, has access to potential subjects, can plan appropriate interventions, and knows the operational resources and constraints of the practice setting (Pollock, 1987; Sneed, 1987). The researcher contributes a more sophisticated knowledge of methodology (Bishop, 1981), support services of a secretary and statistical consultant, and access to potential funding sources (Sneed, 1987). The collaboration yields a diverse perspective, varied expertise, and shared responsibility.

The advantages of collaborative research are many. While the clinical nurse specialist takes an active part in the generation of new knowledge, research liaisons and professional collegiality develop concurrently. Participation in a project in particular and research in general permits the clinical nurse specialist to rapidly translate research results into improved professional clinical practice versus the lengthy time otherwise required for new findings to diffuse to the clinician (Barnard, 1980; King, Barnard, & Hoehn, 1981). The clinical nurse specialist who has a research-based practice fosters scholarly inquiry, improves clinical judgment, focuses on patient care outcomes, and initiates and uses clinical nursing research. The academic researcher who collaborates with the clinical nurse specialist develops relevant and useful practice-based research (Brodish, Chamings, & Tranbarger, 1987; Pollock, 1987) while working toward the tenure requirement of research and publication, and has greater client and practice setting access. While a collaborative team has unique and separate roles, the combined effort helps to bridge the perceived or real gap between the separate roles of the clinical nurse specialist and academic researcher.

The few disadvantages of collaborative research are mostly attributable to any type of joint venture. Differences in time allocation in general can be a source of strain, especially as the academic researcher is apt to have more control over a schedule, whereas the clinical nurse specialist's time is determined by patient priorities. Any collaborative effort should include discussion in the planning stages and, at any later point, of the issues of commitment, accountability, ownership, and listing of authors. The clinical nurse specialist who participates in any clinical research project related specifically to the specialty practice area must be aware of the potential contamination of research results through premature translation of perceived outcomes into practice.

The outcomes of collaboration in the conduct of clinical research are relevant practice-based research, increased research productivity, contribution to the scientific knowledge base of the profession, and improved professional practice. Clinical nurse specialists have not failed to fulfill the research obligation of the role completely, but the research that has been published to date has been limited and has been primarily *descriptive*. It has focused on the role of the clinical nurse specialist and its utilization, attitudes about the role and its implementation, the effect of the role on practice characteristics of the generalist nurse, and how the role is operationalized and the associated problems encountered. Few studies have been published which look at or attempt to measure the clinical nurse specialist's effect on patient care outcomes. (See Chapter 4 for a more extensive discussion.)

ADMINISTRATOR AND CLINICAL LEADER

The manner in which a clinical nurse specialist exercises the administrator component of the role may range from leadership functions which are integrated into the role, to functioning as "an administrator for direct care programs in an area of specialization" (ANA, 1986b, p. 4). The clinical nurse specialist who integrates leadership and management functions into the role is active in determining institutional health care policy, guides or participates in quality assurance activities, provides input into performance appraisals, chairs interdisciplinary committees or manages projects, or acts as an advisor to administrators about clinical issues. The clinical nurse specialist can also design and direct clinical programs, while exercising the four primary role components and maintaining a primarily client-care focus (see Chapter 5). When directing a client-care program that also involves staff supervision, there is disagreement among clinical nurse specialists as to the effectiveness possible in direct client care due to difficulty with time allocation between managerial and clinical priorities (see Chapter 3). In fact, clinical nurse specialists value the administrative role the least (Topham, 1987).

Case management is a method of client care health delivery that has generated enthusiasm for the clinical nurse specialist role. It is a model that continues to evolve and will require further definition. The clinical nurse specialist has the preferred educational preparation and practice experience to address the issues of health assessment, resource assessment, planning and delivery of health care services, and advocacy that characterizes case management (American Nurses' Association, 1988). The goals of case management, whether within institutions or in private practice, are continuity of care, especially with clients whose care is multifaceted, provision of personalized care along a continuum, and cost containment (American Nurses' Association, 1988)—all integral elements of high priority in clinical nurse specialist practice. In today's health care environment that favors an efficient and cost-effective delivery system which meets or exceeds established standards, clinical nurse specialists can be exemplary case managers.

SUMMARY

The clinical nurse specialist integrates the primary role components of expert clinician, educator, consultant, and researcher. The authors have proposed role marker trajectories to indicate the changes that occur in the integration of these primary role components as the clinical nurse specialist develops in the role. The emphasis is on client-based practice. The person who has been educated for the clinical nurse specialist role is given a foundation that provides that person with the versatility and flexibility for not only the clinical nurse specialist role but multiple other possibilities. The person who has previously functioned as a clinical nurse specialist and who does choose an alternative position brings a wealth of experience and knowledge to that new functional role. As a nurse educator or nurse administrator, the former clinical nurse specialist can significantly enhance the educational preparation or utilization of clinical nurse specialists. Ultimately, it is the clinical nurse specialist who successfully integrates advanced clinical practice, consultation, education, and research and maintains client-based practice as the primary focus, who promotes the viability and visibility of the role.

REFERENCES

American Nurses' Association. (1976). The scope of nursing practice—description of practice—clinical nurse specialist. Congress for Nursing Practice. Kansas City, MO: American Nurses' Association.

American Nurses' Association. (1980). *Nursing: A social policy statement.* Kansas City, MO: American Nurses' Association.

American Nurses' Association. (1986a). *Facts about nursing 86–87.* American Nurses' Association Publication, #D84. Kansas City, MO: American Nurses' Association.

American Nurses' Association. (1986b). *The role of the clinical nurse specialist.* Kansas City, MO: American Nurses' Association.

American Nurses' Association. (1986c). *Clinical nurse specialists: Distribution and utilization.* Kansas City, MO: American Nurses' Association.

American Nurses' Association. (1988). *Nursing case management.* Kansas City, MO: American Nurses' Association.

Armacost, B. (1973). On becoming a nurse-manager of psychiatry. In J. Riehl & J. McVay (Eds.), *The clinical nurse specialist: Interpretations.* New York: Appleton-Century-Crofts.

Baker, P.O. (1987). Model activities for clinical nurse specialist role development. *Clinical Nurse Specialist, 1,* 119–123.

Baker, C., & Kramer, M. (1970). To define or not to define: The role of the clinical specialist. *Nursing Forum, 9,* 41–55.

Barnard, K.E. (1980). Knowledge for practice: Directions for the future. *Nursing Research, 29* (4), 208–212.

Barrett, H. (1972). The nurse specialist practitioner: A study. *Nursing Outlook, 20,* 524–527.

Barron, A.M. (1983). The CNS as consultant. In A. Hamric & J. Spross (Eds.), *The clinical nurse specialist in theory and practice.* Orlando, FL: Grune & Stratton.

Beare, P. (1988). The ABCs of external consultation. *Clinical Nurse Specialist, 2,* 35–38.

Beecroft, P., & Papenhausen, J. (1987). Editorial opinion. *Clinical Nurse Specialist,* *1,* 149.

Beecroft, P., & Papenhausen, J. (1985). [CNS survey]. Unpublished research.

Bishop, B.E. (1981). A case for collaboration. *Nursing Outlook, 29* (2), 110–111.

Blake, P. (1977). The clinical specialist as nurse consultant. *Journal of Nursing Administration, 7* (10), 33–36.

Brodish, M.S., Chamings, P.A., & Tranbarger, R.E. (1987). Fostering a research focus for the clinical nurse specialist. *Clinical Nurse Specialist, 1* (3), 99–104.

Caplan, G. (1970). *The theory and practice of mental health consultation.* New York: Basic Books.

Christman, L. (1987). The future of the nursing profession. *Nursing Administration Quarterly, 11,* 1–8.

Christman, L. (1965). The influence of specialization on the nursing profession. *Nursing Science, 3* (6), 446–453.

Cooper, D.M. (1983). A refined expert: The clinical nurse specialist after five years. *Momentum, 1,* 2.

Cronenwett, L.R. (1986a). The research role of the clinical nurse specialist. *Journal of Nursing Administration, 16* (4), 10–11.

Cronenwett, L.R. (1986b). Research contributions of clinical nurse specialists. *Journal of Nursing Administration, 16* (6), 6–7.

Dirschel, K. (1976). The conception, gestation, and delivery of the clinical nursing specialist. In R. Rotkovich (Ed.), *Quality patient care and the role of the clinical nursing specialist.* New York: Wiley.

Donoghue, M., & Spross, J. (1985). A report from the first national invitational conference: The oncology clinical nurse specialist role analysis and future projections. *Oncology Nursing Forum, 12,* 35–37.

Edlund, B.J., Hodges, L.C., & Poteet, G.W. (1987). Consultation: Doing it and doing it well. *Clinical Nurse Specialist, 1,* 86–90.

Everson, S. (1981). Integration of the role of clinical specialist. *The Journal of Continuing Education in Nursing, 12* (2), 16–19.

Felder, L.A. (1983). Direct patient care and independent practice. In A. Hamric & J. Spross (Eds.), *The Clinical Nurse Specialist in Theory and Practice,* pp. 59–71. Orlando, FL: Grune & Stratton.

Fenton, M.V. (1985). Identifying competencies of clinical nurse specialists. *Journal of Nursing Administration, 15,* 31–37.

Fife, B., & Lemler, S. (1983). The psychiatric nurse specialist: A valuable asset in the general hospital. *Journal of Nursing Administration, 13* (4), 14–17.

Fralic, M.F. (1988). Nursing's precious resource: The clinical nurse specialist. *Journal of Nursing Administration, 18,* (2) 5–6.

Gleason, J., & Flynn, K. (1987). The surgical clinical nurse specialist as consultant in a tertiary care setting. *Clinical Nurse Specialist, 1,* 129–132.

Gortner, S.R. (1980). Nursing research: Out of the past and into the future. *Nursing Research, 29* (4), 204–207.

Gresham, M. (1983). Joint appointments. In A. Hamric & J. Spross (Eds.), *The clinical nurse specialist in theory and practice* (pp. 129–148). Orlando, FL: Grune & Stratton.

Hamric, A. (1983). Role development and role function. In A. Hamric & J. Spross (Eds.), *The clinical nurse specialist in theory and practice* (pp. 39–56). Orlando, FL: Grune & Stratton.

Hendrix, M., & La Godna, G. (1982). Consultation: A political process aimed at change. In J. Lancaster, & W. Lancaster (Eds.), *The nurse as a change agent*. St. Louis: C.V. Mosby.

Hodgman, E.C. (1983). The CNS as researcher. In A.B. Hamric & J. Spross (Eds.), *The clinical nurse specialist in theory and practice* (pp. 73–82). Orlando, FL: Grune & Stratton.

Holt, F.M. (1984). A theoretical model for clinical specialist practice. *Nursing and Health Care, 5*, 445–449.

Holt, F.M. (1987). Executive practice. *Clinical Nurse Specialist, 1*, 116–118.

Jackson, B. (1973). Hospital administrators need to know about clinical nurse specialists. *Supervisor Nurse, 4*, 29–35.

Jacox, A. (1974). Nursing research and the clinician. *Nursing Outlook, 22* (6), 382–385.

James, W. (1958). *Talks to teachers*. New York: W.W. Norton and Co.

Johnson, J.E., Fuller, S.S., Endress, M.P., & Rice, V.H. (1978). Altering patients' responses to surgery: An extension and replication. *Research in Nursing and Health, 1* (3), 111–121.

King, D., Barnard, K.E., & Hoehn, R. (1981). Disseminating the results of nursing research. *Nursing Outlook, 29* (2), 164–169.

Kinsella, C.R. (1973). Who is the clinical nurse specialist? *Hospitals, 47*, 72–80.

Kohnke, M. (1978). *Case for consultation in nursing: Designs for professional practice*. New York: Wiley.

Lange, F. (1979). The multi-faceted role of the nurse consultant. *Journal of Nursing Education, 8*, 30–34.

Laureau, S.C. (1985). The nurse as clinical consultant. *Topics in Clinical Nursing, 2*, 79–84.

McGann, M.R. (1975). The clinical nurse specialist: From hospitals to clinic, to community. *Journal of Nursing Administration, 5*, 33–37.

Malone, B.L. (1986). Evaluation of the clinical nurse specialist. *American Journal of Nursing, 86* (12): 1375–1377.

Montemuro, M.A. (1987). The evolution of the clinical nurse specialist: Response to the challenge of professional nursing practice. *Clinical Nurse Specialist, 1, 1* (3): 106–110.

Munro, B.H. (1987). The research role of the clinical nurse specialist. *Clinical Nurse Specialist, 1* (1), 7.

Noll, M. (1987). Internal consultation as a framework for clinical nurse specialist practice. *Clinical Nurse Specialist, 1*, 46–50.

Oda, D, Sparacino, P., & Boyd, P. (1988). Role advancement for the experienced clinical nurse specialist. *Clinical Nurse Specialist, 2* (4), 167–171.

Peplau, H. (1965). Specialization in professional nursing. *Nursing Science, 3* (4), 268–287.

Pollock, S.E. (1987). Clinical nursing research: The needed link for unifying professional nursing. *Clinical Nurse Specialist, 1* (1), 8–12.

Poteet, G.W. (1987). Consultation. *Clinical Nurse Specialist, 1*, 85.

Redman, B.K. (1980). *Process of patient teaching in nursing*. St. Louis: Mosby.

Reiter, F. (1966). The nurse-clinician. *American Journal of Nursing, 66*, 274–280.

Robichaud, A.M., & Hamric, A.B. (1986). Time documentation of clinical nurse specialist activities. *Journal of Nursing Administration, 6*, 31–36.

Sills, G.M. (1983). The role and function of the clinical nurse specialist. In N.L.

Chaska (Ed.), *The nursing profession: A time to speak* (pp. 563–579). New York: McGraw-Hill.

Sisson, R. (1987). Co-workers perceptions of the clinical nurse specialist role. *Clinical Nurse Specialist, 1,* 13–17.

Smith, M. (1974). Perceptions of head nurses, clinical nurse specialist, nursing educators, and nursing office personnel regarding performance of selected nursing activities. *Nursing Research, 23* (6), 505–511.

Sneed, N.V. (1987). Collaboration as a means to achieving the clinical nurse specialist research role expectations. *Clinical Nurse Specialist, 1* (1), 70–74.

Stevens, B. (1976). Accountability of the clinical specialist: The administrators viewpoint. *Journal of Nursing Administration, 6,* 30–32.

Styles, M.M. (1987). Nursing today and a vision for the future. *Nursing Economics, 5,* 103–117.

Tarsitano, B.J., Brophy, E.B., & Snyder, D.J. (1986). A demystification of the clinical nurse specialist role: Perceptions of clinical nurse specialists and nurse administrators. *Journal of Nursing Education, 25,* 4–9.

Topham, D.L. (1987). Role theory in relation to roles of the clinical nurse specialist. *Clinical Nurse Specialist, 1,* 81–84.

University of California at San Francisco (1986). Proposed developmental role markers. Department of Nursing Services.

Walker, M. (1986). How nursing service administrators view clinical nurse specialists. *Nursing Management, 17,* 52–54.

Werner, J.S., Bumann, R.M., & O'Brien, J.A. (1988). Clinical nurse specialization: An annotated bibliography. *Clinical Nurse Specialist, 2,* 14–15.

Wyers, M.E.A., Grove, S.K., & Pastorino, C. (1985). Clinical nurse specialist: In search of the right role. *Nursing and Health Care, 6,* 203–207.

chapter three

Acquiring, Implementing, and Evaluating the Clinical Nurse Specialist Role

Diane M. Cooper
Patricia S.A. Sparacino

The dynamic nature of role implementation is influenced by setting, specialty, experience, level of expertise, co-workers and, perhaps most significantly, the philosophy of and the relationship one establishes with one's peers and immediate supervisor. This chapter will address the issues and process of securing a position as a clinical nurse specialist. Additionally, the placement of the clinical nurse specialist within an organization will be presented, noting the advantages and disadvantages of both staff and line positions. A framework for role implementation, suggested role development markers, and guidelines for developing a role description are also included. The chapter concludes with a discussion of approaches to time management and suggestions for evaluation of the clinical nurse specialist.

SECURING A POSITION

Securing the right position is not an easy task for anyone. The greater the level of expertise, experience, and clarity regarding what one desires in a job, the more critical this already difficult task can become. Much has been written in recent years to assist the job applicant, particularly the professional, in the mechanics of applying for a job. Studies have been done and strategies cited which are thought to increase the likelihood of attaining a desired position. Issues such as the importance of preparing a clear, concise, and professional resume, of selecting the "proper" attire for the interview, and of being prepared with salient questions have been described in both lay magazines and professional journals (O'Connor, 1984). The importance of the basic amenities surrounding the job interview process itself should not be underestimated; however, they will not be reiterated here. On the contrary, this section of the chapter will focus specifically on issues germane to the clinical nurse specialist interested in attaining the optimal position. Although it is true that an increasing number of clinical nurse specialists are assuming or creating positions outside of hospitals, the fact remains that over half are employed in hospital settings. Because of this, the focus of this portion of the chapter will be directed primarily toward clinical nurse specialist job applicants seeking positions within a department of nursing in a hospital. Even so, many of the issues discussed here should be considered by clinical nurse specialists interested in securing a position in any environment, and therefore the usefulness of the comments is not limited by employment setting.

Preliminary Tasks and Preparatory Questions

Prior to filling out an application or scheduling interviews, the individual interested in obtaining a position as a clinical nurse specialist must delineate clearly the type and desired goals of the position sought. This preparatory effort at clarity regarding the scope of a position is mandatory for the novice clinical nurse specialist, but equally crucial for experienced clinical nurse specialists seeking positions outside their current place of employment. The amount of time spent and the degree of precision one has about what it is one wants in a position could be described, in most cases, as a predictor of the "fit" and level of satisfaction ultimately experienced in the position selected (del Bueno & Price, 1987).

A series of questions regarding the clinical nurse specialist role demands a significant expenditure of time and thought in the early stages of the job-seeking process. If clinical nurse specialists grapple with each of these questions and log the answers in *writing*, they will be able, based on the answers, to include as well as exclude certain job offerings. The position-seeking clinical nurse specialist can, through analysis of materials sent by potential employers, discussion with current or past employees of the institution and, if possible, impromptu observational visits to the institution in question, begin to separate out those places of employment whose philosophies are congruent with one's own and therefore warrant more intensive investigation. Similarly, the well-prepared clinical nurse specialist can more quickly determine which offerings appear to require no further pursuit.

The following are a series of questions aimed at assisting the job-seeking clinical nurse specialist in clarifying expectations about the potential employment situation. Although some of the questions could be answered during the interview in ways the applicant never could have imagined, it is important that the clinical nurse specialist be clear about the desired answers prior to that time. Similarly, in formulating responses to the questions, it is important for the clinical nurse specialist to determine which questions, if any, have a range of acceptable anwers, as well as those on which no compromise is possible. Through such an analytical process the essential aspects of the position sought are revealed. In addition, nonnegotiable issues (for example, must be affiliated with a school of nursing) that must be addressed in the search process are identified.

In organizing one's goals for a future position, innumerable questions covering every minute detail could be listed. The series of questions that follows, while not exhaustive, are suggested because of their potential for provoking clarity in the mind of the clinical nurse specialist regarding the "essentials" of a position. The questions cluster around several topics and will be presented in that manner.

Setting and Role Format. The following questions might assist the applicant in determining the type of setting and role format desired.

1. What setting would be most compatible with my level of experience, specialty, degree of specialization, and future goals?
2. If I choose to practice within an institution, is a tertiary care setting, a military hospital, or a community hospital setting what I desire? Am I clear about why such a setting is preferred?
3. Do I desire to function in a line or a staff position?
4. Would I prefer a setting in which a generic job description of the clinical nurse specialist has been formulated?
5. Would I prefer to write my own role description?
6. Whom do I want my client to be? (the patient, the staff nurse, both?)

Level of Scholarship Within Nursing. Levels of scholarship vary from setting to setting. One cannot assume that because a hospital is not a teaching hospital, affiliated directly with a university and its school of nursing, that scholarly activity does not occur. On the other hand, with the increasing emphasis on clinical/faculty collaboration, one would expect that the potential for a scholarly atmosphere in nursing is present within settings with such affiliations. If the clinical nurse specialist desires to work in a milieu where research is ongoing, publications by nursing staff frequent the literature, and time and support are available for inquiry into issues of concern to the practice of nursing, then the questions that follow should be pondered. Subsequent to answering these questions, and as one singles out specific institutions for interview, one would be well served by requesting a list of the publications authored by members of the nursing staff of the institution in question, as well as an overview of ongoing nursing research. If this information is not provided, that also constitutes an important piece of evaluation information. The level of scholarship in nursing within the environment can be determined by answering the following questions.

1. How important to me is a position in a setting in which there are affiliations with a school of nursing?
2. Do I want to work in a setting in which nursing faculty and clinical nurse specialists collaborate or have potential for collaborating in nursing research?
3. Do I want to precept graduate students in nursing?
4. Would I prefer a position in which there would be the opportunity for a faculty appointment with a school of nursing?
5. Is it important to me that nursing research be in process within the department of nursing *prior* to my accepting the position?
6. What clerical and administrative support would I consider necessary for clinical nurse specialists undertaking nursing research projects?
7. Do I want to work in a setting where the expectations of clinical nurse specialists as regards nursing research are explicit, or more general?
8. If I am interested in conducting nursing research, would I expect acknowledgment of this activity through monetary or other rewards?
9. Is the level of educational preparation of the individual to whom I report important to me?

History and Status of the Position in the Organization. It is vitally important that a clinical nurse specialist assuming a new position be assured of some degree of security and longevity in the position. This is not to infer that individuals hiring clinical nurse specialists can predict the future or that they can predict the success in the role of each clinical nurse specialist hired, but rather, it is important that clinical nurse specialists enter a fairly stable environment when they assume new positions. Ascertaining the security of the clinical nurse specialist position within an organization is difficult, particularly when current philosophies differ about maintaining and increasing the number of these nurses.

The following questions have been designed to assist the job-seeking clinical nurse specialist to evaluate the degree of stability of the clinical nurse specialist position within an organization.

1. Do I desire to function within an organization in which the clinical nurse specialist position has been in place for some time, or would I prefer a setting in which the role has been newly implemented?
2. Where would I like to see the clinical nurse specialist on the organizational chart, or need the position be noted there at all?
3. To whom do I think the clinical nurse specialists should report? (director of nursing, assistant director of nursing, head nurse, etc.)

4. If nursing is a significant force within the institution, to whom do I think the highest ranking nursing executive should report?
5. Who should be responsible for the evaluation of clinical nurse specialists?
6. If I asked what the future projections for the use of the clinical nurse specialist were, how precisely would I want the question answered?
7. Where do I think the clinical nurse specialist should be on the pay scale and what kind of an interval between a clinical nurse specialist's salary and a non-master's-prepared clinician would I accept?
8. What kind of relationship between the medical staff and nurses with advanced preparation would I expect within the organization?
9. Do I desire to work in a setting where reward systems for the clinical nurse specialist are clearly established?
10. Do I desire to see advanced nursing practice clearly articulated in the philosophy of the department of nursing?
11. How timely do I think documents such as the organizational chart, statement of philosophy, generic job description of the clinical nurse specialist, and other nursing documents affecting the role of the clinical nurse specialist should be? (i.e., how recently should they have been written or updated?)
12. Would it be of significance to me how long the individual to whom I will report has been in the position, as well as their intentions for remaining in the position?

Alternative Practice Arrangements. An increasing number of clinical nurse specialists are moving out of traditional hospital settings and into private or independent practice settings (see Chapter 13; Rew, 1988). Because these settings and the expectations of the clinical nurse specialists in them differ from those in hospitals, new and different questions aimed at assisting the clinical nurse specialist seeking such a nontraditional position need to be developed. Clinical nurse specialists presently in independent or private practice positions could formulate a list of pertinent questions and explain the rationale behind them. In doing so, clinical nurse specialists making the transition from hospital to private or independent practice could be better prepared for and increase their potential for securing the optimal position. Although some of the questions listed above could be used to assist in the process, those that follow more specifically address the unique aspects of the independent or private practice clinical nurse specialist. Anyone interested in securing such a position or, for that matter, any clinical nurse specialist should be knowledgeable about the state's Nurse Practice Act, especially with regard to regulations about advanced nursing practice.

1. If I move into an independent practice setting, are my referral sources sufficient in number and are they stable enough?
2. Has a need for the nursing services I desire to supply been identified as necessary to the community?
3. Do I have the economic base and the support systems available to sustain me in this endeavor?
4. If I am entering into independent practice with other practitioners, are we personally clear about our goals, reimbursement mechanisms, partnership issues, and so on? Have these been spelled out legally?

Some clinical nurse specialists have been employed full time by physicians outside the hospital setting. The clinical nurse specialist who is hired directly by a physician must have a clear understanding of the role of a nurse in order to execute the role of the clinical nurse specialist and avoid the potential for becoming the physician's assistant or "scut" worker. The clinical nurse specialist employed by the physician in private practice must clearly negotiate the role prior to accepting it, as well as review and clarify role implementation at regular intervals (see Chapter 13). It is imperative that this clinical nurse specialist establish strong peer relationships with other clinical nurse specialists in the community at large or clinical nurse specialists in similar job situations in order to provide both peer support and ongoing input and validation of the appropriateness of role implementation. Issues such as office space, percentage of share in the practice, and time to attend meetings and pursue scholarly activities also need to be considered long before the clinical nurse specialist appears for the first day of work.

Finally, some astute hospital-based physicians, particularly in academic settings, have recognized the value of clinical nurse specialists and have elected to employ them (see Chapter 7). Shrewd nursing directors have utilized this set of circumstances to their benefit by supporting a certain percentage of the clinical nurse specialist's time while the physician, or a department within medicine, assumes the remainder. Such an arrangement is enhanced when the clinical nurse specialist reports to the director of nursing, who then is able to provide support, feedback, and peer relationships within nursing for the clinical nurse specialist. Again, the clinical nurse specialist in this situation must be exquisitely clear about the physician's expectations and evaluate the appropriateness of the tasks to be accomplished for a nursing role.

Although the list of questions one should ask oneself prior to job interviews could go on, clarity regarding the answers to those listed here should be a priority. Only after reflecting on the answers and assessing places of employment where the potential for congruence is high, should one approach selected institutions regarding openings. As an early step, documents should be solicited from selected institutions and examined for congruence with one's own expectation. Requesting this material can serve to identify situations where successful employment is more likely. Reviewing documents such as the generic job description of the clinical nurse specialist, the organizational chart of the department of nursing, and the philosophy of the nursing department can provoke additional questions that will need to be addressed during the interview itself. If the employing agency does not provide such information, this neglect provides the applicant with a significant piece of information.

Self-appraisal

Formulating a self-appraisal list regarding one's qualifications, as well as predicting what it is one might be able to accomplish in positions under consideration, also can assist the applicant in the preliminary period. Additionally, the scrutiny of a self-appraisal affords the clinical nurse specialist applicant a greater sense of self-worth, direction, and ability to articulate goals in subsequent discussions and during the interview itself. Given the fact that any professional should formulate yearly goals and a 3- to 5-year plan, one should reflect early on how a specific job might assist in goal attainment.

Experienced Clinical Nurse Specialist

When the experienced clinical nurse specialist is in the situation of looking for a new position, there are several special considerations. If the clinical nurse specialist has occupied a position for several years or has held several different positions as a clinical nurse specialist, in addition to assessing the questions previously listed, time should be taken prior to seeking a new position to reflect on past accomplishments. A significant task, frequently avoided when one seeks new employment, is to determine specifically why one is leaving the current position. In order to ensure that all aspects of this issue are addressed, the clinical nurse specialist should be able to identify the positive aspects of the current position, as well as its limitations. Only when the clinical nurse specialist is clear about the reason(s) for leaving and what is being "given up" will it be clear what is being sought. There is no "perfect" job, and the grass is never "greener."

If the experienced clinical nurse specialist has kept records of interactions with patients and, better still, effect on patient outcomes, these data should be tabulated and organized clearly and concisely. Such information has the potential for marketing a clinical nurse specialist to a potential employer and further supports the "worth" of one clinical nurse specialist applicant over another.

Geographic Assessment

Another issue necessary to consider is the geographic location acceptable in potential positions. The new clinical nurse specialist graduate often feels so appreciative of recognition that a position in any part of the country might be taken without sufficient evaluation. The novice clinical nurse specialist especially needs to be aware of the combined effects of moving into a new role and to a new geographic location at the same time. Often this set of circumstances leaves the individual alone and without familiar support systems if and when problems arise. This is not to say that there have not been cases where novice clinical nurse specialists moved great distances in order to secure their first position and did so successfully, but issues surrounding support systems and lack of familiarity with new communities also need to be considered prior to scheduling face-to-face interviews. Evaluating the geographic location in regard to setting one's five-year goals, however, would assist both the novice and the experienced clinical nurse specialist to assess in a thoughtful, organized manner a position that would involve moving to a new region. Implications in relation to planning for future graduate work, affiliation with a university or school of nursing, opportunities for collaborative research, among others, all need to be taken into consideration whether the position is across town or across the country.

Identifying Potential Positions

There are various means by which the clinical nurse specialist can become aware of potential positions. Friends and colleagues may inform one of an opening by word-of-mouth. The same level of rigorous scrutiny as that used in assessing any other potential employment opportunity must be applied in this situation.

More recently, with an increase in the number of conferences directed specifically at clinical nurse specialists, there is an additional opportunity to hear of interesting and challenging positions. Hospitals frequently use this recruiting mechanism for seeking interested applicants due to the prolonged interval between submitting an advertisement to journals and its appearance. Pertinent journals, however, should not be dismissed as an unlikely source of interesting positions. Agencies go to great expense to advertise in them and frequently do so in order to ensure a wide range of applicants.

Using the services of a search firm can streamline the process of determining which interview to pursue, and particularly for the individual currently occupying a position as a clinical nurse specialist, such an approach affords inroads, leg work, and guaranteed confidentiality that would be difficult under any other set of circumstances. If a search firm is utilized, however, the process of identifying positions with high potential is made possible only if one is able to clearly delineate all the particulars desired in a job to the individual conducting the search on one's behalf. Realistically, no matter how one goes about learning about job openings, one should not expect to acquire the "perfect" position immediately. The process is often time-consuming.

Although not the normal course of events, experienced clinical nurse specialists have been known to approach a specific institution in which they desired to practice in spite of the absence of advertised job openings. When the clinical nurse specialists were able to clearly articulate what they could accomplish in terms of patient care outcomes, there have been cases where nursing administrators have hired them. Therefore, one should not let the absence of an advertised position deter one from proposing that a position be created. Obviously, such an applicant must be assertive, able to clearly articulate the advantages of creating such a position, and be prepared for lengthy and serious discussion. This latter method of job seeking demands energy and perseverance; it is not recommended for the faint-hearted or easily discouraged.

Frequently, graduate schools and universities have bulletin boards that post position descriptions available locally and across the country. This approach affords the applicant some background information and time to inquire regarding the record of the potential place of employment.

In some cases, newly graduated clinical nurse specialists assume positions in institutions where they have worked as staff nurses. This transition reduces a number of unknowns faced by clinical nurse specialists. Moving from one position to another in the same institution is not without its difficulties, however, particularly if the clinical nurse specialist is assuming a newly established position. It behooves the clinical nurse specialist applicant in this situation to interview for the position in the same manner as any other candidate. The clinical nurse specialist should insist that the full interview process be undertaken. If clarifying role expectations through a formal interview process is judged superfluous by the employer, then one should be concerned not only about the value being ascribed to the position, but also the potential for being successful in it.

The Interview

It is important that the clinical nurse specialist, whether novice or experienced, be extremely selective about which interviews are actually pursued. Not only is it exhausting and expensive to undertake numerous interviews, but such an approach can expose one to confusion and sometimes it is a waste of time. If discretion is employed in choosing appropriate interviews and the preparatory tasks suggested in this section of the chapter are completed, one should schedule only those interviews that exhibit high potential for congruence between the way in which the applicant envisions the role and the employer's expectations.

If several sites are selected in which to interview, it is helpful to ask the same or similar questions during the interviews. Even within a single interview, asking the same questions of the various individuals involved is helpful, for such an approach affords the interviewee greater opportunity to detect conflict or philosophical disagreements among key individuals, and thereby to make comparisons.

During the interview itself, the clinical nurse specialist applicant should be critically assessing the type of questions asked by the interviewer(s), the mix of individuals included in the process, the tone of the questions, and the candor with which questions are answered. One would be concerned if clinical nurse specialists, nurse managers, staff nurses, as well as physicians and hospital administrators were not included on the interview schedule. Additionally, the optimal interview day should include a tour of the environment in which one might eventually be employed, as well as time to peruse materials, such as nursing care plans and procedure manuals.

Most crucial of all, however, is the quality of time spent with the director of nursing, and in cases where this person is not the immediate supervisor, the individual who will be. Again, the type of information these individuals seek and the candor with which they respond to questions are important and should be assessed by the applicant as the interview unfolds. More crucial than that analysis, however, is close and continuous monitoring by the clinical nurse specialist applicant of the Gestalt, the "feeling tone," and the gut reaction to these individuals (del Bueno & Price, 1987). Despite the large number of people with whom one interacts as a clinical nurse specialist, perhaps none is more pivotal than the individual to whom one reports. Therefore, besides evaluating this individual's philosophy of nursing and strategies for implementing and supporting the role of the clinical nurse specialist, it is also important to evaluate one's visceral response to the human being.

Through it all, it is necessary for any clinical nurse specialist applicant to realize that scrutiny by the applicant is as important as scrutiny by the potential employer. Interviewing can be exhausting. It demands an enormous expenditure of energy on the part of the applicant. It is an active process. The healthy employment environment has little to hide and desires a good fit between its employees and the institutional goals; consequently these employers expect and look for candidates equally concerned about scrutinizing them.

The Choice

Making the final selection of a position is always a difficult task, particularly for the individual who is offered several enticing opportunities. There are multiple factors that go into the final decision one makes, and every choice rejects others. The clinical nurse specialist who has taken the time to prepare and carry out the interview(s) in a deliberate and methodical manner, however, should have far less difficulty with the final choice than the one who approaches the task in a "laissez faire" manner. Ideally, immediately following or even during the interview, the applicant should note in writing the responses of the interviewers. Additionally, it is advantageous to summarize one's overall reaction to the experience. Although these tasks may seem tedious at the time, they are invaluable sources of information, which could easily be forgotten if several interviews occurred over a period of time. Reviewing one's "transcript" of each interview, particularly in those situations where the final decision rests on selecting between two seemingly optimal situations, can often make the decision much easier by providing a comparison of crucial strengths or weaknesses in each of the positions.

Having reassessed the congruence between the answers to the questions the applicant prepared and those provided by the individuals with whom one interviewed, the clinical nurse specialist should reflect on the following questions and then make a decision in a timely fashion.

1. Is the director of nursing supportive of the role of the clinical nurse specialist?
2. Is there clarity regarding the expectations of the clinical nurse specialist within the leadership of the department of nursing?
3. Do the institution's expectations of the clinical nurse specialist role coincide with expectations outlined by me prior to the interview?
4. Is there a peer network for the clinical nurse specialist(s) within the institution or within the community at large?
5. Are the head nurses within the institution, particularly those with whom I will interact, supportive of the role of the clinical nurse specialist?
6. Are clinical nurse specialists supported by the medical staff?

Pragmatics and Perquisites

The philosophical notions underlying the clinical nurse specialist role cannot be underestimated; ultimately, most clinical nurse specialists are satisfied or dissatisfied in their positions because of the beliefs held by their employers about nursing, advanced practice, and how the role of the clinical nurse specialist should be implemented. Even when philosophies between the clinical nurse specialist and the potential employer appear aligned, the job-seeking clinical nurse specialist, particularly the experienced specialist, must be clear about issues surrounding one's appointment, including salary, benefits, and perquisites. If the clinical nurse specialist is not being represented by a search firm that will carry out this investigation, the clinical nurse specialist must investigate the range of salaries within the community for clinical nurse specialists, nurse managers, executives, and other business and professional individuals. This information provides a context from which the clinical nurse specialist can establish salary requirements. It is essential that the applicant be prepared to engage in salary and benefits negotiation. Among the factors that should be considered during these negotiations are percentage of total compensation comprised by the benefit package, that is, does the benefit package consist of 10 percent of total salary cost or 50 percent? If the benefit package is only 10 percent, the applicant must determine what it will cost to provide essential benefits for oneself and for one's family. The base salary request should be framed within this context. Other issues to be considered during preliminary negotiations include clinical nurse specialist office space, financial support to attend professional meetings, clerical support, parking facilities, library resources, time provided for scholarly pursuits, expectations regarding nonpatient-care activities, level and type of committee membership expectations/opportunities, degree of flexibility in time management, and moving expenses/salary advances (S. Ellerbe-O'Donnell, 1988, personal communication).

No matter how perfect the choice of a new job, problems will present themselves. The individual who has carefully reflected on goals, organized priorities, and selectively sought out positions where the potential for a good fit is more likely, however, will not only select the right position but will grow in the position selected. Too often, nurses in general and clinical nurse specialists in particular have not approached the job search in the serious and pragmatic manner it warrants. Increasingly, as positions become less available and employers become more selective, clinical nurse specialists must incorporate the marketing skills already embraced by our fellow professionals in business. Incorporating such strategies ultimately will assist qualified clinical nurse specialists to stand out over their less qualified peers. Securing the appropriate position as a clinical nurse specialist is a crucial aspect of one's career development, as well as a determinant of one's overall satisfaction as a professional. A great deal of preparation and thought needs to be put into the process in order to prevent negative and unsatisfactory experiences.

The career-minded professional devotes a great deal of time and energy in a job. The wrong position can drain one's energy and stifle creativity. The right job is not only rewarding, but can springboard the individual occupying it to accomplishments never dreamed possible. The patients, nursing staff, physicians, and employer deserve to have satisfied clinical nurse specialists available to them; such a scenario is likely to occur when time and effort have been expended on getting the "best fit."

PLACEMENT OF THE CLINICAL NURSE SPECIALIST WITHIN THE SYSTEM

One of the clinical nurse specialist issues that has generated the most debate and disagreement is the appropriate placement of the clinical nurse specialist within the nursing as well as organizational system. Due to its individualized evolution, the clinical nurse specialist role is an organizational anomaly which does not necessarily fit logically into the institutional management system (Niessner, 1979; Parkis, 1974a, 1974b; Stevens, 1976). With the evolution of the role, there has been disagreement among clinical nurse specialists themselves as to what are the definition and responsibilities of the role (Roberts, 1987). With this disagreement comes individualized role definitions, variability among clinical nurse specialists regarding actualization of their roles, and confusion about role similarities and dissimilarities (Disch, 1978; MacPhail, 1971). Disagreement also results in conflicting prevailing expectations of administrative and clinical colleagues. Further, with disagreement comes confusion about whether a nurse whose functional capabilities have been expanded to assume tasks formerly carried out by physicians is, thus, a clinical nurse specialist (Cahill, 1973).

The key issue is the relationship of clinical nurse specialist role implementation to the primary issues of professional versus administrative authority. Every competent clinical nurse specialist, by virtue of expert knowledge and clinical expertise, should be accorded professional authority. The crux of the debate is the issue of whether administrative authority should be a part of the clinical nurse specialist position. Administrative authority should be granted by virtue of the job description and role placement within the organization (Stevens, 1976).

The 1980 American Nurses' Association (ANA) document, *Nursing: A Social Policy Statement*, took a necessary stance when addressing the issue of clinical nurse specialist authority:

> When nurse specialists are employed in health care settings, descriptions of their position and functions ought not to be standardized. The work rules for the specialist must be jointly determined and negotiated. . . . the emphasis should be on developing negotiated positions and organizational arrangements that are most likely to result in freedom and responsibility for maximum use of the abilities of the particular specialist in the particular health care setting (pp. 26–27).

Because of the diversity of organizational arrangements available, the clinical nurse specialist role can be variously utilized in positions whose responsibilities demand flexibility and multiple allegiances: private practice, either solo or in conjunction with allied health professionals or other clinical nurse specialists, or collaborative or joint practice with physicians. It is with departments of nursing service, however, that the greatest strength and control may lie for the support of the role in its purest form. This is dependent on administrative commitment. If lacking administrative commitment, the role is subject to changes in implementation that dilute and weaken effectiveness.

Staff Versus Line Position

Presently clinical nurse specialists are placed within the organizational system in a staff position, whether by preference or by design. A survey conducted in 1984 and sponsored by the American Nurses' Association Council of Clinical Nurse Specialists (ANA, 1986a) elicited responses from 2512 clinical nurse specialists surveyed, for a response rate of 74 percent. Of the 2327 clinical nurse specialists who responded to the question about organizational position in their primary employment setting, 72 percent were in a staff position and 13 percent in a line position.

The clinical nurse specialist in a staff position has freedom from administrative tasks and derives power by virtue of clinical expertise and knowledge. It is clinical competence and expert knowledge that create the referent power. The staff position allows a multidimensional functional position that can directly improve patient care by direct intervention and that can indirectly improve patient care by collaboratively working with other clinical nurse specialists, members of the health care team, and administrators in the areas of consultation, education, and research (Beeber & Scicchitani, 1980). Particularly when serving in a consultative capacity, a nonadministrative position offers less of an overt threat and hence the consultee is more apt to ask for assistance (Blake, 1977; Everson, 1981; Jackson, 1973).

The disadvantage of the clinical nurse specialist in a staff position is the lack of formal authority. Being in a staff position necessitates the building and testing of professional authority. The utilization of the clinical nurse specialist by staff nurses, physicians, and other members of the health care team becomes dependent upon each person's understanding not only of the role and its functions, but also their perception of how patient needs will benefit from the clinical nurse specialist's intervention (Crabtree, 1979; Stevens, 1976). Because the professional authority can be so dependent upon the whims and determinations of others, the lack of formal authority can thwart the efforts of a clinical nurse specialist, limit accountability, and cause frustrations to mount higher. Subsequently the clinical nurse specialist in a staff position feels that any attempt to measure effectiveness through patient care outcomes may not produce valid results as access to patients is so dependent upon the perception of need and referral by others (Stevens, 1976).

On the other hand, the clinical nurse specialist with administrative or line authority traditionally has combined the clinical practice component of the role with the assumption of the role of head nurse, supervisor, or assistant or associate director of nursing (Butts, 1974; Crabtree, 1979; Fagin, 1967). The advantage that a clinical nurse specialist has in such a position is that when patient care has been evaluated and the implementation of alternative approaches determined as necessary to improve the quality of patient care, the line position grants the necessary authority to enforce clinical decisions (Barrett, 1972; Castronovo, 1975; Johnson, Wilcox, & Moidel, 1967). This concept of an authority role is seen as facilitating the process of affecting change but also makes available the reward power to hold staff accountable and to counsel and discipline when staff are noncompliant in enacting recommendations (Edwards, 1971; Niessner, 1979, Odello, 1973). This approach is frequently viewed as desirable by nursing administration as it is deemed cost effective, allowing one person to theoretically function as both supervisor and clinical nurse specialist.

Beeber and Scicchitani (1980) view the clinical nurse specialist role as most effective in improving patient care delivery when that person is placed in a unit-based line position. Their rationale is that when a staff person sees the clinical nurse specialist coping with the usual number of nonclinically-related demands and still effectively implementing changes in patient care, then the clinical nurse specialist as well as the recommendations made will be accepted by staff. The understanding is that a clinical nurse specialist who understands the administrative problems of administering patient care will be more effective in working with the nursing team in the resolution of nursing care problems.

The primary disadvantages of the clinical nurse specialist being in a line position is that it is extremely difficult to apportion time equitably between managerial and clinical responsibilities. Some authors feel that administrative responsibilities detract from clinical responsibilities and thus limit time and energies the clinical nurse specialist can devote to direct patient care (Parkis, 1974a, 1974b; Stevens, 1976). Another disadvantage of the line position is that it is highly improbable that the clinical nurse specialist has had graduate preparation in both nursing administration and an area of clinical specialization and so will not be equally prepared to function in both capacities at an advanced level. Likewise, if the clinical nurse specialist in the authoritative position is required to evaluate staff performance, staff may be reluctant to seek clinical assistance with skills or acquisition of theory, as such a request may be seen as a lack of knowledge rather than seeking improvement and hence may jeopardize advancement opportunities (Beeber & Scicchitani, 1980; Crabtree, 1979).

Although one may have preferences as to whether the clinical nurse specialist in a staff position is more effective than one in a line position, or vice versa, the key issue should be that the clinical nurse specialist's expectations and those of the organization should fit in a position that allows for cooperation, collaboration, flexibility, and congruence (del Bueno & Price, 1987). A satisfactory arrangement may be a staff position with sufficient line authority to add power to the clinical nurse specialist role and to implement change (Roberts, 1987). While there have been no studies evaluating which organizational position is best, both the clinical nurse specialist and the organization should be aware of the advantages and disadvantages of both staff and line positions for the clinical nurse specialist and of the placement of the position within the organizational hierarchy. The desired goal is improved patient care outcomes.

ROLE DESCRIPTION

Role Titles

Over the years, role titles have increased in length and, in many cases, decreased in providing information about what it is the title bearer actually does. Clinical nurse specialists are fortunate to have had the generic title they bear described by the profession. In spite of the fact that the average citizen lacks an understanding of the educational requirements and clinical competence of clinical nurse specialists, an increasing number of nurses and other members of the health care team are aware of what clinical nurse specialists do. Each clinical nurse specialist is, by definition, a master clinician of a particular area of nursing practice. As such, the clinical nurse specialist needs to select descriptors of the particular speciality that are (1) succinct, (2) easily understood by a wide range of individuals, from lay people to physicians, (3) commonly recognizable or identifiable across settings, and (4) more focused on phenomena of concern to the practice of nursing and less on medical/ surgical diagnoses or physiological systems.

In choosing a title, the clinical nurse specialist should state in two or three words what it is that is done in practice. These terms could, most likely, form the basis of the title selected. Additionally, clinical nurse specialists need to reassess their titles at intervals. Often, as one's practice evolves, the focus of the speciality is clarified or becomes more precise (see Chapter 10). Similarly, situations can arise during one's tenure where the development of new technologies or the provision of new services result in the clinical nurse specialist addressing new patient populations or aspects of care. Whenever significant changes occur in the focus of the clinical nurse specialist's activities, and these changes are assessed as permanent, the clinical nurse specialist's individualized title also must change.

Professional Role Descriptions

In 1987, Sisson undertook a study investigating the perceived contributions of clinical nurse specialists in a university hospital. After interviewing 120 individuals, including head nurses, directors, staff nurses, and physicians, Sisson found, among other things, that in general all respondents desired increased time in patient care by clinical nurse specialists. Additionally, the data revealed that when interviewees were asked what it is that a clinical nurse specialist does that is *not* helpful, "most respondents indicated that they did not understand the specific role components" of the clinical nurse specialist (p. 15). One of Sisson's conclusions was that "the lack of the ability of most personnel to identify all the role functions of the clinical nurse specialist would imply that the practicing clinical nurse specialist needs to educate other hospital personnel as to the specific activities which are part of this role" (p. 17). Obviously, one way of educating staff regarding the role of the clinical nurse specialist is with a well-developed role description.

Also in 1987, Chambers, Dangel, Germon, Tripodi, and Jaeger reported on the task of rewriting the generic job description of clinical nurse specialists used by their institution. They set out on this task "to promote internal understanding of the role and for recruitment" purposes (p. 124). The authors cited the fact that over a period of years the number of clinical nurse specialists employed by the institution had grown, and that these increased numbers resulted "in variations in role implementation" creating "confusion among hospital personnel," thus "revision of the job description was identified as a method of eliminating this confusion" (p. 124).

Each of the articles cited above emphasizes the importance of clinical nurse specialists being able to communicate clearly to others what it is they do. Although there are numerous ways of describing the scope of one's practice, all should emanate from a well-written, easily understood role description. Role descriptions are written in various lengths, depending on the degree of analysis of the various facets of the position, and serve various purposes, from fulfilling a requirement to reflecting the way in which a specific individual identifies goals or the manner in which a position has evolved. Perhaps it could be said that the length of the job description is a reflection of the clarity one has about the role. One nursing executive encourages the clinical nurse specialists employed in her institution to hone and refine their individual role descriptions to the point where they are one page long (H. Ripple, 1982, personal communication); such precision has the potential of increasing staff's understanding of the clinical nurse specialist's role and thereby increasing patient referrals.

The remainder of this section of the chapter will focus on some of the significant components of both the generic and individualized role descriptions of the clinical nurse specialist.

General Guidelines and Rationale

The task of completing a role description requires time, reading, forethought, and numerous revisions. In spite of this, the task of formulating a role description is well worth the effort for the clinical nurse specialist who successfully accomplishes the task, whether as a member of a peer group writing or revising a generic role description or as an individual developing or revising an individual speciality role description. Most often clinical nurse specialists work in settings where other clinical nurse specialists are employed. As Chambers et al. (1987) pointed out, increased numbers of clinical nurse specialists, coupled with varying specialities and emphases in role implementation, can create confusion among other members of the health care team concerning appropriate use of the clinical nurse specialists, both as individuals and as a group. Additionally, clinical nurse specialists themselves can face the dilemma of being unable to describe in a succinct, objective, and more general way how the role of the clinical nurse specialist is implemented in their institution when recruiting new candidates.

Without a generic job description, it is also difficult in settings where more than one clinical nurse specialist is employed to counsel clinical nurse specialists having difficulty implementing the role, or to ensure a more equitable approach to the clinical nurse specialist evaluation process. For these reasons, it is wise for clinical nurse specialists to develop a generic job description where none exists, or to revise those in situations where they have become outmoded. Such efforts should include input and reaction from staff nurses, head nurses, and especially one's supervisor, as well as the director of nursing, if they are not the same individual.

Generic Role Description

The generic role description of the clinical nurse specialist should be as clear and concise as possible. Lengthy documents, whatever their quality or intent, are more easily ignored. The language used should be understandable to all who might read it. Although Brown (1983) suggested that clinical nurse specialist role descriptions "have limited value when explaining the role to physicians and other department heads" (p. 168), one cannot ensure that these individuals, as well as residents, newly-employed nursing staff unfamiliar with the role, and other ancillary members of the health care team, will not read them. Consequently, it is to the advantage of the group authoring the generic role description to have it read by a number of employees, including non-nurses who are potential patient-referral sources.

The generic role description should be based on the statement on *The Role of the Clinical Nurse Specialist* (ANA, 1986b). Similarly, it should acknowledge and not deviate from the state's Nurse Practice Act regarding advanced nursing practice. The generic role description should also be consistent with the philosophy of the department of nursing regarding patients, institutional goals, and nursing practice as expressed in documents such as the Mission Statement or the Philosophy of the Department of Nursing.

Within the context described above, the generic role description begins by stating briefly who clinical nurse specialists are and what services they provide in that setting. This statement should be broad enough to cover all the clinical nurse specialists employed by the department, including those whose client may be other than the patient, for example the psychiatric liaison clinical nurse specialist, whose primary client may be the nursing staff who care for the patients (see Chapter 12).

Following this initial paragraph, the clinical nurse specialists' activities usually are listed grouped by role components. Such an arrangement can range from dividing the role into the classic four components of clinician, teacher, consultant, and researcher (see Table 3–1) or more than four components (Girouard & Spross, 1983; Heine, 1988).

In addition to citing examples of the activities undertaken by clinical nurse specialists in a generic fashion, the role description includes a clear statement identifying the clinical nurse specialist's clients in the particular institution, a statement of the reporting relationship of the clinical nurse specialist, a list of the qualifications required for the position, and a statement of the time frame during which clinical nurse specialists are available (e.g., 8 hours, 24 hours). Table 3–1 provides one example of an institution's generic job description of the clinical nurse specialist.

TABLE 3–1. UNIVERSITY OF CALIFORNIA, SAN FRANCISCO DEPARTMENT OF NURSING SERVICE: POSITION DESCRIPTION

Title: Clinical Nurse Specialist in a tertiary care teaching medical center.

Role Definition: A clinical nurse specialist is a professional nurse who, as a result of graduate education and in-depth clinical experience in a defined area of nursing practice, possesses the advanced knowledge and clinical skills necessary to provide expert nursing care in the defined areas of specialization. The major role functions of the clinical nurse specialist include education, consultation, clinical practice, and research. The primary responsibility of the clinical nurse specialist is the direct application of clinical expertise to patients and families being managed in a tertiary care teaching medical center. The clinical nurse specialist has responsibility for the quality of standards of nursing care for a specified patient population. The clinical nurse specialist evidences self-direction and accountability in the development of this role within the medical center.

Lines of Authority: Staff position responsible to the Director of the Department of Nursing Service.

Method of Evaluation: Negotiated with the Director of the Department of Nursing Service.

Qualifications

1. Current license to practice professional nursing in the state of California
2. Master's degree in nursing from an accredited program in clinical specialization
3. Demonstrated clinical competence and in-depth knowledge in specialty area
4. Demonstrated effective leadership, teaching, research, and communication skills

(Continued)

TABLE 3–1. (Continued)

Role Description

I. Provides direct nursing care to select groups of patients/families in area of specialization
   A. Identifies patient population through own selection and/or referral and for that population:
      1. assesses health status and identifies health care needs
      2. develops or facilitates the development of comprehensive nursing care plans
      3. provides expert nursing care
      4. provides instruction in disease, process, and medical plan
      5. provides counseling and crisis intervention as necessary
      6. facilitates and formulates the implementation of the discharge plan
      7. documents actions in patient chart
      8. assumes ongoing responsibility for nursing care management
      9. fosters continuity of care within the health care system
   B. Serves as a patient/family advocate in the health care system
II. Serves as a consultant to nursing staff, physicians, and other health care providers in area of specialization
   A. Consults with health care providers within the hospital and community regarding standards of nursing practice
   B. Plans and/or participates in interdisciplinary patient care conferences/rounds
   C. Assists nursing staff to solve patient care problems
   D. Secures a non-salaried clinical appointment to the School of Nursing
   E. Represents area of specialization clinically on hospital-wide committees
   F. Represents hospital in community activities related to the area of specialization
   G. Serves with other clinical nurse specialists in an advisory group to the Director of Nursing
   H. Establishes standards for nursing practice in consultation with nursing administrative leadership
III. Contributes to the ongoing education and professional development of nursing staff and students in area of specialization
   A. Consults with nursing administrative leadership concerning educational requirement of nursing staff
   B. Participates with Department of Nursing Education in meeting learning needs of nursing staff
   C. Provides individual and small group instruction in nursing care techniques and procedures
   D. Presents lectures, seminars, or conferences
IV. Maintains current knowledge and competency in area of specialization and in professional practice
   A. Attends relevant conferences and workshops
   B. Participates in professional organizations
   C. Utilizes other clinical nurse specialists for ongoing support and feedback
   D. Facilitates the use of clinical nurse specialists within the organization
V. Contributes to the expansion of the body of knowledge in nursing within area of specialization
   A. Evaluates and disseminates research findings
   B. Utilizes research findings in own practice and encourages staff to do the same
   C. Initiates and participates in nursing research
   D. Contributes to the literature

Components of Individual Role Description

In those settings where a current and acceptable generic description exists, the individual clinical nurse specialist's role description detailing particular contributions to patient care evolves from it. If a generic job description does not exist, there is perhaps no better time to complete one than at the time one is formulating an individualized description. If the director of nursing is implementing the position of a clinical nurse specialist in an institution where previously no such position existed, it is helpful to formulate the specific job description with input from key individuals well in advance of advertising for the position (Brown, 1983).

Because the individualized description of the particular clinical nurse specialist's activities is more focused and specific, it is more streamlined than the generic. Often the entire procedure requires time—time to write, time to reflect, and time to modify—in order that the role description is a true reflection of what it is the individual does. There are many formats for actually laying out a role description. Although creativity should be encouraged in the presentation, some attention to uniformity aids staff in knowing where to look for the information they need. In this regard, it is helpful for the clinical nurse specialist group to decide on the format to be used in preparing the individualized role description or if such uniformity is desirable.

Suggested components are described below. Whatever is included should focus on clear description of what the particular clinical nurse specialist can do for and with patients, nursing staff, and others in order to promote referrals and contribute to quality patient care.

Personal Philosophy of Nursing Practice. Stating one's philosophy affords the opportunity for personal reflection. More importantly, adding this brief but powerful piece of information to the role description gives staff, who may not know the clinical nurse specialist, the opportunity to understand the clinical nurse specialist's thinking and beliefs about patients and nursing care on a deeper level (M. Boyd, personal communication, 1981). When possible, this statement should consist of no more than two or three sentences (see Table 3–2). By articulating one's personal philosophy of nursing, the clinical nurse specialist becomes more than an abstract title or member of a group different from other nurses; in the experience of the authors, such descriptions have been known to stimulate discussion and act as an impetus for patient referrals by nursing staff. After realizing the alignment between their philosophies and those expressed by the clinical nurse specialist, the nurses in question were more ready to seek and evaluate the input of the clinical nurse specialist in specific patient situations.

TABLE 3-2. UNIVERSITY OF CALIFORNIA, SAN FRANCISCO DEPARTMENT OF NURSING SERVICE

Position Description for:
Patricia Sparacino, MS, RN
Cardiovascular (Surgical) Clinical Nurse Specialist

General Description

The Clinical Nurse Specialist in cardiovascular surgery is a professional nurse who, as a result of graduate education and in-depth clinical experience, possesses the advanced knowledge and clinical skill necessary to provide expert nursing in cardiovascular surgery. The major role functions of the Clinical Nurse Specialist include clinical practice, education, consultation, and research. The primary responsibility is direct application of clinical expertise to the patients and families being managed in the acute care setting. The Clinical Nurse Specialist evidences self-direction and accountability in the development of this role within the Medical Center.

Minimum Qualifications

Current license to practice professional nursing in the state of California. Master's degree in nursing. Demonstrated clinical competence and in-depth knowledge in cardiovascular surgical nursing. Demonstrated effective leadership, teaching, and communication skills.

Responsibility/Accountability

Responsible for maintaining the knowledge and abilities essential to the performance of stated behaviors. Staff position responsible to the Director of the Department of Nursing.

Personal Philosophy of Nursing

My goal in nursing is to support and promote patient independence by means of aiding the patient and family. "Patient independence" is the patient's ability to adapt to altered physiological demands and modified role functions without jeopardizing established role functions and relationships of interdependence.

The means by which to reach this goal are to employ creativity and to carefully balance demands. The responsibility for this creativity lies in the Clinical Nurse Specialist who choreographs the health care team approach to ensure and honor excellence in the delivery of patient care. This responsibility requires precision of discipline and constant attention to the creative melding of the delivery of optimal patient care, patient and family education, and patient-care-oriented research.

Role Description

A. Patient Care
    1. Participates directly in delivering patient care
        a. Provides preoperative, postoperative, and discharge teaching to selected and/or referred adult cardiothoracic and vascular patients
        b. Provides selected nursing care for specific patients
            1) plans and delivers care for complex adult cardiothoracic and vascular patients
            2) maintains clinical expertise
            3) provides role modeling for nursing staff to establish and maintain a standard level of quality patient care
            4) role models advanced nursing skills
        c. Counsels families of critically ill or dying patients
        d. Supports and facilitates continuity of patient care between nursing units, through transfer to another institution, or directly to home
        e. Translates current and new findings into usable information or approaches for patients, families, and/or staff

TABLE 3–2. (Continued)

Role Description (Cont.)

  2. Participates indirectly in delivering patient care
    a. Establishes standards of patient care
      1) updates standardized nursing care plans
      2) continually updates guidelines for patient teaching
      3) integrates American Heart Association/American Nurses' Association standards of care for cardiovascular surgical patients
    b. Oversees the quality of care delivered to all patients, and monitors patients progress
    c. Assists nursing staff in planning care for complex or unusual patients, and serves as a resource in identifying nursing diagnoses
    d. Collaborates with physicians and health care team members in planning, implementing, and evaluating comprehensive care in order to assure coordination of care for cardiothoracic and vascular patients
    e. Serves as a liaison between surgeons, patients, families, nurses, and health team members
    f. Participates in planning patient care during physician and/or nursing rounds
    g. Conducts patient care conferences and nursing rounds on a regular basis
B. Consultation
  1. Acts as nurse consultant to other disciplines in the area of cardiothoracic and vascular surgical nursing
  2. Participates in formulating and implementing policies, procedures, and standards necessary to provide high quality care to cardiovascular surgical patients
  3. Participates in hospital committees related to clinical practice
  4. Provides information to nursing staff about cardiothoracic and vascular disease processes, surgical procedures, therapies, and/or special equipment
  5. Acts as a resource to Nursing Administration for clinical issues of cardiothoracic and vascular patients, and for problem resolution
C. Education
  1. Independently and/or in collaboration with Nursing Education
    a. Assists the nursing staff in identifying learning needs
    b. Utilizes adult teaching/learning principles in providing informal and formal educational opportunities
    c. Presents lectures, seminars, or conferences related to cardiovascular surgery
  2. Contributes to the ongoing educational and professional development of students and guests in the area of specialization
  3. Provides instruction in new modes of therapy, equipment, and nursing care techniques and procedures
  4. Fosters an educational environment in which sharing of expertise and differing perspectives of other health care team members is encouraged
  5. Obtains and maintains a non-salaried faculty appointment in the School of Nursing
D. Research
  1. Initiates and collaborates in clinical nursing research regarding cardiothoracic and vascular patients
  2. Contributes to the nursing literature
  3. Utilizes research findings to assist nursing staff to improve quality of care for cardiothoracic and vascular surgical patient
  4. Acts as a resource for nursing staff conducting research
E. Professionalism
  1. Assumes responsibility for maintaining current knowledge and competency in area of specialization

(Continued)

TABLE 3–2. (Continued)

Role Description (Cont.)

    a. Develops annual plan for own professional development
    b. Utilizes direct patient care experiences to maintain clinical knowledge and skill
    c. Attends relevant conferences and workshops
  2. Facilitates the use of Clinical Nurse Specialists within the institution
    a. Utilizes other clinical nurse specialists for ongoing support and feedback
    b. Utilizes other clinical nurse specialists as resources for clinical problem resolution
  3. Participates in departmental, hospital, and/or university committees
  4. Promotes the image of nursing through professional, political, and/or community activities
  5. Demonstrates courtesy and follow-through in all telephone communications by maintaining telephone standards as established by the medical center
  6. Ensures a professional, helpful working environment by upholding the house standards as adopted by the Medical Center

From the Medical Center at the University of California, San Francisco, copyright © 1981. Reprinted with permission.

Definition of Patient Population. Defining the specific patient population for whom the clinical nurse specialist will provide services is an essential component of the role description. Numerous clinical nurse specialists, even those with years of experience in the role, have had difficulties in their positions because they have never clearly defined the patient population with whom they are qualified and wish to work. If clarity regarding the patient population is accomplished in the role description, it not only facilitates referrals, consultations, and so on, but additionally, it assists the clinical nurse specialist in focusing the area of practice. In an institution where there are several clinical nurse specialists, clarity regarding the patient population one consults with can assist other clinical nurse specialists to know when to suggest that staff contact a colleague, thereby facilitating patient care. In addition, particularly in tertiary centers where numerous clinical nurse specialists are employed and areas of practice overlap, clarity and communication regarding the patient population one is specialized to function with can reduce friction and misunderstanding in those situations where "territoriality" could be a problem. If nurses do not know what clinical nurse specialists do, they will not call them; if they are confused about areas of practice, especially between clinical nurse specialists who address similar populations, they will seek out the clinical nurse specialist who has more clearly defined the population and the role.

Accountability. Because of the lack of clarity of some individuals regarding "what" the clinical nurse specialist is, it is important that the role description briefly explain one's position in the organization. With this in mind, stating to whom one is accountable becomes an important part of the role description. Such clarification is particularly necessary if the clinical nurse specialist is the only one in an organization, or the role is new to the setting. It is important to remember that reporting lines make a strong statement regarding the stature of a position within an organization. If the clinical nurse specialist reports to the most executive nurse within the organization, this indicates the significance of the clinical nurse specialist position within the organizational hierarchy and can add a "vote of confidence."

Descriptors of Implementation of Role Components. Classically, the clinical nurse specialist role has been defined in terms of four components: educator, researcher, clinician, and consultant (Hamric & Spross, 1983). Because of the potential for confusion by staff, due to varying modes of role implementation by clinical nurse specialists, it is important to give some precise and concrete examples of actual activities within each component.

List of Types of Situations for Which You Are Available. In the early phase of role implementation, a list with easily recognizable examples of types of interactions in which the clinical nurse specialist would like to be involved, or has been involved successfully, greatly aids staff in knowing when it is appropriate to call the clinical nurse specialist. If the role of the clinical nurse specialist is established in the institution, this list may not be necessary, especially for those clinical nurse specialists who have been in the setting for some time; it would certainly be of benefit to newcomers. Again, such a list facilitates utilization of the specialist by the staff.

Hours Usually Worked and How One Can Be Reached. Information regarding hours worked is often viewed as too obvious to include in a role description, but a clear statement of availability, as well as how to reach the clinical nurse specialist, greatly increases the possibility of being called. In some institutions, where there are numerous specialists, cards listing the specialists' names, their specialities, and their beeper or office numbers are posted near the unit phones; this approach increases the possibility that timely referrals will occur (see Chapter 5).

Utilizing a Role Description

Though formulating a clearly delineated role description is a task that should be completed prior to interviewing for a position, modifications must occur once a position is obtained. Obviously, the master's-prepared nurse would be assisted greatly if such a task were an integral part of the assignments necessary for completion of the graduate program. Increasingly, this is becoming a trend, and faculty are to be commended for such sound expectations. The process of making minor adaptations is also aided by having written the original description succinctly and in a thought-provoking manner.

Role descriptions need to be shared with nursing staff, one's immediate supervisor, and others. In one setting, the clinical nurse specialists have required that the individual role description of newly employed clinical nurse specialists be presented to the specialist's peers prior to it being presented to the director of nursing or immediate supervisor. The author is encouraged to present the role description to the supervisor only after giving an in-depth explanation and receiving critique and clarification by the other clinical nurse specialists regarding the specifics of what it is the clinical nurse specialist intends to do in the position, how it will be carried out, what outcome measures will be used for evaluation purposes, and how realistic self-expectations are in relation to the "markers" established by the group. Such an approach facilitates clarity in writing style, format, and ability to succinctly articulate one's role. The interchange between the clinical nurse specialists and the individual presenting the role description provides a forum for clarification of philosophies about role implementation and allows the presenting individual's peers to be clear and supportive about the scope of the new or newly employed clinical nurse specialist's practice.

Once the individualized role description has been accepted by one's immediate supervisor, the next step is to share the role description with nursing staff on those units with which the clinical nurse specialist will be most closely affiliated. Usually a brief description and a short period of questions and answers will suffice for the first visit. It is wise to leave a copy of the role description or to personally affix it in a prominent place on the unit where staff members can review it at their leisure.

Although it is usually unnecessary to share copies of the role description with physicians with whom the clinical nurse specialist will interact, it is important to set up appointments with them in order to explain the role as envisioned, or to discuss changes that have occurred, and to answer questions, reduce anxiety, promote interaction, etc. Frequently these brief meetings with medical staff serve as positive reminders of one's availability for patient care and collaborative efforts.

Job descriptions stated clearly and succinctly enable staff and others to determine quickly the appropriate use of the clinical nurse specialist and the appropriate clinical nurse specialist to call. An orderly approach to the process and periodic review facilitates utilization of the clinical nurse specialist in patient care situations and results in improved patient care, ultimately leading to increased recognition of contributions to quality care.

A FRAMEWORK FOR ROLE IMPLEMENTATION

The concept of "role" is a dynamic representation of behavior determined by cultural, personal, and situational factors operating in a given situation (Sarbin & Allen, 1968). Traditional social learning theory states that the person who is enacting a role is guided by certain criteria and inferences: correct role selection, congruence between the manifest behavior and the normative standards, and legitimate role occupation (Sarbin & Allen, 1968). Role acquisition involves complex interactional learning, specifically the implicit and explicit expectations involved in the knowledge and skills that are associated with the behavioral, attitudinal, and valuational standards ascribed by society (Gross, Mason, & McEachern, 1958; Thornton & Nardi, 1975). Role acquisition, whether as a novice or an experienced clinical nurse specialist in a new position, requires passage through developmental stages (Thornton & Nardi, 1975).

Oda (1977, 1985) has applied the role development process to define phases of role implementation in nursing specialization (Figure 3–1). The phases are:

1. *Role identification* is the introduction phase. Whether the clinical nurse specialist is assuming a new position with no predecessor or role model, is negotiating for a new position, is assuming a role for which the predecessor had a different concept, or is

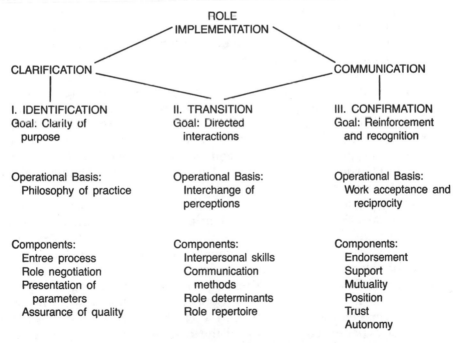

Figure 3–1. Role development process in nursing specialization. (*From Oda, D.S. (1985). Community health nursing in innovative school health roles and programs. In S.E. Archer & R.P. Fleshman (Eds.), Community health nursing. Boston: Jones & Bartlett Publishers, Inc., p. 376. Reprinted with permission.*)

acquiring a role with multiple reporting mechanisms, clear identification of role purpose and function is essential. The first step
of this process is writing a role description (see Role Description
section). This identification process assumes particular importance when there are multiple and conflicting role expectations,
requiring clarity about what one will and will not do. Through
ongoing communication and clarification of role parameters, the
quality of practice will be protected and the flexibility maintained.

2. *Role transition* is the implementation phase. As the clinical nurse
   specialist's role is implemented, clearly articulated goal-directed
   interactions help the specialized role to fit with the particular
   staff and institution. By validating perceptions and modifying
   one's approach, the clinical nurse specialist as clinician establishes
   clinical credibility, as consultant assists others in their roles, as
   educator motivates others to learn, and as researcher utilizes
   valid data to improve nursing practice and collaborates in nursing research.

3. *Role confirmation* is reached when there is organizational support
   for the role. Once the clinical nurse specialist gains support and
   positive recognition for the role, continued clarification and communication is needed to maintain acceptance of the role by staff
   and others, and to maintain the resulting reciprocal, and interdependent working relationships.

Role implementation, then, goes through a series of stages, with the
greatest time and energy expended in the early phases when the individual is mastering the role itself. As the phases are completed, role
performance becomes more effective and flexible as the individual develops in interdependence and fusion with role activities and role identification (Thornton & Nardi, 1975; Turner, 1978). It is almost as if the
person becomes the role.

Practically applied, the phases of role development become a framework for specific role activities and priorities. The experienced clinical
nurse specialist in a new practice setting will have previously developed
expertise in each of the role components, while the novice clinical nurse
specialist will need considerable guidance in the phases of role implementation. While there are differing estimates as to timing of role tra-
jectory (Baker, 1987; Baker, 1973; Cooper, 1983; Holt, 1987; University
of California, San Francisco, 1986), the clinical nurse specialist, whether
novice or experienced, must spend the first six months of practice in a
new setting establishing credibility. Markers of role development derived
from personal experience and opinion can serve as a guide for role
evolution (Table 2–2) (Baker, 1987; Cooper, 1983; Holt, 1987; University of California, San Francisco, 1986).

One example has been presented in Chapter 2, but there are many perspectives as to what elements of each component comprise developmental role markers. While the individual clinical nurse specialist might look at the original models and select which approach is most appropriate to the practice setting, we are proposing a model based on the integration of several perspectives (Table 2–2).

TIME MANAGEMENT

The goal of time management is to provide control over priority allocation in the various components of the role, bringing clarity to a multifaceted process, guidance in determining yearly goals with outcome criteria, and refinement of one's specialty. A weekly or monthly summary of the diverse activities associated with the role documents and validates productivity, records the percentage of time spent in each area of responsibility, and provides an overview of trends. A quarterly or yearly report of activities becomes a valuable method for quantification, interpreting the role, determining role effectiveness, documenting impact, and gaining administrative support.

Most methods of clinical nurse specialist activity documentation are practice-specific, developmental in format, and only intermittently used. Brown, and Wilson (1987) suggested a method for monitoring time management which uses the calendar and a list-making system as key strategies. This system is a necessary part of activity documentation as it is proactive and predictive. Calendars and master lists or daily lists serve as items for recall and can provide a comparison of planned versus completed activities. A periodic analysis can aid in the identification of role satisfiers and dissatisfiers, as well as assist with reordering of priorities.

A retrospective time study of activities has been similarly described as a step in evaluating clinical nurse specialist effectiveness (Baker, 1987; Robichaud & Hamric, 1986; Topham, 1987; University of California, San Francisco, 1986). By documenting both anticipated time allocations per role component and then comparing it to actual time expenditure, the clinical nurse specialist can re-evaluate goal-setting appropriateness and efficiency. The difference between predicted and actual time expenditure can substantiate the need to shift allocations because of changing practice setting needs (i.e. an influx of new staff, a new client population). Two studies have reported time spent within each role component (Robichaud & Hamric, 1986; Topham, 1987). A limitation of both these studies was a lack of data about phases of role development. Varying allocations of time per role component may be related to years of experience in the role and presumably the phases of role development (Table 3–3). Another important outcome in the process of time

TABLE 3–3. TIME SPENT WITHIN DEVELOPMENTAL ROLE MARKER CATEGORIES

	Year 1	Year 2	Year 3	Year 4	Year 5+a
Clinical Practice					
Predicted	50–75%	40–75%	30–40%	20–30%	
Actual	29%	27.5%	52.2%	39.9%	
Consultation					
Predicted	10–20%	15–25%	15–30%	20–40%	
Actual	14.3%	6.5%	10.6%	6.8%	
Education					
Predicted	10–20%	15–25%	15–25%	10–20%	
Actual	38%	56.3%	22.9%	31.3%	
Research					
Predicted	1–4%	5–10%	10–30%	20–40%	
Actual	1.38%	3%	5.9%	6.8%	
Other					
Actual	19.6%	5.3%	11.1%	14.2%	

aAt the time these data were collected, information was not available about 5+ years
Adapted from University of California, San Francisco (1986).

documentation is the means to achieve congruence between administrative expectations of the clinical nurse specialist role and actual time the clinical nurse specialist spends.

EVALUATION

A regular process of clinical nurse specialist evaluation is a professional responsibility, reviewing professional growth and measuring the impact made on improving client-care outcomes (Davis, Greig, Burkholder, & Keating, 1984; Morath, 1988). The primary evaluation processes are *self-evaluation, peer review, administrative review,* and *certification.* The clinical nurse specialist is *self-accountable* for practice and therefore should evaluate progress according to the individualized role description and yearly personal goals and objectives. This method of evaluation is limiting, as self-evaluation is more often subjective rather than objective. Self-evaluation alone can prevent the clinical nurse specialist from examining alternative methods for improvement. In the process of *peer review,* a peer or a group of peers can provide objective as well as subjective critical appraisal as to the attainment of a colleague's behavioral objectives. Peers can also comment on visibility, impact, and style of interaction. A peer may be overly critical and may tend to be more subjective than objective, but a peer is better able to evaluate a clinical nurse specialist colleague than someone else not as familiar with the expectations of the clinical nurse specialist role. Peer review in a group process is costly in terms of time spent away from client care, but it can be as effectively accomplished by letter or evaluation form (see Chapter 12, Appendix). The *administrative review* is the completion step of the evaluation process. In the administrative review the focus is on outcomes and the determination of overall performance, combining comments provided by peers, physician colleagues, consumers, head nurses, and staff, with outcomes of goals and objectives. This process allows the opportunity for communication and mutual development of future goals, so that congruence of expectations by the administrator, organization, and clinical nurse specialist can be achieved.

Another component of evaluation, in addition to the processes of peer, self, and administrative review, is *outcome evaluation*. Examples of outcome evaluation are patient-care outcomes (Edlund & Hodges, 1983) and program evaluation (Morath, 1988). Patient-care outcomes evaluate criteria such as client/family feedback, complications associated with nursing care, incident reports, nursing audits, length of hospital stay, and recidivism. Program evaluation assesses productivity, program management, impact of a clinical program on the system, outcomes, and consistency of quality care.

Yet another method of evaluation is *certification*. Certification is a voluntary, self-regulatory function which is meant to validate qualifications and assure quality in knowledge and practice. Professional certification is based on preexisting standards of practice in a defined clinical area and is developed by peers in professional or specialty associations (Cipriano, 1986). Certification is offered by the American Nurses' Association, with eligibility requirements based on experience or education, or both. Different examinations are available for generalists and specialists. A number of the speciality nursing organizations also offer certification.

The tools for evaluation provide documentation. Documentation of clinical nurse specialist activities, particularly when severe budgetary cutbacks and reduction in personnel are a current challenge, is one method of clarifying and strengthening the role and substantiating clinical nurse specialist utilization, impact and, presumably, cost effectiveness (Hamric, 1983; Malone, 1986). Examples of tools for evaluation are:

- Time study of activities in patient care (direct and indirect), consultation, education, and research
- Volume indices (number of client caseloads, classes taught and number attending, number of consultations) (see Chapter 7)
- Liaison activities (i.e., community service, departmental and institutional committees, public relations)
- Letters or evaluation forms from peers, staff, and physician colleagues (see Table 12–6 in Chapter 12 for sample forms)
- Updated curriculum vitae
- Completed yearly goals and objectives

- New yearly goals and objectives
- Updated position description, as necessary
- Client education materials developed within the past year
- Title and representative samples of procedures or nursing standards and criteria for client care developed within the past year
- Articles published
- Research completed or in progress:
    proposals developed
    funding sought/awarded

SUMMARY

The clinical nurse specialist role is threatened by a variety of factors, including fiscal constraints, the sometimes difficult fit of an autonomous role in a bureaucratic system, and the lack of successful and uniform measurements of clinical nurse specialist impact on client care outcomes. The clinical nurse specialist seeking a position will be better prepared by following the well-outlined recommendations. Success will be influenced by congruence between clinical nurse specialists and administrators about definition and purpose of the role. The role will achieve greater stability and effectiveness through development according to stages and reasonable time frames within which to accomplish goals and objectives. Finally, the evaluation of both quality care and the clinical nurse specialist who plans, coordinates, and delivers it will provide sound data for measuring impact.

REFERENCES

American Nurses' Association. (1980). *Nursing: A social policy statement.* Kansas City, MO: American Nurses' Association.

American Nurses' Association. (1986a). *Clinical nurse specialists: Distribution and utilization.* Kansas City, MO: American Nurses' Association.

American Nurses' Association. (1986b). *The role of the clinical nurse specialist.* Kansas City, MO: American Nurses' Association.

Backshieder, J. (1971). The clinical nurse specialist as a practitioner. *Nursing Forum, 10* (4), 359–377.

Baker, P.O. (1987). Model activities for clinical nurse specialist role development. *Clinical Nurse Specialist, 1* (3), 119–123.

Baker, V.E. (1973). Retrospective explorations in role development. In J. Riehl & J. McVay (Eds.), *The clinical nurse specialist: Interpretations.* New York: Appleton-Century-Crofts.

Barrett, J. (1972). The nurse specialist practitioner: A study. *Nursing Outlook, 20* (8), 524–527.

Beeber, L., & Scicchitani, B. (1980). Should the clinical nurse specialist be free of administrative responsibility? *Perspectives in Psychiatric Care, 18* (6), 250–269.

Blake, P. (1977). The clinical specialist as nurse consultant. *Journal of Nursing Administration, 7* (10), 33–36.

Brown, M.M., & Wilson, C. (1987). Time management and the clinical nurse specialist. *Clinical Nurse Specialist, 1* (1), 32–38.

Brown, S.S. (1983). Administrative support. In A.B. Hamric & J. Spross (Eds.), *The clinical nurse specialist in theory and practice* (pp. 149–170). Orlando, FL: Grune & Stratton.

Butts, P. (1974). The clinical specialist vs. the clinical supervisor. *Supervisor Nurse, 5* (4), 38–44.

Cahill, I. (1973). The development of maternity nursing as a specialty. In J. Riehl & J. McVay (Eds.), *The clinical nurse specialist: Interpretations.* New York: Appleton-Century-Crofts.

Castronovo, F. (1975). The effective use of the clinical specialist. *Supervisor Nurse, 6* (5), 48–56.

Chambers, J., Dangel, R., & Germon, K., et al. (1987). Clinical nurse specialist collaboration: Development of a generic job description and standards of performance. *Clinical Nurse Specialist, 1*, 124–127.

Cipriano, P.F. (1986). Certification: Self-regulation for specialty practice. In *Patterns in specialization: Challenge to the curriculum.* New York: National League for Nursing.

Cooper, D. (1983). A refined expert: The clinical nurse specialist after five years. *Momentum, 1* (3), 1–2.

Crabtree, M. (1979). Effective utilization of clinical specialists within the organizational structure of hospital nursing service. *Nursing Administration Quarterly, 4*(1):1–11.

Davis, D.S., Greig, A.E., Burkholder, J., & Keating, T. (1984). Evaluating advanced practice nurses. *Nursing Management, 15* (3), 44–47.

del Bueno, D.J., & Price, M.S. (1987). Interviewing for a CNS position? Ask the right questions. *Clinical Nurse Specialist, 1* (4), 179–184.

Disch, J. (1978). The clinical specialist in a large peer group. *Journal of Nursing Administration, 8* (12), 17–20.

Edlund, B.J., & Hodges, L.C. (1983). Preparing and using the clinical nurse specialist. *Nursing Clinics of North America, 18* (3), 499–507.

Edwards, J. (1971). Clinical specialists are not effective—why? *Supervisor Nurse, 2* (8), 38–41, 45, 47, 51.

Ellerbe-O'Donnell, S. (1988). Personal communication.

Everson, S. (1981). Integration of the role of clinical specialist. *The Journal of Continuing Education in Nursing, 12* (2), 16–19.

Fagin, C. (1967). The clinical specialist as supervisor. *Nursing Outlook, 15* (1), 34–36.

Girouard, S., & Spross, J. (1983). Evaluation of the CNS: Using an evaluation tool. In A.B. Hamric & J. Spross (Eds.), *The clinical nurse specialist in theory and practice* (pp. 207–233). Orlando, FL: Grune & Stratton.

Gross, N., Mason, W., and McEachern, A. (1958). *Explorations in role analysis.* New York: Wiley.

Hamric, A.B. (1983). A model for developing evaluation strategies. In A.B.

Hamric & J. Spross (Eds.), *The clinical nurse specialist in theory and practice*. Orlando, FL: Grune & Stratton.

Hamric, A.B. & Spross, J. (Eds.). (1983). *The clinical nurse specialist in theory and practice*. Orlando, FL: Grune & Stratton.

Heine, C.A. (1988). The gerontological nurse specialist: Examination of the role. *Clinical Nurse Specialist, 2*(1):6–11.

Holt, F.M. (1987). Executive practice role. Editorial. *Clinical Nurse Specialist, 1* (3), 116–118.

Jackson, B. (1973). Hospital administrators need to know about clinical specialists. *Supervisor Nurse, 4* (9), 29–34.

James, W. (1958). *Talks to teachers*. New York: W.W. Norton and Co., Inc.

Johnson, D., Wilcox, J., & Moidel, H. (1967). The clinical nurse specialist as a practitioner. *American Journal of Nursing, 67* (11), 2298–2303.

MacPhail, J. (1971). Reasonable expectation of the nurse clinician. *Journal of Nursing Administration, 1* (5), 16–18.

Malone, B.L. (1986). Evaluation of the clinical nurse specialist. *American Journal of Nursing, 86* (12), 1375–1377.

Morath, J.M. (1988). The clinical nurse specialist: Evaluation issues. *Nursing Management, 19* (3), 72–80.

Niessner, P. (1979). The clinical specialist's contribution to quality nursing care. *Nursing Leadership, 2* (1), 21–30.

O'Connor, P. (1984). Resumes: Opening the door. *Nursing Economics, 2*, 428–431.

Oda, D.S. (1977). Specialized role development: A three-phase process. *Nursing Outlook, 25*, 374–377.

Oda, D.S. (1985). Community health nursing in innovative school health roles and programs. In S.E. Archer & R.P. Fleshman (Eds.), *Community health nursing* (pp. 368–393). Monterey, CA: Wadsworth Health Sciences.

Odello, E. (1973). The clinical specialist in a line position. *Supervisor Nurse, 4* (9), 36–41.

Parkis, E. (1974a). The management role of the clinical specialist. (Part 1). *Supervisor Nurse, 5* (9), 44–51.

Parkis, E. (1974b). The management role of the clinical specialist. (Part 2). *Supervisor Nurse, 5* (10), 24–35.

Rew, L. (1988). AFFIRM the role of the clinical specialist in private practice. *Clinical Nurse Specialist, 2*, 39–43.

Roberts, L.R. (1987). Clinical nurse specialist: Line or staff using Lewin's field theory to resolve the issue. *Clinical Nurse Specialist, 1* (1), 39–44.

Robichaud, A.M., & Hamric, A.B. (1986). Time documentation of clinical nurse specialist activities. *Journal of Nursing Administration, 16* (1), 31–36.

Sarbin, T., & Allen, V. (1968). Role theory. In G. Lindzey & E. Aronson (Eds.), *Handbook of social psychology* (pp. 488–567). Reading, MA: Addison-Wesley.

Sisson, R. (1987). Co-workers' perceptions of the clinical nurse specialist role. *Clinical Nurse Specialist, 1*, 13–17.

Stevens, B. (1976). Accountability of the clinical specialist: An administrator's viewpoint. *Journal of Nursing Administration, 6* (2), 30–32.

Thornton, R., & Nardi, P.M. (1975). The dynamics of role acquisition. *American Journal of Sociology, 80* (4), 870–885.

Topham, D.L. (1987). Role theory in relation to roles of the clinical nurse specialist. *Clinical Nurse Specialist, 1* (2), 81–84.

Turner, R.H. (1978). The role and the person. *American Journal of Sociology, 84* (1), 1–23.

University of California, San Francisco Medical Center. (1986). Clinical nurse specialists: Role markers for the clinical nurse specialist. (Unpublished) Presented by M. Inturrisi, & D. Oda, *CNS role development and evaluation*, at UCSF Conference, Create the Future Now, February 12–13, 1987, San Francisco, CA.

chapter four

Review of Research Relevant to the Clinical Nurse Specialist Role

Patricia S.A. Sparacino

There is a wide variation in master's-level preparation in research methodology. Thus there is debate as to whether the clinical nurse specialist's familiarity with the research process is sufficient for independent use of the research framework to address a clinical problem (Hodgman, 1983). Generally, clinical nurse specialists are expected to evaluate research findings and determine whether those findings are appropriate for implementation in the clinical setting. The issue of what level of preparation provides which degree of precision and research sophistication was briefly discussed in Chapter 1. It is imperative that the clinical nurse specialist be involved in nursing research, whether as initiator or collaborator, to develop new nursing innovations and to help improve the general practice of nursing (Peplau, 1965).

An extensive review of the literature reveals that most of the research relevant to clinical nurse specialists has dealt with the role and its implementation and the effect of the role on practice characteristics of the generalist nurse. Very few studies have focused on the direct effect of clinical nurse specialist interventions on patient care outcomes. Likewise, there have been few publications of clinical trials suggesting new ways to approach patient care in which the author or co-author is acknowledged as a clinical nurse specialist. The research discussed in this chapter was selected according to historical significance, merit, or impact.

ROLE UTILIZATION

The aspect of the clinical nurse specialist role that has been most extensively studied has been the description of problems encountered in the utilization of the role. Baker and Kramer (1970) investigated the areas of title designation, role functions and authority, and accountability.

Their survey revealed that title designations are numerous and not limited to "clinical nurse specialist," that the function of the role is to improve patient care but that opinions are divergent as to the actual activities involved. There was divided opinion among respondents about authority and accountability (line vs. staff) and to whom the clinical nurse specialist directly reports. Another descriptive study by Barrett (1971) reported the attitudes of physicians toward the clinical nurse specialist role. Surgeons reported that the presence of a clinical nurse specialist was directly related to a high quality of patient care and that patient care was better when the clinical nurse specialist directly administered the care. Davidson and associates (1978) surveyed 200 psychiatrists to explore their attitude toward the master's-prepared psychiatric nurse clinician; psychiatrists who had positive attitudes about utilization of the role had knowledge of the role and prior contact with a master's-prepared psychiatric nurse clinician.

Aradine and Deynes (1972) reported findings that illuminated the broad scope of activities and pressures that have hampered the full utilization of the role. As identified in this study, patient care comprised the initial major involvement by the clinical nurse specialist, but involvement in other consultative, administrative, and educational activities broadened over subsequent time periods. The result was that in the areas of research and writing for publication there was a small degree of involvement and a point of perceived pressure.

The negative relationship between perceived administrative support and clinical nurse specialist job dissatisfaction was the significant finding of the sampling of 208 clinical nurse specialists by Shaefer (1973). An interesting result of Shaefer's study was that the findings of previous studies, which had suggested a curvilinear relationship between career length and job satisfaction, could not be replicated.

ROLE IMPLEMENTATION

Attitudes about the role and its implementation have been documented by Boucher (1972), Bruce (1972), and Smith (1974). Boucher and Bruce explored the understanding and acceptance of the clinical nurse specialist role components by various health care providers and the value ascribed to certain role functions. Educators, nursing administrators, and clinical nurse specialists agreed that the clinical nurse specialist is perceived as an educator and researcher with practitioner expertise. In their valuation of the role, educators and nursing administrators highly valued the components of educator and practitioner with research competencies but minimally valued involvement with change planning or implementation. The clinical nurse specialists, interestingly enough, valued the role components of educator and practitioner but valued their change agent capabilities higher than the research component of the role.

Smith (1974) also described perceptions of the activities of the clinical nurse specialist role. The important finding of this study was the lack of unanimity by any category of inpatient nursing personnel about their own functions or the functions of anyone else. Head nurses viewed clinical nurse specialists predominantly as consultants whereas clinical nurse specialists perceived their primary role functions as consultant and researcher. The clinical nurse specialist as clinician involved in direct client care was ranked third by head nurses but fourth by clinical nurse specialists themselves.

CLINICAL NURSE SPECIALISTS' IMPACT ON NURSING STAFF

Several researchers have examined the effect of the clinical nurse specialist on practice characteristics of nursing staff, and therefore presumably on the improvement of patient care. In 1970, Georgopoulos and Christman described a research project in progress in which the clinical nurse specialist role was introduced into three patient care units, while three comparable control units were managed by the traditional head nurse. Two aspects of this study were subsequently reported by Georgopoulos and Jackson (1970) and Georgopoulos and Sana (1971). They found that the patient care units led by clinical nurse specialists demonstrated an increase in evaluative nursing statements (factual data associated with judgments, conclusions, reasons, or relationships), while the units led by head nurses emphasized descriptive nursing statements (facts, actions, or instructions). Likewise, the experimental units demonstrated a more clinical or patient-centered approach while the control units maintained a more managerial or staff-focused approach. Georgopoulos and Sana (1971) then reported on the influence of the clinical nurse specialist on the qualitative-evaluative nursing information given in intershift reports. It was again found that, on the basis of the evaluative statements which emphasized managerial versus clinical concerns, there was an inverse relationship between the groups. The data supported Georgopoulos and Christman's original hypothesis that nursing practice is measurably superior when influenced by clinical nurse specialist leadership.

Also with the intent to study the effect of the clinical nurse specialist on nursing staff and nursing practice, Ayers, Padilla, Baker, and Crary (1971) placed clinical nurse specialists with responsibilities for patient care, consultation, and education on patient units. The study systematically described the integration of the clinical nurse specialist with staff and patients and described their experiences and acceptance.

At the conclusion of the study, the control units showed overall the least increase in clinical insight. The clinical nurse specialists more experienced in the role were more accepted, but nonetheless they all had to deal with ambiguities in responsibility and role. The study also revealed that the cognitive and emotional phases of the development of the role were those of orientation, frustration, implementation, and reassessment. One clinical nurse specialist in the study perceived the four phases as being cyclic and repetitive. There was agreement that the clinical nurse specialist's authority should concern clinical nursing issues and not administrative ones.

In a study designed to investigate the influence of the clinical nurse specialist on the improvement of nurse-dependent patient responses, Girouard (1978) examined whether the availability of a clinical nurse specialist would influence nurses to do more preoperative teaching. Although there was no difference between the experimental and control groups in opinions or claims about doing preoperative teaching and documenting it, the experimental groups did, in fact, provide significantly more preoperative teaching and provide more documentation about the teaching in the kardex. However, neither experimental nor control groups demonstrated a significant increase in the amount of patient teaching documented in the nursing notes.

CLINICAL NURSE SPECIALISTS' IMPACT ON PATIENT OUTCOMES

The area of research which has been relatively limited and yet is most essential is the measurement of the effect of clinical nurse specialist intervention on patient care outcomes. The studies that have been published have not always utilized a clinical nurse specialist whose clinical speciality was the same as the patient population being studied. The pioneer of studies was that of Little and Carnevali (1967) who conducted an exploratory study to determine variations in patient response to illness when patient-centered care was given by clinical nurse specialists. Psychiatric clinical nurse specialists cared for patients with pulmonary tuberculosis, and patient response to illness was measured by behavioral as well as physiological data. The patient responses of improvement in radiological and bacteriological results, length of hospital stay, involvement in self-care, and deviant behaviors did not correlate with the patient-centered care given by the psychiatric clinical nurse specialists. Future studies would have more validity if they utilized a clinical nurse specialist whose area of clinical expertise is the same as the patient care problem in question.

A study by Murphy (1971) examined the effect of different nursing care approaches (customary care given by staff nurses in addition to that given by the clinical nurse specialist) to cardiac surgical patients. Partially because of methodological problems, the positive impact of the additional care by the clinical nurse specialist could not be supported by the data. The study did identify the most common postoperative complications. Murphy discussed the inadequacies of the study and projected a conceptual model for further studies of the impact of the clinical nurse specialist.

Pozen and associates (1977) looked at the effect of a rehabilitation clinical nurse specialist's intervention with myocardial infarction patients and found that the experimental group had a better rate of early return to work, decreased smoking, and tested as having an increased knowledge of heart disease. However, the clinical nurse specialist did not have an effect in reducing anxiety.

In a study specifically designed to compare the teaching effectiveness of clinical nurse specialists and non-master's-prepared nurses, Linde and Janz (1979) examined the effect of a structured comprehensive teaching program on knowledge and compliance of cardiac surgical patients. The significant finding was that not only did all the patients increase their knowledge test score after receiving the postoperative patient education program, but that the patients taught by the clinical nurse specialists had significantly higher knowledge test scores at the time of hospital discharge than did the patients taught by non-master's-prepared nurses.

Another relatively neglected but increasingly essential area of research is that which relates clinical nurse specialist intervention and cost containment. Two pioneering studies are those of Brooten and associates (1986) and Neidlinger, Kennedy, and Scroggins (1987).

In an experimental study that utilized master's-prepared clinical nurse specialists for the four activities of parent education, infant care continuity between nursing units and home, home visits, and coordination between health care providers, Brooten and associates (1986) demonstrated a net savings of $18,560 per infant in the experimental group. The randomized, controlled clinical trial addressed the problem of the risks of lengthy hospitalization to very low birthweight infant health and development and the associated high cost of care. The outcomes studied were infant status, parental concerns, and program savings. The study is well designed and the significant results demonstrate no difference between the early discharge experimental group and control groups in the number of rehospitalizations or acute care visits or in the measures of physical and mental growth. The interventions by master's-prepared clinical nurse specialists resulted in significant cost savings.

A study completed at Scott and White Hospital in Texas (Kennedy, Neidlinger, & Scroggins, 1987; Neidlinger, Kennedy, & Scroggins, 1987) demonstrated that the effect of a gerontological clinical nurse specialist spending an average of 80 minutes in comprehensive discharge planning per elder in the experimental group resulted in 1) a shorter length of stay, 2) delayed readmission to the acute care hospital, and 3) a computed savings of $35,000 generated by the experimental group. The limitations of the study were that the research was based in one hospital and the intervention delivered by one clinical nurse specialist, with the computed savings based on the single hospital's expenses and prospective payments by Diagnostic Related Groups (DRGs). Such an outcome needs to be replicated by others in other settings to confirm the impact of clinical nurse specialist intervention on both patient care outcomes and program savings.

SUMMARY

Much of the literature that describes the role or its implementation is anecdotal; it is paramount that, as there is increasing clarity in the definition of the role, there be research conducted by clinical nurse specialists themselves that extends beyond description and branches into experimental hypothesis testing related to clinical care and patient outcomes. It is the professional obligation of the clinical nurse specialist to contribute to the further development of a scientific basis of nursing practice and to improve specialty practice through scientific inquiry and research. The clinical nurse specialist role is in an optimal position to bridge the gap between academics and nursing practice through research.

REFERENCES

Aradine, C., & Deynes, M.J. (1972). Activities and pressures of clinical nurse specialists. *Nursing Research, 21* (5), 411–418.

Ayers, R., Padilla, G.V., Baker, V.E., & Crary, W.G. (1971). *The clinical nurse specialist: An experiment in role effectiveness and role development.* Duarte, CA: City of Hope National Medical Center.

Baker, C., & Kramer, M. (1970). To define or not to define: The role of the clinical specialist. *Nursing Forum, 9* (1), 41–55.

Barrett, J. (1971). Administrative factors in development of new nursing practice roles. *Journal of Nursing Administration, 1* (4), 25–29.

Boucher, R. (1972). *Similarities and differences in the perception of the role of the clinical specialist,* Vol. I. Kansas City, MO: American Nurses' Association.

Brooten, D., Kumer, S., Brown, L.P., et al. (1986). A randomized clinical trial of early hospital discharge and home follow-up of very-low-birth-weight infants. *New England Journal of Medicine, 315* (15), 934–939.

Bruce, S. (1972). *Valuation of functions of the role of the clinical nursing specialist,* Vol. II. Kansas City, MO: American Nurses' Association.

Davidson, K.R., Donovan, K.B., & Gilman, C.S., et al. (1978). A descriptive study of the attitudes of psychiatrists toward the new role of the nurse thera-pist. *Journal of Psychiatric Nursing and Mental Health Services, 16* (11),. 24–28.

Georgopoulos, B., & Christman, L. (1970). The clinical nurse specialist: A role model. *American Journal of Nursing, 70* (5), 1030–1039.

Georgopoulos, B., & Jackson, M. (1970). Nursing kardex behaviour in an exper-imental study of patient units with and without clinical nurse specialists. *Nurs-ing Research, 19* (3), 196–218.

Georgopoulos, B., & Sana, J. (1971). Clinical nursing specialization and in-tershift report behaviour. *American Journal of Nursing, 71* (3), 538–545.

Girouard, S. (1978). The role of the clinical specialist as change agent: An experiment in preoperative teaching. *International Journal of Nursing Studies, 15* (2), 57–65.

Hodgman, E.C. (1983). The CNS as researcher. In A.B. Hamric & J. Spross (Eds.), *The clinical nurse specialist in theory and practice* Orlando, FL: Grune & Stratton (pp. 73–82).

Kennedy, L., Neidlinger, S., & Scroggins, K. (1987). Effective comprehensive discharge planning for hospitalized elderly. *The Gerontologist, 27,* 577–580.

Linde, B., & Janz, N. (1979). Effect of a teaching program on knowledge and compliance of cardiac patients. *Nursing Research, 28* (5), 282–286.

Little, D., & Carnevali, D. (1967). Nurse specialist effect on tuberculosis. *Nursing Research, 16* (4), 321–326.

Murphy, J. (1971). If p (additional nursing care), then q (quality of patient welfare)? In M. Batey (Ed.), *Communicating nursing research* Boulder, CO: West-ern Interstate Commission for Higher Education, pp. 1–12.

Neidlinger, S., Kennedy, L., & Scroggins, K. (1987). Effective and cost efficient discharge planning for hospitalized elders. *Nursing Economics, 5,* 225–230.

Peplau, H. (1965). Specialization in professional nursing. *Nursing Science, 3* (4), 268–287.

Pozen, M.W., Stechmiller, J.A., Harris, W., et al. (1977). A nurse rehabilitator's impact on patients with myocardial infarction. *Medical Care, 15* (10), 830–837.

Shaefer, J. (1973). The satisfied clinician: Administrative support makes the difference. *Journal of Nursing Administration, 3* (4), 17–20.

Smith, M. (1974). Perceptions of head nurses, clinical nurse specialists, nursing educators, and nursing office personnel regarding performance of selected nursing activities. *Nursing Research, 23* (6), 505–511.

part two

Experts in Action

The nine chapters in Part II illustrate clinical nurse specialists in action, working with different age groups in different specialties in a variety of health care delivery settings. In this introduction to Part II we have posed core discussion questions to aid in the comparison of role implementation and impact of each clinical nurse specialist. At the end of each chapter specific questions will highlight aspects of that chapter. The questions can be used by faculty and students in graduate programs to stimulate discussion about the variety of ways in which the clinical nurse specialist role can be implemented, as well as to identify the commonalities inherent in the clinical nurse specialist role. Clinical nurse specialists in practice, whether novice or experienced, can use the discussion questions to stimulate peer review as well as self-evaluation, thus promoting one's own thoughtful development of the clinical nurse specialist's role.

The core questions that can be applied to all the chapters are:

1. How would you document the impact of the clinical nurse specialist in the case presented in order to support the development of additional clinical nurse specialist positions in the same setting or the creation of the clinical nurse specialist role in another practice setting? How could the interventions of the clinical nurse specialist be evaluated? What would be relevant outcome measures?
2. Where would you place this clinical nurse specialist in the phases of role development? Substantiate your answer with an analysis based on the content presented in Chapters 2 and 3.
3. What factors in this setting have facilitated or obstructed the implementation of the clinical nurse specialist role? Identify the strategies used by the clinical nurse specialist to deal with these factors. Give an example of how these strategies could be used in your practice.
4. In relation to the role and setting described, discuss the importance of 1) a clear role definition, 2) communication skills, 3) interpersonal style, 4) administrative support, and 5) peer support.

5. What is your assessment of the clinical nurse specialist's success in integrating the four role components and setting time priorities among them?

6. Based on what this clinical nurse specialist has demonstrated thus far, speculate how she might contribute to the future of the nursing profession in regard to 1) restructuring the profession, 2) providing for authority, homogeneity, and unity in the specialties, 3) drawing new recruits into the field, 4) developing a research base for practice, and 5) responding to ethical dilemmas related to cost containment efforts and the nursing shortage. (Refer to Chapter 14.)

7. How could this story be adapted for the public media to portray a new professional image of nursing: dynamic, caring, well-educated, ethical, scholarly, assertive, powerful, and independent?

chapter five

The Oncology Clinical Nurse Specialist in a Tertiary Care Referral Center

Deborah Welch-McCaffrey

The oncology clinical nurse specialist is often beset with a stressful clinical dilemma. Although entitled a "specialist," this advanced practitioner is required to be a "generalist" since the disease of cancer can affect any organ system. Thus the requirement of "knowing a little about a lot" is a reality, along with the requirement to be holistic in orientation and to integrate psychosocial needs of both the family and patient into one's clinical repertoire. The four practice components that oncology clinical nurse specialists should be expert in, and thus a resource for, include physical status management, patient/family education, resource facilitation, and psychosocial support (Welch-McCaffrey, 1986). Add to this knowledge base a need to be cognizant of organizational issues that affect the utilization of the oncology clinical nurse specialist, and one has quite an ongoing job of assessment, education, and role assertion. This chapter will describe my practice in a tertiary care referral center and includes a depiction of the types of specialist interaction, factors that influence these interactions, and the evaluation of the effectiveness of my role. A case study will be used to describe my clinical experiences as an oncology clinical nurse specialist.

Case Study

ES was one of 222 consultations referred to me in 1984. She was a "difficult" patient in many ways. Only 40 years old, she entered the hospital for a routine hysterectomy for treatment of uterine fibroids. At surgery, she was found to have widely disseminated metastatic cancer, presumed primary of the ovary; however, this could never be definitively stated by pathology. She was engaged to be married, had one of the most extensive networks of friends I have ever seen, and was revealingly articulate in her coping style and need to understand exactly where she stood with the cancer. Because of the extent of the cancer at initial diagnosis, ES would require systemic chemotherapy. It was stated to her, however, that this would only palliate her disease and almost certainly would not cure it.

Around the time of initial diagnosis, I had many individual sessions with ES, discussing the nature of cancer and what was known about her specific case. Complicating the reality of the physicians' inability to cite any specific figures for survival for ES was her need to decide about her future, specifically her plans for marriage, coupled with her need to avoid becoming "a burden" on a new husband. Many of these issues were articulated in the presence of ES's fiancé.

Once the chemotherapy regimen was known, discussion about side effects and their management, impact of the regimen on ES's lifestyle, and outlining predictors of response became the focus of conversation. Whenever possible, I encouraged the nursing staff to remain in the room and to hear first-hand not only the content of the conversation but the way in which the conversation was directed. When direct role-modeling was not an option (usually because of nursing staff time constraints and responsibilities to other patients), ES's primary nurse was sought out and the specifics of the interaction were discussed.

Often, my interaction with the staff had other agendas besides the transmission of information about a specific patient-centered conversation. There was significant staff identification with ES. Because of her age, sex, outgoing manner, and unfortunate clinical dilemma, the staff had an ongoing need to talk about their feelings associated with her terminal condition, her family's reaction to her condition, the staff's feelings of helplessness, and their desire to optimize ES's care, since they expected her to progress in a rapidly downhill course. As ES returned monthly for chemotherapy, this need for staff catharsis became magnified, and periodic meetings with each shift of nurses were planned to discuss feelings, sometimes termed "sharing and caring" conferences.

Symptom management suggestions were ongoing interventions in ES's case. A close alliance occurred between the staff and myself in attempting to ameliorate chemotherapy-related nausea and vomiting and chronic pain. Suggestions were discussed on a one-to-one basis. It was the staff's stated responsibility to translate these joint symptom management decisions to the nursing kardex and to the other nursing shifts. As an additional resource, articles describing the rationale for these decisions were kept in the front of ES's chart, especially if they were questioned by the attending or house staff. For the most part, the physician's staff were receptive to new strategies for symptom management as suggested by the nursing staff.

The amount of time spent with ES during her hospitalizations was very cyclical, depending upon the nature of her problems and the need for intensive contact with the nursing staff. Initially, when she was first diagnosed, there were lengthy interventions with ES, her fiancé, her family, and the nursing staff, who quickly became attached to ES. During her six months of chemotherapy, contact decreased in time and focused on the control of symptoms associated with her chemotherapy regimen. At this time ES was also not as interested in discussing psychosocial issues and the possibility that she might die soon, as she was holding onto the hope that the treatment might work, and therefore she wanted to focus on this hope.

When ES returned to the hospital with gastrointestinal obstructive problems, all this changed. It became evident that the cancer was progressing despite chemotherapy. ES knew this, wanted to talk about it, and wanted to help her family deal with her dying. My interventions at this time became more intensive and included individual support for the patient, family meetings, wound management, and aggressive symptom management to control pain and emesis. ES's family was also encouraged to attend our family support group, which was cofacilitated by myself and an oncology counselor, a master's-prepared non-nurse. In addition to peer support, the family support group also offers families the chance to ask questions about cancer and its treatment. I continue to feel that an ideal pair of group facilitators to lead this type of group session is made up of a clinical nurse specialist and a counselor or social worker. Individuals often exhibit anxiety, much of which is generated from either misinformation or a lack of information. The clinical nurse specialist is able to interpret, explain, or provide the rationale for questions focusing on a specific cancer-related entity, thus reducing some or all of the anxiety. The role of the oncology clinical nurse specialist in psychosocial problems is also a critical one, as the identification of possible physiological etiologies to coping problems and behavioral changes can be readily considered. The presence of hypercalcemia and other metabolic changes, brain metastases, and the use of corticosteroids in the course of cancer are just some examples of these contributing factors (Welch-McCaffrey & Dodge, 1988). As ES's condition deteriorated, my identification of these factors contributing to her confusion helped the family cope with her mental status changes.

With ES, collaboration was a necessity as the staff nurse group, as in many cases, became the instrument for ongoing assessment and follow-up on teaching and support. Initially, the group established a division of work. The teaching of wound and stoma care and the administration of ES's chemotherapy became the staff's responsibility. Joint endeavors by the nursing staff and myself included toxicity management, the provision and monitoring of leukopenic care, and general daily assessment. Psychosocial support was my major responsibility with ES, particularly as her condition worsened and depression ensued. There were also multiple family members who needed supportive interventions. Although responsibilities were divided, this did not imply that those not deemed directly responsible did not intervene in those areas. It meant that the general responsibility for establishing optimum care in that area was allocated and overseen by either the staff or myself.

Because ES was seen as a "difficult" patient in the psychosocial realm, her care provided examples for looking at nursing measures to deal with psychosocial problems. During lengthy periods of reverse isolation, ES became very depressed. She had been extremely active all her life, not used to sitting and waiting, and these periods of isolation and prolonged waiting for marrow recovery and wound healing depressed her greatly. It was during these times that ES would not talk; she would lie on her bed with a gravely sullen facial expression and make little eye contact.

Each time I visited ES, I shared my impressions with the nursing staff. Having comfort with silence, commenting on ES's outward appearance, and gentle prompting of her feelings at appropriate times seemed to work best with her. Her depression was difficult, not only for the staff but also for her family, who felt helpless, out of control, and at times angry at ES for not being more verbal with them, like her old self. ES died on the night shift with one family member present, unlike the rest of the day when multiple family members took turns with their vigil visiting. I made contact with ES's husband and parents by phone the next day, as well as three months following her death. Cards were sent and several staff, plus myself, attended a memorial service for her. This completion of care for ES and her family was important for those of us who grew to know her well.

CLINICAL NURSE SPECIALIST INTERVENTION

Method of Patient Selection

ES's referral came from a staff nurse from the unit where all the gynecologic oncology patients are admitted. This particular staff nurse has consistently been good at identifying patients and families who required the oncology clinical nurse specialist's intervention. It is important to assess the staff nurse group's prior exposure to clinical nurse specialists and receptiveness to this role. Having had prior experience on the staff nurse's part often helps pave the way for a better understanding of appropriate referral making and using the clinical nurse specialist as a resource.

Initially, when I entered this system, there were no other clinical nurse specialists. I was the first, and the staff of this 770-bed tertiary-care referral center had had no prior experience with the clinical nurse specialist role. Thus, even though several weeks of personalized and group introductions were made throughout the hospital, there was still a need to remind staff that I was available as a resource. To help, I devised cards (Fig. 5–1) that were kept on all the medical-surgical floors in the area where nurses charted. My idea to do this was shared at a nursing directors' meeting, where the key nursing managers met weekly to address issues affecting their nursing care areas. By soliciting their feedback and support up front, no resistance to this idea prevailed. On these cards were the criteria for referral to the oncology clinical nurse specialist. Ongoing informal interactions with head nurses and key staff nurses helped me to form critical alliances with the units having cancer patients.

During my initial period of orientation, I also identified and solicited discussion with team members who might perceive my clinical expertise as threatening or overlapping their territory. I met with key oncologists and pharmacists concerning symptom management, social workers, counselors and discharge planners regarding psychosocial support and resource mobilization, dieticians concerning nutritional needs,

Deborah Welch RN, MSN
Oncology Clinical Nurse Specialist
Extension 3390
Pager 8303
Leave message at 2076, 2077

Offers assistance in:
* **Patient Care:**
  — Psychosocial support for patient and family
  — Toxicity management
  — Patient education concerning treatment
  — Nutritional problems
  — Pain management
* **Nursing Education:**
  — Inservices
  — Patient care conferences

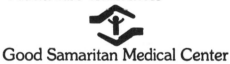

Good Samaritan Medical Center

Figure 5–1. Card Describing Oncology Clinical Nurse Specialist Services.

and technicians who were involved in intravenous care and radiation therapy. We discussed role perceptions, possible conflicts, and conflict resolution strategies, if necessary. This anticipatory "up front" approach has worked effectively in dealing with role conflict issues.

Criteria for Patient Case Load

Our tumor registry identified 1200 patients in 1984 as having received a diagnosis of cancer in our institution. That can be broken down to 100 patients per month, a significant population and, in fact, the greatest number per hospital in the southwest. One oncology clinical nurse specialist could hardly interact with the majority of these patients.

Usually, the larger the patient population, the smaller the impact of the clinical nurse specialist. Spross and Hamric (1983) recommended that there be three to five clinical nurse specialists for each 100 patients in a large teaching hospital. Thus, when there is only one clinical nurse specialist in a given specialty for a large population of patients, the clinical nurse specialist can impact directly on only a very small percentage of patients.

The philosophy of our nursing department is that the clinical nurse specialist should be a resource hospital-wide and should not remain unit-based. Thus, although we have a 30-bed designated general oncology unit and a 15-bed gynecology/oncology unit, I receive referrals from many units throughout the hospital.

In looking at last year's descriptive data of referral patterns, the 222 consultations came primarily from medical nursing units where the majority of oncology patients are admitted. Consultations are tallied after logging information from cards I use as reference for patients I see (Figure 5–2). These are identified as initial consultations (I have never met the patient before) and return consultations (patients previously known to me). Thus, not all the consultations are with new patients.

Patient _____

Location _____

Attending _____

Type Ca _____

_____

Past Hx _____

_____

Current Rx _____

_____

Family _____

_____

Phone _____

Address _____

Referral Source _____

Reason _____

Other Problems _____

_____

_____

_____

Figure 5–2. Patient Information Card

Criteria for Appropriateness of Method or Type of Intervention

There is no uniform standard or patient/problem profile that must be met before my intervention is deemed appropriate. Rather, staff characteristics such as experience within the specialty of oncology nursing and stability or turnover on the unit are considered when requests for my services are made. Hence, if a consult is placed from the pulmonary unit where there has been major turnover, the unit is staffed primarily with new graduates, and they are asking me to intervene with an anxious patient and family told within hours of a new diagnosis of oat cell lung cancer, that would be an appropriate referral. However, an objective look at the clinical milieu and individual staff is required if there is no transference of skill to the staff after six months of similar ongoing referrals characterized by continued mentoring and teaching the staff about lung cancer and its treatment and crisis intervention techniques. For units with experienced staff, interventions should primarily be with complex oncology patients (i.e., intensive multisystem problems, severe symptom distress, any new or unusual patient disease-type or symptomatic complaint) or for problems whose solutions require housewide changes in nursing practice, application of nursing research findings, or generation of a new nursing intervention.

Reviewing information tallied from my patient cards helps me analyze reasons for referral, source of referral (person referring and unit), additional problems identified by the oncology clinical nurse specialist, and types of intervention employed. The compilation of this information has a direct effect on my goal setting. When I describe where my referrals are coming from, I can identify gaps as well as strong points. For example, in reviewing referrals for the first half of 1985, I noted a persistent problem with establishing a referral base from one of the general surgical floors. Thus, I targeted some change strategies in this area in an effort to develop the key head nurse in that area as an ally rather than a barrier to my interventions there. In dealing with this problem on previous occasions, I have found the strategies of dealing directly with the head nurse's reasons for not promoting my use as a resource, educating the staff, implementing oncology nursing walking rounds on the unit, and including the staff in establishing oncology nursing guidelines for the entire hospital (rather than just the oncology unit) has helped increase referrals. This clinical impression can be substantiated with actual figures from descriptive statistics of referral patterns showing changes in frequencies following deliberative goal setting.

Analyzing these data helps me not only to log the types of interventions but also to quantify the time spent in clinical practice (Figure 5–3). The end result is then compared to my goals established in role delineation. Am I spending more or less time in clinical practice than originally negotiated?

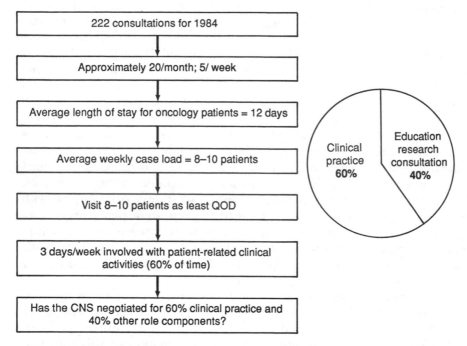

Figure 5–3. Analyzing referral patterns with reference to quantification of clinical time.

Clinical Nurse Specialist and Patient Communication

The amount of time spent with each patient/family unit varies greatly depending upon the nature of the problem, availability of other resources, and the expertise of the staff. Depending upon the problem I visit the patient from at least every other day to many times daily. If the titration of an effective narcotic regimen is necessary to control cancer-related pain, then it is imperative that this be evaluated every 24 hours. If the patient has just been told of the diagnosis of cancer, both the patient and the family need time with the oncology clinical nurse specialist. Thus daily visits are often necessary. When a patient is undergoing a diagnostic work-up and it remains unclear what type of cancer the patient has or the extent of disease present, then daily visits may or may not be necessary. When there are many unknowns, talking about the "ifs" with many people sometimes may confuse the patient more. Therefore visits every other day may be sufficient.

When the problem needing assistance involves support and counseling, the one-to-one approach is necessary. When staff have time, I encourage them to join me as I interact with the patient/family unit. If they cannot, I share with them important elements of our interaction. There are also times when patient contact is minimal and the staff are the main instrument of intervention. For example, if a consultation to advise on the treatment of stomatitis is requested, an initial assessment visit with the staff nurse can be done, recommendations jointly discussed, and follow-up and reassessment can become the responsibility of the staff.

Clinical Nurse Specialist and Health Care Team Communication

Ongoing communication is a must among all team members involved in the patient's care. The time in which clinical nurse specialists interact with patients is often a small portion of the patient's total day, and thus the clinical nurse specialist often learns much from staff input. They are the contributors of valuable information to the clinical nurse specialist's data base for the evaluation of clinical problems. It may be a temptation to remain an independent practitioner; however, the full nursing story cannot unfold without interaction with the entire staff. This open, clear, ongoing pattern of communication promotes the acceptance of the clinical role as well. Hence, interpersonal skills with staff as well as with patients and families are critically important competencies for successful oncology clinical nurse specialist functioning (McGee, Powell, Broadwell, & Clark, 1987).

Interventions by the clinical nurse specialist should be characterized by a deliberative analysis of care (Siehl, 1982). The ongoing validation of effectiveness and asking the question, "Is there a better way?" are the hallmarks of clinical nurse specialist intervention. The use of the nursing process in charting helps the nursing staff learn from this deliberative analysis of care. I find it necessary to communicate my interventions with patient/family units to both the nursing and medical staffs. Hence, the approach I have taken to charting is to leave a note in the medical progress notes and refer them to the details of the account in the nursing notes (e.g., Oncology Clinical Nurse Specialist Note/Please see Nurses' Notes). This way both the nursing staff and the physicians are made aware of my impressions and interventions.

Interdisciplinary team work often provides an ideal setting for teaching by the clinical nurse specialist. In discussing ES at one team meeting, I chose to elaborate on coping strategies of cancer patients, following the dietician's perception of ES being scared on this particular morning. This information was presented in the hope that the staff nurses, in particular, could expand their assessment skills, be able to read patient cues, and then validate if in fact what they were perceiving was indeed what the patient was feeling.

It is not unusual for the non-nursing interdisciplinary team members to identify patients that would benefit from my intervention. I feel that, at many conferences, the rehabilitation team members that we include in our team have been particularly helpful in showing the oncology staff how to use resources and work together. It has probably been the rehabilitation specialty alone that has paved the way for the promotion of teamwork and collaboration in meeting the many needs of both patients and families dealing with chronic illness.

When a non-nursing team member identifies not only a patient for me to see but also lists the specific reasons and interventions that might be helpful, I then ask the nursing staff to validate if this in fact would be an appropriate referral. The nursing staff must be included in the decision making. I do this for several reasons.

First, although clinical nurse specialists are indeed nurses, the staff nurse group may still perceive them as outsiders since they are not staff nurses (Girouard, 1983). Territorial issues may then surface. The staff may feel that these are "their" patients and want to control who does and does not interact with them. Second, if the appropriateness of the referral is not discussed and the clinical nurse specialist acts independently, the staff may perceive the identification of the clinical nurse specialist as a resource for the patient to be a value judgment by the referral source, that the staff is not delivering optimum nursing care. Resistance rather than collaboration can then become the norm.

IMPACT OF CLINICAL NURSE SPECIALIST INTERVENTION

Method of Evaluating Patient Outcomes

One measure of acceptance and evaluation of my interventions in the case of ES was the increase in requests for my assistance with problems other than those initially identified. For example, the initial request to see this patient was for assistance with helping the patient/family cope with the initial diagnosis of the cancer and their related need for accurate and updated information regarding antineoplastic therapies. However, as these initial psychosocial and patient/family educational needs were met, the staff continued to identify further needs that related to symptom management with which I could help. The staff also identified additional patients on their unit for my consultation.

On an individual basis, the success to which the oncology clinical nurse specialist manages symptom distress can be measured by Likert-type scales. I often have patients document by Likert scale the degree to which they have pain, feel nausea, are anxious, etc. (McCorkle & Young, 1978). Then, after planning a variety of interventions to ameliorate the severity of symptom distress, I have patients reevaluate their status and thereby have subjective and objective documentation of improved patient well-being as a result of my problem solving. When the plan for the relief of symptom distress is documented in the patient's chart and the patient indeed experiences relief from the problem—and this is charted as such—not only do the nursing staff but also the physician staff become aware of my interventions. I have also noted that another measure of acceptance of my problem solving occurs when the physician's staff chart in their notes the contributions that I have made to the patient's care and when interventional suggestions are ordered "as recommended by the oncology clinical nurse specialist."

With each individual patient/family unit with whom I interact, the patient and I jointly identify outcome criteria specific to symptom management, patient education, psychosocial support, and resource mobilization. The Oncology Nursing Society in collaboration with the American Nurses' Association has written *Standards for Cancer Nursing Practice* (Oncology Nursing Society & ANA, 1987), which can serve as a reference for the measurement of behavioral outcomes that promote optimum functioning throughout the course of cancer. Although not easily measurable, subjective reports from the patient and family account for important validation of the degree to which the clinical nurse specialist "makes a difference." Letters and cards describing the clinical nurse specialist's contributions to individualized care should not be tossed in the basket, but rather kept as written documentation. This input from consumers of health care is becoming increasingly important as administrators and marketing executives are becoming acutely aware of those factors that make people choose one health care agency over another. The Oncology Nursing Society's statement on *The Scope of Advanced Oncology Nursing Practice* (1987) identified that advanced cancer nursing practice is best defined as expert competency and leadership in the provision of care to individuals with an actual or potential diagnosis of cancer. The challenge confronting oncology clinical nurse specialists now as well as in the future is our ability to document the difference our practice makes on select aspects of agency functioning and quality of patient care (Yasko, 1985).

Method of Evaluation of Cost Effectiveness

In general, evaluation encompasses a comprehensive review of oncology clinical nurse specialist endeavors that focus on upgrading the quality patient care outcomes and a determination of one's effectiveness as a change agent. Ideally, the clinical nurse specialist's personal reflections on alterations in patient and organizational functioning should be supplemented by written documentation and supported by feedback from other team members who have witnessed the clinical nurse specialist's leadership role in directing the necessary change effort.

The discussions of patient care between the oncology clinical nurse specialist and the nursing staff provide the impetus for improving nursing care. In ES's case, from discussions of her care needs evolved the need to revise and then publicize an updated version of consistent leukopenic care housewide. With guided questioning on my part, staff were assisted with developing their own attitude of clinical inquiry about the state of leukopenic care at our hospital. They began to ask, with my help: Are we being consistent? Are we doing all we should? Are we teaching patients accurately? What more should we be doing? This is a good example of the clinical nurse specialist's role as a change agent in quality assurance projects. The presence of the clinical nurse specialist spearheading this clinical questioning promotes continued analysis of patient care and therefore creates an ongoing thermometer reading of what is and what ought to be. In ES's case, when she became infected while neutropenic, this clinical problem elicited ongoing discussion about the nature of infection and nursing measures to treat it. It was important for the staff themselves to be a part of the problem identification. When staff participate in identifying problems, they gain ownership of the problem, increase their cooperation in problem solving, and more readily accept the clinical nurse specialist role.

Rodgers (1973) described steps in planning for change that have implications for clinical nurse specialists in their role as change agent. These steps include:

1. Identify the problem
2. Collect sufficient data to accurately diagnose the problem
3. Make inferences and judgments
4. Plan an intervention on the basis of the above inferences and judgments
5. Intervene
6. Evaluate the change process and the solution

This type of more rigorous approach to planning for change is a necessary one as clinical nurse specialists continually strive to improve their skills in problem solving and evaluation. It is this general skill of evaluation that I believe forms the foundation of effective and successful clinical nurse specialist practice.

My practice is hospital-wide as opposed to unit-based. I evaluate my referral patterns yearly to see which nursing units routinely identify problems that require my attention and place a consultation with me. After my first year in the institution, it became obvious to me that one unit was not referring many patients. Thus, following Rodger's steps, I did the following:

1. Identified a unit with a significant number of newly-diagnosed cancer patients making few referrals to the oncology clinical nurse specialist
2. Validated my perception by looking at monthly admission census data on cancer patients at our hospital

3. Made inferences that a situation requiring change existed knowing (a) there were significant numbers of cancer patients admitted to this unit, (b) many newly-diagnosed cancer patients have a crisis situation to deal with and many questions regarding their predicament, and (c) many nurses feel ill-equipped to handle the emotional aspects at this time, or have inadequate time to spend with patients and families to help in this adjustment
4. Planned a meeting to discuss this with the head nurse; mutually decided on offering an inservice on my role and the institution of weekly oncology nursing walking rounds
5. Did the above for six months
6. Evaluated change in referral patterns; saw individual consultations increase; saw increased evidence of charting on the psychosocial and educational needs of patients and their families; heard subjective reports by nurses of their increased comfort in caring for cancer patients

One aspect of the change effort missing from Rodger's (1973) model is that concerning the need to reinforce the change. Lewin (1947) termed this "refreezing" after an old behavior is "unfreezed" and the person "moves" toward a new set of behaviors. Refreezing is needed to stabilize the new situation. In the above-mentioned example, I did three things to reinforce the new behavior. They included:

1. Gave one-to-one positive feedback when appropriate
2. When a patient or family directly commented on the high standard of nursing care they received in terms of emotional support and teaching, I responded by writing a letter of support to the head nurse and copied it to the director
3. I remained visible and available, to informally discuss patients on the unit

Documentation of these changes as one component of evaluation is of paramount importance in clinical nurse specialist practice.

At Good Samaritan Medical Center, our clinical nurse specialist group has devised a comprehensive model to evaluate our practice. This model is based on the premise that no one tool or approach can systematically address all aspects of our practice. Thus, in addition to the customary quantitative approach to clinical nurse specialist evaluation, we combine reporting of peer review, patient/family feedback, results of hospital-wide quality assurance projects, and nursing research endeavors that focus heavily on practice-related problems. Also included is descriptive information on our involvement with the corporate level of agency functioning, where we help to identify trends with a futuristic approach and how these trends will have both a quality and financial impact. A summation of revenue we have generated through educational programs and consultations is also included as a critical part of our cost effectiveness.

ROLE OF THE CLINICAL NURSE SPECIALIST IN THE PRACTICE SETTING

My position is a staff position, which reports to the director of medical nursing. All of the clinical nurse specialists at my institution report to area directors; thus we have different direct supervisors. When I first started out in my position, this placement caused problems and even now, periodically, still does.

Because the oncology unit comes under the jurisdiction of medical nursing, it was deemed that my likely position would be there as well. However, this caused ownership issues, as it was perceived that I "belonged" to medical nursing. The director of nursing's philosophy (and mine as well) was that I should not be unit-based but hospital-wide in my interventions with patients, families, and staff. This was supported by the admission data noting that cancer patients were consistently admitted throughout the hospital to myriad speciality services. When it came time to evaluate my referral base during my second year of practice, an obvious lack of referrals came from the general surgery, gynecologic surgery, and radiation therapy areas, whom I later found to perceive my services as being medical unit-based. Work with individual head nurses and other area directors helped address this misconception and devise change strategies to reverse this problem. Thus effective clinical nurse specialist intervention that is hospital-wide mandates multiple interactions with a variety of nursing leaders.

The introduction of a clinical nurse specialist into a system can elicit threat responses, and a nurse leader may perceive her territory as being invaded. A key person in any problem identification and/or change effort is the head nurse (Kwong, Manning, & Koetters, 1982). The more the clinical specialist can become a close ally with the head nurse, the more one can expect motivation to change and improve nursing care. The clinical nurse specialist–head nurse relationship should be fostered and cultivated as an ongoing process. If there is any lesson to be learned from years of practice as an oncology clinical nurse specialist, it is that you can never function independently and that the support of head nurses is critical.

How does the clinical nurse specialist influence the head nurse to make changes that have quality assurance or cost implications? Probably the two most important techniques are through sharing information and advocacy. Increasing the head nurse's awareness about new knowledge with implications for a particular patient population can promote improved delivery of care. Sharing journal articles and important points from conferences, as well as translating nursing research into workable practice guidelines enhance change. With the clinical nurse specialist functioning as the information broker, a specialized unit or entire hospital can benefit from the integration of new knowledge. For example, after a discussion with the geriatric clinical nurse specialist about the problem of falls in the elderly and the related implications for geriatric cancer patients, I discussed this problem with the oncology head nurse. We then agreed on the importance of the problem as both a quality and cost problem (with increased length of stay) and pursued the option of devising a fall prevention protocol for the elderly cancer patients in our designated oncology unit. We are now in the initial stages of research formulation and program planning.

As another example of advocacy, involvement with product evaluation committees in institutions can alter expenditures when quality is evaluated by clinical nurse specialists and head nurses, who may collaboratively decide on optimum product use that is also cost efficient. The choice of infusion lines, dressing kits, and alternatives to the promotion of immobility-related pressure sores by the head nurse and clinical nurse specialist have critical implications in the prevention of iatrogenic effects of treatment and hospitalization. Enhancing creative use of new products by nursing staff is thus another avenue for head nurse–clinical nurse specialist collaboration instead of competition.

Resistance is an issue that all clinical nurse specialists must deal with at some point in their career. It may be present for a variety of reasons. These reasons may stem from staff characteristics or may be provoked by the clinical nurse specialist. An initial assessment of the nursing staff's receptivity to your role and an ongoing reflection (with help) of your own interpersonal style identify sources of resistance. Clinical nurse specialist colleagues, head nurses, and other team members can offer valuable feedback on personal and interpersonal barriers to effective practice.

With one resistant nursing staff, I saw a need to share information regarding the management of chemotherapy extravasation. They did not perceive this as a need. Over time I identified one of the leaders of "the resistance" and began using her as a resource for myself concerning hospital routine and standard nursing practices. Gradually, and in an informal style, I began to share information with her regarding extravasation and to include her in various groups working on new projects, especially writing nursing standards. Eventually, as the issue of chemotherapy administration guidelines arose, this staff nurse became an instrumental ally in sharing information regarding extravasation management and the need to identify nursing standards for it. I think a major issue here was establishing the fact that there can still be staff nurse leaders and a clinical nurse specialist who work together, not in a mutually exclusive manner.

Hamric (1983) identified the need to provide anticipatory socialization for clinical nurse specialists. She stated that students need to understand the inevitability of encountering resistance and they also need to learn some strategies to use in overcoming it. Lawrence (1969) noted that the key to the problem of resistance is to understand its true nature. He said that what people resist most is not technical change but social change, the change in human relationships that results.

Change interferes with existing alliances and, if there is relative satisfaction with the current system, resistance predominates. When one nurse is given the title of specialist, this may threaten and alienate staff nurses who feel they are doing an excellent job at giving specialized care (Hamric, 1983). This problem can be perpetuated by a lack of staff involvement in the needs identification for a specialist. If the staff were not included in the planning to hire a specialist, when the specialist arrives on the scene the staff may perceive his/her entry as a value judgment by administration that their care has not been optimum. Thus, reasons for resistance may be in place even prior to the clinical nurse specialist's entry into the system.

Reasons for resistance are plentiful and require more elaborate discussion than can be done in this chapter. However, what is most important is the understanding that resistance should be expected and dealt with in an ongoing direct manner. If resistance is not dealt with, subversive tactics become the norm and no effective change can result.

Only when steps are taken to counter resistance will the clinical nurse specialist be able to succeed in all aspects of the role. Some signs that the process of acceptance is occurring include:

1. Staff making time to discuss issues with the specialist (Girouard, 1983)
2. Staff explaining to patients and new staff what the clinical nurse specialist's role is and how to utilize the clinical nurse specialist (Hamric, 1983)
3. Hearing evidence of the staff emulating the clinical nurse specialist, quoting verbatim or paraphrasing what the clinical nurse specialist said
4. Charting that reflects the clinical nurse specialist's advice or teaching
5. Increase of direct referrals to the clinical nurse specialist
6. Increase in requests for teaching services
7. Staff interested in going on to graduate school to become a clinical nurse specialist

Probably one of my most memorable examples of a staff nurse's acceptance and comprehension of my role occurred after a lengthy series of exchanges concerning an elderly man with advanced cancer of the prostate with bone metastasis. This nurse surprised me with her revelation,

"Now I know what the difference is between you and me . . . it's not just that you know more, it's also the depth and scope of what you know and you know just how to say it."

RESEARCH IN PRACTICE

Selection of Research

Research endeavors by the oncology clinical nurse specialist often are directed to clinical practice dilemmas encountered in daily activities. Questions concerning the major elements of practice (e.g., patient teaching, psychosocial support, symptom management, resource mobilization) are plentiful (Welch-McCaffrey, 1986). Involvement in nursing research can reach many levels, from interpreting research findings to orchestrating, as a principal investigator, a funded nursing research project. Quality assurance projects can also be viewed as less formal research endeavors. By attempting to identify and problem solve, however, quality assurance work becomes critical in improving patient care.

As an oncology clinical nurse specialist, I work closely with the oncology head nurse on our unit-based quality assurance program. We mutually, along with the staff, identify indicators of quality care and methods to evaluate that quality. The staff assumes the responsibility for the actual monitoring activities which, for example, may include an evaluation of documentation or observation of behaviors, depending on the quality indicator being monitored (e.g., patient teaching activities, psychosocial support, leukopenic care). Thus, in these activities, I function more as a consultant on quality care rather than as the actual surveyor of that care.

Another factor that may affect the choice of nursing research topic is one's current emphasis in clinical practice. I have recently identified elderly cancer patients at high risk for many problems associated with cancer treatment. Thus, I am gathering descriptive data on their hospital and discharge needs as compared to other age groups. I have also encouraged the staff to devise an organized bereavement support program for families of cancer patients who have died. As a result, I am fostering their interest in collecting data on grief support needs of acutely bereaved families. Thus, as a researcher and as a promoter of research activities among the staff, I keep active in nursing research endeavors.

Time Allocation

In my current position, my first research interest centered around an issue that related to a clinical practice dilemma that took up a great deal of time (i.e., the nursing care of the patient receiving chemotherapy), and my proposed solution to many problems associated with that clinical practice issue (e.g., the provision of a structured chemotherapy certification course). The research associated with this educational program was done on a good deal of personal time, as I was doing this during my first two years of practice, years often requiring a heavy focus on clinical practice and high unit visibility to establish competency with the staff. I chose, however, to evaluate the short-term and long-term effects of this course on knowledge retention and nursing care activities (Welch-McCaffrey, 1985). The evaluation of this course's impact on patient care revealed positive effects and therefore, as a secondary benefit, the evaluation substantiated the impact of the oncology clinical nurse specialist's problem assessment and intervention planning on improving patient care activities.

Now in my eighth year as the oncology clinical nurse specialist at this particular institution, my role delineation has changed in that there is less time spent in direct clinical practice and more time devoted to educational, consultative, and research pursuits. Yearly, time for each aspect of clinical nurse specialist practice is negotiated. As longevity increases, the aspects of my role other than clinical practice and direct care increase in time allocation. As the staff become more knowledgeable and more adept at problem solving, the complex patient forms my case load and more global programmatic nursing issues become a focus. I have also been able to substantiate the need for an additional oncology clinical nurse specialist and the creation of a more formal cancer center at our medical center.

My research interests must be in synchrony with my practice. Currently I am investigating informational needs of newly-diagnosed cancer patients, the results of which will have implications for patient education programs and my community teaching activities. The provision of an organized patient teaching program may also be a calling card for consumers of health care who are now picking health care agencies based on their range of services, experience in the specialty, humanistic and holistic approaches, and cost effectiveness.

Impact on Patient Care

I see a need to keep in touch with health care trends that affect my ability to function optimally as an oncology clinical nurse specialist (Welch-McCaffrey, 1987). This mandates ongoing flexibility in a role designed to foster creativity and innovation (Starck, 1983). Thus, I must remain cognizant of the need to be a resource to the hospital in general. Some ways in which I can positively impact patient care, plus be an advocate to administrators, include helping to translate nursing costs per diagnostic related group, interface with the home care market, function as a coordinator of care as specialization increases, plan unique consumer-oriented programs that focus on the specialty of oncology, and generate revenue as a result of my specialized services (Donoghue

& Spross, 1984; Paulen, 1985; Yasko, 1985). Planning new innovative delivery of nursing care is a prime market for clinical nurse specialists. Currently I am in the process of developing a nurse-directed clinic for breast cancer patients, that will hopefully enhance the care of patients during the phase of initial diagnosis of a breast malignancy. Evaluation efforts will focus on decreased length of stay, patient satisfaction, and the reduction of psychological and symptom distress.

SUMMARY

As an oncology clinical nurse specialist, one of my primary roles is to help identify what is and what ought to be (Siehl, 1982). One of the most challenging aspects of this role is to be a generalist while at the same time being a specialist. Benner (1985) described this challenge well when, in defining the expertise of the oncology clinical nurse specialist, she noted that "the oncology clinical nurse specialist offers a hybrid of practical knowledge gained in front-line practice, and the most sophisticated skills of knowledge utilization, that is, applying the latest theories and technical innovation in practice." In addition to having advanced knowledge about cancer care, the oncology clinical nurse specialist must possess an astute awareness of one's practice environment, effective interpersonal skills, and a collaborative, team approach in reaching one's goals.

Periodically throughout my career as an oncology clinical nurse specialist, I have reflected on my motivation to take on this role, as well as why I have continued with it. Although there have been many times marked with frustration and outright anger, I can remember an equal number of times marked by success and a sense of completion over an idea, project, nursing care guideline, or hospital-wide policy that I generated. I think it is the free reign of creativity, the challenge of working with complex interpersonal issues, and knowing I am helping to make the illness of cancer just a bit easier to deal with that fuels my ongoing interest to remain a motivated and committed oncology clinical nurse specialist.

SPECIFIC QUESTIONS

1. What are the similarities and differences between this role as a "generalist" specialist and the subspecialization discussed in Chapter 10?
2. Describe how you could use the strategies developed by this author for introducing and implementing the clinical nurse specialist role in a new setting.

3. This author developed a thorough and proactive method of documentation and record keeping. How can you adapt these methods to your practice setting?
4. Describe a situation in which you have encountered resistance to your role. What was the outcome? Compare the strategies you used with those described in this chapter.
5. In relation to the role and setting described, discuss the importance of the clinical nurse specialist functioning as a catalyst for change.

REFERENCES

Benner, P. (1985). The oncology clinical nurse specialist: An expert coach. *Oncology Nursing Forum, 12* (2), 40–44.

Donoghue, M., & Spross, J.A. (1984). The future of the oncology clinical nurse specialist. *Oncology Nursing Forum, 11* (1), 74–78.

Girouard, S. (1983). Theory-based practice: Functions, obstacles and solutions. In A.B. Hamric, & J. Spross (Eds.), *The clinical nurse specialist in theory and practice*. Orlando, FL: Grune & Stratton.

Hamric, A.B. (1983). Role development and functions. In A.B. Hamric, & J. Spross (Eds.), *The clinical nurse specialist in theory and practice*. Orlando, Fla: Grune & Stratton.

Kwong, M., Manning, M.P., & Koetters, T.L. (1982). The role of the oncology clinical nurse specialist: Three personal views. *Cancer Nursing, 5* (6), 427–434.

Lawrence, P.R. (1969). How to deal with resistance to change. *Harvard Business Review, 47* (1), 4–6.

Lewin, K. (1947). Frontiers in group dynamics: Concept, method and reality in social science, social equilibria and social change. *Human Relations, 1*, 5–41.

McCorkle, R., & Young, K. (1978). Development of a symptom distress rating scale. *Cancer Nursing, 1* (5), 373–378.

McGee, R.F., Powell, M.L., Broadwell, D.C., & Clark, J.C. (1987). A delphi survey of oncology clinical nurse specialist competencies. *Oncology Nursing Forum, 14* (2), 29–34.

Oncology Nursing Society. (1987). The scope of advanced oncology nursing practice. *ONS News, 2* (2), 1.

Oncology Nursing Society and ANA. (1987). *Standards for oncology nursing practice*. Kansas City, MO: Oncology Nursing Society and ANA.

Paulen, A. (1985). Practice issues for the oncology clinical nurse specialist. *Oncology Nursing Forum, 12* (2), 37–39.

Rodgers, J.A. (1973). Theoretical considerations in the process of change. *Nursing Forum, 12* (2), 160–174.

Siehl, S. (1982). The clinical nurse specialist in oncology. *Nursing Clinics of North America, 17* (4), 753–761.

Spross, J., & Hamric, A.B. (1983). A model for future clinical specialist practice. In A.B. Hamric & J. Spross (Eds.), *The clinical nurse specialist in theory and practice* (pp 291–306). Orlando, FL: Grune & Stratton.

Starck, P. (1983). Factors influencing the role of the oncology clinical nurse specialist. *Oncology Nursing Forum, 10* (4), 54–58.

Welch-McCaffrey, D. (1985). Rationale, development and evaluation of a chemotherapy certification course for nurses. *Cancer Nursing, 8* (5), 255–262.

Welch-McCaffrey, D. (1986). Role performance issues for oncology clinical nurse specialists. *Cancer Nursing, 9* (6), 287–294.

Welch-McCaffrey, D. (1987). 2001: An oncology nurse odyssey. *Innovations in Oncology Nursing, 3* (4), 1, 12.

Welch-McCaffrey, D., & Dodge, J. (1988). Acute confusional states in elderly cancer patients. *Seminars in Oncology Nursing, 4*(3), 208–216.

Yasko, J. (1985). The predicted effect of recent health care trends on the role of the oncology clinical nurse specialist. *Oncology Nursing Forum, 12* (2), 58–61.

chapter six

The Clinical Nurse Specialist Consultant in a Community Hospital

Diana L. Nikas

Most clinical nurse specialists work in large medical centers. Although nurses and patients in smaller hospitals have many of the same needs, the hospitals frequently cannot afford clinical nurse specialists for all services, nor do they require these services full time. With this in mind, I marketed myself as a critical care clinical nurse specialist consultant to small and medium-sized hospitals. The following case study illustrates how I implemented the clinical nurse specialist role on a part-time, consultation basis in a medium-sized community hospital.

Case Study

SP was a 20-year-old female in her second year of college. Ten days prior to admission in September, she had had flu-like symptoms and an upper respiratory tract infection. Two days prior to admission, SP noticed some weakness in her legs and some tingling sensations. The day before admission the weakness became more pronounced, and she experienced a mild amount of difficulty breathing. She was admitted to the intensive care unit (ICU) with a preliminary diagnosis of impending respiratory failure secondary to Guillain-Barre Syndrome (GBS) (Anderson & Siden, 1982; Gracey, McMichan, Divertie, & Howard, 1982; Prydum, 1983).

Over the next week, SP's weakness progressed to complete respiratory paralysis and paralysis of all extremities and motor cranial nerves (CN). She required intubation and mechanical ventilation. Motor cranial nerve dysfunction resulted in the inability to move her eyes through their normal range of movement (CN III, IV, VI), inability to open and close her eyes (CN III, VII), loss of muscles of mastication (CN V), loss of muscle of expression (CN VII), loss of gag and swallow reflexes (CN IX, X), and inability to move her tongue (CN XII).

SP's complete motor and respiratory paralysis led to a state of total physical dependency. Additionally, because SP was conscious and alert but was intubated and unable to move the muscles of her face or eyes, she was unable to communicate. This made her fearful and anxious. The nursing staff was unsure how to approach her.

After about three weeks, SP's paralysis began to reverse and she began to regain some ability to communicate, first with eye signals, then by nodding or shaking her head, then with facial expressions. This allowed us to develop a communication system using an alphabet board and eye signals. This was a tedious and frustrating system that required a great deal of patience on the part of both SP and the nursing staff. As her ability to communicate improved, so did the complexity of her care.

As SP began to slowly regain motor strength, she also began experiencing irritating and uncomfortable paresthesias. Although these sensory abnormalities are not uncommon in patients whose nerves are regenerating, there is no specific and consistently successful nursing or medical intervention. Because SP described these sensations as painful, the nursing and medical staff decided to treat them with morphine. SP also continued to display fear and anxiety. This was treated with diazepam. Due to the complex nature of her condition and communication difficulties, a psychiatric consultation was called. The psychiatrist determined that she was depressed and put her on tricyclic antidepressant medication. These medications had the potential for leading to complications.

SP became very dependent and demanding. Because of feelings of frustration with her condition and her perceived slow improvement, she had periods of acting out and periods of withdrawal. She occasionally complained about the "pain" in her extremities and autonomic discomfort (e.g., hot flashes and tachycardia).

SP's family consisted of her 9-year-old brother, her mother, and maternal grandparents. Her father had died a couple of years earlier. Her mother was an intelligent woman who worked part-time as a secretary. She was attentive to SP and cooperative with the nursing and medical staff. She asked questions and wanted to participate in SP's care. SP's brother and maternal grandparents also visited often. Mrs. P's involvement with SP's care left Mrs. P little time and energy to spend with her young son. This situation was complicated by the feeling of abandonment the son had been experiencing since the death of his father 2 years earlier.

CLINICAL NURSE SPECIALIST INTERVENTION

Method of Patient Selection
I worked 16 hours per week as a critical care clinical specialist in a 340-bed community hospital with fifteen critical care beds in two adjacent units. Referrals for the patients I followed came from a number of sources. The two major ways I selected patients were by request of the nursing staff or by assessing a need as I became familiar with the patients. The head nurse, the critical care supervisor, and occasionally the medical social worker also asked me to consult on specific patients (Hamric & Spross, 1983).

Criteria for Patient Case Load
Patients I followed usually met one or more of the following criteria (Edlund & Hodges, 1983):

1. Diagnosis not often seen in this community hospital
2. Real or potential complications
3. Complex medical or nursing diagnoses, or both
4. Real or potential complex psychosocial problems of patient or family, for example, family of suicide victim
5. Patients who were long-term, for example, spinal cord injury

Criteria for Appropriateness of Method/Type of Intervention

Because of my part-time position, I usually followed three or four patients who met the above criteria and consulted with the nursing staff on many of the other 10 to 12 patients in the unit. This arrangement also allowed me to carry out the other roles of the clinical specialist, such as providing some formal didactic educational programs, consulting with nursing staff on other units, and acting as a liaison with nursing management regarding policies and procedures in the ICUs.

SP met a number of the above criteria. She was selected because of the complex nature of her care and the collaborative approach that was developed to deal with her problems. The diagnosis of GBS is not common in most acute care settings, including this community hospital. Only a few nurses had ever cared for a patient with GBS, and the nurses expressed concern regarding their ability to meet this patient's needs. SP also had a potential for developing complications. These complications included potential for infection, that is, atelectasis and pneumonia secondary to her altered respiratory function, and need for respiratory therapy (i.e., intubation, mechanical ventilation, suctioning, inability to deep breathe and cough to clear secretions); alteration in skin integrity secondary to paralysis and bedrest; autonomic nervous system (ANS) dysfunction manifested by cardiac arrhythmias, labile blood pressure, altered temperature perception; altered nutritional status secondary to inability to eat due to cranial nerve paralysis; and other complications of prolonged immobility, such as sleep disturbance and sensory disturbance.

SP met the third criterion also. She had complex nursing diagnoses that included altered sensory perceptions manifested as pain secondary to altered nerve function. This was a particularly difficult diagnosis to treat because the paresthesias typical of GBS are not responsive to the usual pain medications. SP was also anxious about her diagnosis and fearful about her prognosis and her day-to-day progress. At times she seemed to resent us and would get angry when we encouraged her and told her how well she was doing.

Because of the suddenness of this devastating event, there was a potential for family disruption and discord. SP derived a great deal of support from her family, especially her mother. Because of the long-term nature of the illness, I saw the need to provide support and guidance for Mrs. P and to assist her in maintaining her home-life for her son and herself. Mrs. P was eager to participate in SP's care, but began to show signs of exhaustion and anxiety when SP became demanding and manipulative.

SP also met the last criterion as she was a long-term patient. Patients typically spend 3 to 5 days in the ICU, with a fair number staying 7 to 10 days. Occasionally, one patient among the fifteen would be in the ICU 2 to 3 weeks or longer. These were usually patients with multiple injuries or complications. SP required intensive care for 6 weeks because of her need for respiratory support due to her inability to ventilate independently.

Critical care nurses who are not experienced in caring for long-term patients are not always able to develop a plan of care that meets the needs of the patient, the family, and their own needs. Because of the complexity of her physical and emotional needs, SP had the potential for becoming a "difficult patient" and the family a "difficult family." As a critical care nurse specialist with a speciality in neuroscience nursing, I had the knowledge and extensive experience with situations similar to SP's and knew that there were ways to circumvent the development of problems.

In order to avoid these problems, I assisted the nursing staff in the development of the following objectives that were dictated, in part, by the periodic nature of my position as critical care clinical nurse specialist:

1. Identify a team of nurses to care for SP
2. Educate the nursing staff regarding the pathophysiology of GBS with autonomic nervous system (ANS) involvement
3. Assist the nursing staff to develop a plan of care to meet the immediate needs of the patient and family
4. Assist the nursing staff to modify the plan of care as SP's condition changed
5. Evaluate SP's physical and psychological responses to her disorder and nursing interventions
6. Assess the family's response to SP's condition, change in condition, and nursing care
7. Consult with physicians regarding the plan of care, particularly the drug regimen
8. Act as a resource to other members of the health care team (e.g., respiratory therapist, physical therapists, medical social worker)
9. Assist the nursing staff to prepare for SP's transfer to the rehabilitation unit

My major role, therefore, was that of consultant. Although I provided some direct care and a considerable amount of education, I could not provide or monitor day-to-day care. Because of this major limitation, I felt it imperative to provide the nursing staff with the tools they would need to carry out the plan of care.

My initial involvement was to assess SP's physical and psychological condition. I talked with the nursing staff about my findings and their experience. Because of the long-term nature of SP's illness, I felt it would be beneficial to SP and for the nursing staff to identify a team of nurses who would be responsible for planning and administering care for SP.

I initially tried to sell the concept of a primary nurse, but the head nurse and some of the staff nurses were not comfortable with this concept. I decided that it was not worth pursuing this idea at that time and decided to modify this concept to a "team" approach. I discussed the idea of identifying a team of nurses to care for SP with the head nurse and the supervisor for critical care. They were willing to support this concept and to make every effort to schedule the identified group of nurses so that they could provide continuous care.

There were two nurses who had had experience with patients with GBS or similar disorders (such as spinal cord injured patients) and who enjoyed the complex and long-term nature of these patients. They were willing to coordinate SP's care and assisted in recruiting other nurses to become part of the team. We had a meeting with the majority of the nursing staff to explain the team concept and hear their ideas and concerns. Because many of the nursing staff preferred short-term patients, they were willing to help develop this concept. Once formulated, we explained our plan to SP, her family, and the physicians. Everyone was supportive of the concept.

As the neuroscience clinical nurse specialist, I had two educational conferences to review the pathophysiology of GBS and the care and complications. Questions and concerns of the nursing staff and other health team members regarding the nature of this disorder and SP's progress and prognosis were addressed. Journal articles describing GBS and ANS involvement were provided.

The team of nurses and I spent time with SP and her family answering questions and keeping them informed of her progress. They wanted to know about the disorder itself and what they could expect over the next days and weeks. They were justifiably concerned about SP's prognosis and the potential length of her recovery.

I saw SP at least twice a day the 2 days per week I was at the hospital. During those visits I evaluated the efficacy of the plan of care and assessed the need for modifications. I met with the nurses caring for SP on each of the 12-hour shifts and reviewed progress and problems. I worked part of the night shift once per week and had excellent rapport with these nurses. This allowed me to assist in communication between staff members and to provide educational material directly to these nurses. I was also able to assist them in planning and implementing nursing care.

Nursing Diagnoses and Desired Outcomes

A plan of care was developed that incorporated routine nursing care of patients with GBS (e.g., identifying signs of ANS involvement and developing appropriate interventions should they occur) while giving special attention to SP's more complex nursing care problems (Edlund & Hodges, 1983). Evaluation of SP's progress was based on outcomes to the problems and diagnoses we had identified. The identified complex nursing diagnoses and desired outcomes included:

1. Knowledge deficit related to the pathophysiological progression of GBS and prognosis

   Desired Outcomes: SP and Mrs. P will communicate understanding of the pathology and prognosis of GBS.

2. Impaired verbal communication related to cranial nerve dysfunction and intubation

   Desired Outcomes: SP will be able to communicate needs and feelings.

3. Alteration in comfort, that is, paresthesias and hot flashes related to abnormal sensory and autonomic nervous system functioning

   Desired Outcomes: SP will report that discomfort was controlled using a combination of medication and noninvasive techniques without narcotics.

4. Fear and anxiety related to loss of ability to move, breathe, or communicate

   Desired Outcomes: Fear and anxiety will be alleviated as reflected by SP's expression of confidence in nursing care and understanding of her condition and prognosis.

5. Impaired adjustment manifested by depression and frustration related to slow recovery from GBS

   Desired Outcomes: Progress toward rehabilitation would not be inhibited by frustration or depression.

6. Powerlessness related to total physical dependency manifested by desire to have constant attention from the nursing staff and her mother

   Desired Outcomes: SP will display independent behaviors by performing activities of which she is capable.

7. Potential complications, specifically musculoskeletal problems, respiratory and urinary tract infections related to immobilization

   Desired Outcomes: There will be an absence of complications, for example, skin breakdown, respiratory or urinary tract infections.

I reviewed routine nursing assessments and interventions with the nursing staff, with the major objective of assisting them in assessing SP for the above problems and developing objectives of care and appropriate interventions. The assessments and interventions are discussed below.

Knowledge Deficit Related to Pathophysiological Progression and Prognosis of GBS. When SP was admitted to the ICU, she had minimal movement of her lower extremities and mild impairment of movement of her upper extremities and respiratory muscles. Over the next 7 to 10 days, her paralysis increased so that she was completely quadriplegic with no respiratory muscle function. This paralysis included the motor cranial nerves leading to loss of eye movement, facial expression, and gag and swallowing ability.

An initial objective was to prepare SP and her family for this progressive loss of function. Patients expect to get better, not worse, after coming to the hospital and submitting to care. It is very frightening for them and their families to experience a worsening of symptoms. It was important to help them anticipate this occurrence and thereby lessen their fear and anxiety. While this increasing loss of function still created fear and anxiety on the part of the patient and family, they admitted that it would have been worse if they had not been aware of the typical course of the disorder.

It was also vital that the nursing staff understand the nature of the progression of GBS so they could anticipate SP's increasing physical needs and respond accordingly. As a result of the classes they had attended, they were able to respond to these changes with calm confidence and to support SP and her family and allay their fears. Most of this fear and anxiety seemed to be related to a knowledge deficit regarding GBS and medical and nursing interventions.

Initially I assessed the level of understanding of SP and her mother about the nature of GBS and its prognosis from the explanations they received from the physician. I found they had a general understanding, but required some detailed explanations about the nature of the disease, the progression of symptoms, and specific nursing and medical interventions, such as intubation, mechanical ventilation, tube feedings, turning, and so on. These explanations were communicated to the nursing staff so they could reinforce this teaching and answer questions.

Impaired Verbal Communication Related to Cranial Nerve Deficits and Intubation. SP's total motor paralysis also resulted in an inability to communicate. Because SP had been able to communicate the first few days she was in the ICU, the nurses were able to get to know her prior to her cranial nerve paralysis. This assisted them to anticipate some of her needs. The problem of communication became paramount when SP was not even able to communicate with facial expressions or eye blinks. During this period of time, which lasted about 2 weeks (almost 3 weeks from admission), communication with SP was unidirectional. It was difficult for the nursing staff to give care to a person who was awake and alert but unable to give them any feedback. We relied on SP's mother for feedback, while at the same time realizing that she, too, required a great deal of support through this difficult time. It was important for the nursing staff, SP, and her mother to remember that the paralysis was temporary and that movement would return, beginning with the most recent motor loss first. This resulted in return of eye movement and facial expression prior to motor return in her extremities.

When SP regained eye movement and facial expression, communication became very complicated. The nurses developed tools to aid in communication and taught SP to use them. An alphabet board was used for complex words and eye signals for yes and no. The nurses worked together and with the family, primarily the mother, to develop consistent patterns of communication. With Mrs. P's assistance, the nurses were able to interpret subtle changes in SP's facial expression and eye movements. This system was successful in large part because of the consistency of nurses caring for SP.

As SP regained more control of facial expression, she was able to mouth words. Again, each step of increasing ability to communicate was a smooth transition owing to continuity of care. SP worked hard to communicate her needs and was usually patient when we had difficulty understanding her. Occasionally she displayed impatience and frustration. The amount of time required for communication alone was significant. For this reason, nurses who cared for SP in the initial weeks of her illness did not have other patient care responsibilities other than assisting with the care of at least one other patient.

Alteration in Comfort: Paresthesias and Hot Flashes Related to Abnormal Sensory and Autonomic Nervous System Functioning. A problem of major concern was that of pain. Patients with GBS typically do not have sensory loss, although paresthesias often develop (Prydum, 1983; Ropper & Shahant, 1984). The paresthesias are usually described as tingling and pins-and-needles sensations and others as muscle cramping described as a "charlie-horse." Some patients experience bursts of electrical shock-like sensations. These sensations have been described as mildly irritating and uncomfortable by some patients and painful and disturbing by others. SP was in the latter category. These uncomfortable sensations developed in the interim between my scheduled times at the hospital.

Because SP had limited ability to communicate, she described these sensations as pain in her legs and arms. The nurses and physicians decided to treat her pain with morphine sulfate (MS) 2 to 4 mg intravenously every 3 to 4 hours around the clock. I was concerned about this regimen because MS is often ineffective in alleviating the pain produced by peripheral nerve problems. Additionally, because of the long-term nature of GBS and these painful paresthesias, I was concerned that the patient may develop a dependency on narcotic analgesics.

I discussed the sequence of events that led to the administration of MS with the nurses. The team of nurses had not known how to assess SP's discomfort and responded to her expressions of pain by requesting a narcotic order from the physician. They told me that the morphine helped SP sleep for an hour or 2, but admitted that she still complained of pain.

The team of nurses and I developed a method of assessing SP's pain that included asking SP to:

1. Describe her pain sensations as graphically as possible
2. Rate the severity of pain from one (least) to ten (worst), and estimate the average intensity
3. Identify factors that affected the pain
4. Evaluate interventions designed to relieve pain, such as positioning, distraction, and medication

Initially, SP had difficulty describing her painful sensations. I assisted her by relating how other patients had described these sensations and asked her to compare those descriptions with her own. She was able to confirm that her extremities felt as if they were "asleep" and described this as pins-and-needles and tingling. She also stated she had periodic shooting pains "like tiny electrical shocks." The shooting pains caused her the greatest discomfort and were the most anxiety producing.

She rated the shooting pains as an eight on the severity scale, mostly because they were unpredictable in frequency and severity. The tingling and pins-and-needles sensations were more constant and less severe, usually three to four on a scale of ten. The constancy of these sensations was irritating and exhausting for SP. She related that lack of sleep and lying in one position for longer than one to one and a half hours seemed to aggravate her discomfort. She typically had more discomfort in the late afternoon and during the night.

I discussed some methods for relieving the pain with SP. She said that being positioned was uncomfortable, but once positioned (which took considerable time and attention), it helped to relieve her discomfort. Because of the diplopia that resulted from cranial nerve dysfunction (CN III, IV, VI), she could not watch television or read. She found music to be a favorable distraction, and her mother brought in a radio and tape deck with some of her favorite music. She also found that gentle rubbing of her skin decreased the discomfort tremendously. This relief lasted minutes to an hour or more. SP admitted that the morphine really did not relieve the pain as much as it allowed her to sleep.

After discussing my findings with the nursing staff, a plan was developed to alleviate SP's pain without the use of morphine, using the methods described above. Her physician agreed to discontinue the morphine order and try aspirin or aspirin with codeine. SP was not altogether pleased with the withdrawal of morphine. The support of her mother and consistency of the nursing interventions assisted her in adjusting quite well for about two weeks.

Then SP had an episode of hysterical and belligerent behavior. The nurses caring for her felt this was due in part to sleep deprivation and requested diazepam to calm her. Repeated doses of diazepam failed to quiet her and morphine was ordered. SP slept for almost 4 hours after receiving morphine.

Although the intervention did not seem appropriate, the objective was attained. Unfortunately, the morphine was not discontinued with that dose and SP continued getting periodic doses for 5 days—for sleep, not pain. I had another conference with the physician and nurses and discussed my concern regarding the use of morphine. It was decided that the use of morphine would be discontinued. This was not difficult as SP's pain was diminishing somewhat and the other interventions were effective. Her difficulty with sleeping seemed to be temporary, and no further problems were encountered.

By having a stable nursing staff caring for SP, the nurses were very knowledgeable of SP's course and were able to build a close relationship with SP and her mother. I encouraged the nurses to include SP and her mother in planning care and to keep them informed of her progress. I also encouraged them to allow SP's mother to participate in care giving. This was accomplished by having Mrs. P participate in pain control measures. She provided diversion for SP by talking to her about daily events and reading to her. Mrs. P also spent time rubbing SP's skin, as this had been identified as a method of controlling her discomfort and was a time-consuming task for the nursing staff. Mrs. P felt that she was helping both SP and the nursing staff by carrying out these activities.

I spent time alone with both SP and her mother with the objective of allowing them to evaluate SP's progress and to voice concerns and ask questions. I related my extensive experience with other GBS patients and assured SP that she was following a typical course, and that her youth and lack of complications would be positive factors in her recovery. The nurses and I gave SP regular feedback on her progress.

Fear and Anxiety Related to Loss of Ability to Move, Breathe, or Communicate, and Impaired Adjustment Manifested by Depression and Frustration Related to Slow Recovery from GBS. The nursing diagnoses of fear and anxiety and impaired adjustment manifested by frustration and depression overlapped and were sometimes difficult to separate. Initially, the fear and anxiety that the patient and families experience is in response to the threatening nature of the disease and concern over the prognosis. Once the progression of symptoms has stopped and the patient has begun to make meaningful recovery, the realization of the long-term nature of the rehabilitation leads to frustration and periods of depression. This is especially true in the impatient young adult who views this disruption of life as unfair and is angry at the impotence in righting this terrible wrong. Communication with SP and her mother revealed their fear of SP's inability to breathe and move and the immediate and long-term significance of these problems.

The nursing staff attempted to alleviate SP's fear and anxiety by offering repeated explanations regarding both GBS and her treatment regimen. They carefully explained everything they were doing to her, even when it was repetitive activities such as suctioning or turning. They encouraged her to give them feedback using the communication system that had been developed.

About 3 weeks into her hospitalization, SP began to regain movement and the ability to communicate. Her fear and anxiety, as is typical of many of these patients, began to be replaced by frustration, alternating with periods of depression. SP frequently became impatient when the nurses had difficulty understanding what she wanted. She became obsessive about her positioning and other aspects of her care. She was very demanding of her mother and often was disrespectful. These periods of acting out alternated with periods of withdrawal and crying. She seemed to resent being told that she was making excellent progress, but she became extremely depressed if she could not exhibit daily progress in her ability to move.

This ambivalent behavior was sometimes difficult for the nurses to understand and accept. This behavior never interfered with her care or progress, however, and we decided that we would offer support and understanding while allowing her to vent her feelings about the dilemma in which she found herself. The nurses and I had periodic conferences to discuss their feelings about caring for SP and her responses to their care.

Her desire to progress rapidly allowed us to move SP toward independence as her physical abilities improved. Even when she moved to rehabilitation, however, SP expressed frustration and a negative attitude that did not parallel her progress.

The team of nurses and I learned to accept this negative attitude when we realized that it did not interfere with her willingness to work toward recovery. We decided that we would continue to communicate the progress we perceived and continue to enforce the behavioral limits we had established. We believed that by acknowledging but not accepting these negative perceptions or behaviors, we helped SP to progress, at least physically.

Powerlessness Related to Total Physical Dependence. During this period, SP also became demanding and somewhat manipulative. The nurses and I decided to include SP's mother in designing a plan to circumvent this behavior. We developed a "generic" set of guidelines for planning care that could serve throughout SP's hospitalization. These included such things as explaining the plan of care to SP and allowing her to make decisions where appropriate. SP then agreed to this plan of care and was expected to adhere to it and participate in it. When SP displayed dependent behavior inappropriately, such as asking to have her mouth suctioned even though she was able to swallow, the nurses were firm and consistent in their approach.

Limits were also set on other behaviors. Sometimes SP would request nursing attention when she knew that once the nurse left the room there would be a specific length of time until the nurse returned. I encouraged the nurses to tell SP how long they would be gone and to return at the specified time. They emphasized to SP that her light was to be used only if she needed help in the interim, and not be used to ask for routine care measures that would be provided at scheduled times.

This "rule" was applied differently at different stages of SP's course. Initially, SP had no way of calling the nurse because of her paralysis. In this case the nurse would frequently put her head in the door and let SP know everything was okay. As SP became more independent, the frequency of interventions decreased and the intervals lengthened. SP did not always like this decreased attention, but the nursing staff was encouraged to maintain these limits. For the most part, this worked quite effectively, although at times SP sulked.

SP sometimes used her physical dependency to manipulate her mother. Initially, Mrs. P tried to respond to all of SP's demands and was coming in more often and staying longer than we had agreed. She was beginning to look tired and stressed and I was concerned that she would jeopardize her health. This was a concern for many reasons, not the least of which was that SP was going to be in the hospital for many months.

When questioned by me, Mrs. P admitted she was very tired (this was about the second week of SP's hospitalization) and was concerned about her son. As we talked, we developed some guidelines for her visits, both in frequency and length, and the activities she would engage in while she was with SP. This gave Mrs. P the rest she needed while also giving her specific objectives for her visits. She began to resist SP's manipulative behavior gently but firmly and became a valuable ally in aiding the nursing staff in dealing with SP's ambivalent behaviors.

Potential Complications Related to Immobilization. The last major problem was prevention of potential complications. This was achieved with great success. SP's skin was beautifully intact when she left for rehabilitation 6 weeks after being admitted to the ICU. She did not develop a urinary tract infection and had only a minor respiratory infection that was responsive to antibiotic therapy. Although I evaluated

SP routinely for signs of complications, outside of my initial conference with the nursing staff in which I identified these potential complications and discussed the nursing interventions necessary to prevent them, I had little involvement with the nursing activity that prevented them.

Clinical Nurse Specialist/Patient Communication

I maintained communication with SP by visiting her at least twice per day (once during the day shift and once on the night shift) 2 days a week. I usually began by assessing her physical progress. Frequently, she would proudly demonstrate her progress. I also evaluated the effectiveness of our plan of care, including SP's psychosocial responses. I visited with SP's mother at least once per week.

Clinical Nurse Specialist/Health Care Team Communication

Communication with those involved in SP's care was vital in assuring continuity of the plan of care, and yet difficult because of the periodic nature of my practice. Communication, therefore, became a priority issue. I made it a point to talk with the primary physician at least once per week. We had not met before because he rarely had patients in the ICU, so I described my position as a critical care clinical nurse specialist consultant and shared my background and experience. He had had little experience caring for patients with GBS and was willing to collaborate in caring for SP.

I met with the team of nurses, head nurse, and supervisor weekly to assess the efficacy of the "team" approach to SP's care. Because of staffing problems, nurses outside the team had been assigned to care for SP on several occasions. When this occurred, SP became anxious and demanding, insisting that her mother stay in her room almost constantly. The relief nurses resented this treatment because they felt that SP was implying that they were not competent; at the same time they admitted that they were not sure how to do some things for SP, such as positioning and communication. This in turn led to resentment toward the team of nurses caring for SP, and the relief nurses concluded that this team of nurses was "spoiling" SP. The relief nurses also felt that SP did not require one-to-one nursing.

These feelings were expressed in a conference that was held to allow the team of nurses and the relief nurses to air their feelings. The critical care supervisor attended the conference to help work out a solution. The group concluded that the team approach to SP's care was working well, but that communication with the rest of the nursing staff had been inadequate. The team agreed that SP no longer required one-to-one care and agreed to take an additional patient. This change was to be communicated to SP via her mother and two of the team nurses, one from the day shift and one from the night shift. Because the acuity of SP's care was decreasing as she improved, other nurses were incorporated into SP's care by having them assist one of the team nurses with SP's care. We also agreed to have a 20-minute conference once per week to discuss SP's care. The objective of this conference was to insure adequate communication between SP's team of nurses and the other staff nurses in ICU in order to diminish discord.

I had two educational conferences for the staff nurses. The respiratory therapists assigned to SP also attended, as did the medical social worker. I also had two articles on GBS that I made available to the nursing staff. I met with the nurses who agreed to be SP's team of nurses, and we discussed logistics and problems. The head nurse and critical care supervisor attended this meeting.

In addition, I had a conference to orient the staff to the team approach to caring for SP. The two primary nurses who would be caring for SP on the day shifts led this conference and addressed questions and concerns regarding this concept. I talked with the nurse on each shift who was caring for SP the days I was at the hospital. We discussed SP's progress and any problems the nurses or SP were having. We reviewed the plan of care and updated it where necessary. I charted my assessments and recommendations, and made suggestions for entries to the nursing care plan to the nurses caring for SP.

I was also a resource to others who participated in SP's care, such as physical therapists and respiratory therapists. They often had questions about GBS and SP's responses to this disorder. While they were familiar with the general features of GBS, they were unfamiliar with autonomic nervous system involvement and responses. They wanted to learn and use the methods we were using to communicate with SP.

Communication with staff was potentially difficult because of my part-time status. Because I had worked with all of the nurses and therapists for one and a half years, I had developed rapport and credibility. My major responsibilities were to the two ICUs and the intermediate care ward, so I was readily available to the staff the days I was there. I had excellent communication and rapport with the critical care supervisor. She was open to ideas and actively supportive. The head nurse was more resistant to new ideas but did not actively block (nor support) my ideas. Because of the nature of this patient, the head nurse was more receptive than usual.

IMPACT OF CLINICAL NURSE SPECIALIST INTERVENTION

We were able to attain all of the goals outlined. Communication became easier as SP regained motor ability. There had been some setbacks in control of pain, primarily complicated by fear and anxiety and the inexperience of some of the nurses in applying noninvasive methods for controlling pain. SP became confident in the ability of the nursing team to care for her, but became fearful again whenever a nurse outside the team was assigned.

Although the team and I did our best to minimize SP's sense of frustration and occasional depression regarding the long-term nature of GBS, we realized that we had limited ability to alleviate these feelings. We could not change the impatience of this 20-year-old woman, which her mother had shared was part of her nature. We actually found that this quality was of benefit in her willingness to work toward recovery, if we could keep it in perspective. This characteristic also allowed us to move SP toward independence as her physical abilities improved.

Method of Evaluation of Effectiveness

By working closely with the nursing staff, I was able to prevent problems and thereby improve patient care (Edlund & Hodges, 1983; Hamric & Spross, 1983; Morath, 1983; Padilla & Padilla, 1979). The team approach worked well in providing effective and continuous nursing care, while preventing complications and minimizing maladaptive behavior. This resulted in a timely move to the rehabilitation unit, where SP could focus on improving her motor ability. Complications such as skin breakdown and infections would have prolonged the stay in the ICU and may have influenced SP's rate of motor return.

SP's 6-week stay in the ICU was not atypical for a patient with GBS (Gracey et al., 1982). She left the ICU off the respirator, with her tracheostomy tube plugged so that she could talk. She was able to eat, so her feeding tube and IVs were removed. She was able to sit in a wheelchair and move herself about in bed, thereby decreasing the potential for skin breakdown. Her urinary catheter was removed and she was able to urinate on her own, thus eliminating another potential source of infection.

SP progressed in her rehabilitation and was able to go home on a visit for the Christmas holidays, nearly 4 months after her admission. She was not able to start back to college in January as she had hoped, but was able to take a couple of classes at the local community college while she continued her rehabilitation. She anticipated going back to her college in the spring quarter.

ROLE OF THE CLINICAL NURSE SPECIALIST IN THE PRACTICE SETTING

I marketed myself as a clinical consultant performing the clinical nurse specialist role in small to medium-sized hospitals. I theorized that many of these hospitals could not afford nor did they need full-time clinical nurse specialists, yet could benefit from what a clinical nurse specialist had to offer. I based this assumption on many years of teaching and talking to staff nurses in community hospitals all over the country.

To my knowledge, the concept of a nurse acting as a clinical consultant had not been done in an acute care setting prior to this. The nursing administrators I first approached were intrigued, yet hesitant. They all asked where I had tried it before, and it became obvious that they did not want to be the first to try an innovative approach. Some expressed concern that a consultant would not have the commitment an employee would have. I pointed out that if I could not demonstrate results, it would be easy to get rid of me by simply not renewing my contract. I also emphasized the need for collaboration in identifying and operationalizing my goals. My written proposal delineated my approach.

Some nursing administrators also expressed concern regarding the difficulty in my gaining the trust and confidence of the nursing staff, since I would only be working 2 days a week and would be viewed as an outsider. I had already recognized this as a major disadvantage to this type of role. The lack of power inherent in staff positions was potentially more profound than usual. Having worked in staff positions most of my career, I had developed some mechanisms for overcoming this lack of line authority. I found that it took about 6 to 8 months to gain the credibility and rapport with the nursing and medical staff that allowed me to influence change.

The other major disadvantage that the nursing administrators and I shared was my inability to follow patients as closely as I would have preferred since I would be there only 2 days a week. It would be necessary to collaborate with the nursing staff as I was working with patients, so that they could provide the follow-up that I would not be able to. I also worked with the nursing staff in devising methods for indirect follow-up.

When I met with the assistant administrator for nursing services in the hospital where I eventually got a contract, my proposal had just been turned down for the fourth time. Although I was discouraged, I was ready to try again as I believed my concept had merit. Because the hospital was 125 miles from my home, I knew nothing about it or the people who worked there. I actually was responding to a 'newspaper advertisement for a critical care clinician.

After my interview with the nursing administrator, I interviewed with the associate director of nursing, the supervisor for critical care, the head nurse, the medical director for the unit, and the associate hospital administrator. Each person had his or her own concerns and needs. After about 6 weeks of interviews and negotiation, I was given a 6-month contract to work sixteen to twenty hours per week.

The salary I negotiated was at a much higher hourly rate than any other nursing employee. Fringe benefits were not included, and I was required to carry malpractice insurance. Travel costs and lodging (since the hospital was 125 miles away, I usually stayed overnight) were also my responsibility. I calculated my hourly salary based on these factors and the base salary for an experienced clinical nurse specialist.

My contract was reviewed every 6 months. At this time the administrator and I discussed my effectiveness in meeting previously agreed-upon clinical and educational goals. Goals that were still relevant or current were continued, and as new needs were identified, new goals were established. On the basis of successful completion of the goals, my contract was renewed for another 6 months. The contract was for clinical work only. Fees for classes (except nursing rounds and patient care conferences) were negotiated separately. The reason for separating the clinical and didactic portion of my role was to avoid the trap of getting involved in giving a lot of classes to the exclusion of clinical work. Typically, they would pay my usual fee for teaching classes and they were responsible for advertising and handouts.

I realized that getting the first 6-month contract was the beginning of some very hard work. At the time, I was on the graduate faculty at a university teaching a critical care clinical nurse specialist program. I had students who were in the second of a 3-semester program. A major advantage of teaching in this program was that it provided me with a peer group of fellow faculty as well as graduate students.

Although none of the students were in clinical nurse specialist positions at the time, all were anticipating these positions within the next year. I shared my experiences with them, including my "successes" and "failures." They were eager to help me problem solve and were able to learn from my experiences. They gained a realistic view of the process of developing the clinical nurse specialist role in a setting where the role had not existed before. This dialogue also helped them to realize that there is no template for implementing the clinical nurse specialist role. I was able to emphasize aspects of the role that were not as amenable to didactic discussion, such as pathophysiology, but were nevertheless critical to the successful implementation of the clinical nurse specialist role.

The issues that I focused on the first few months in my new role included how to gain support for the changes I wanted to make; how to deal with resistance, sabotage, or hostility; the importance of role modeling professionalism and problem solving; the importance of making sure that the necessary people knew what I was doing; getting to know and getting known by people who had an impact on my role, such as physicians, nurses on other units, social workers, respiratory therapists, physical therapists, nursing educators, and secretaries. Initially, I spent much time explaining my role to these people as well as to the nursing staff with whom I was working.

My relationship with the nursing administrator and the associate director for nursing was excellent. We met every other week, sometimes just the administrator and I, often all three of us. After about 6 months, the associate director and I began meeting alone, but I continued to meet with the administrator about once per month.

The associate director and I discussed my goals and plans. She shared unit problems with me and often asked for my input. She sometimes asked me to work with the critical care supervisor on projects or problems involving the critical care units or the step-down unit. We worked well together and we both gained from our relationship.

The medical director for critical care was another key person with whom I developed a relationship. Because my major focus initially was to build relationships with the nursing staff, I had neglected to keep the medical director informed about my activities. The nursing administrator reminded me of the importance of this, and I quickly worked to rectify the situation. I began to meet with him on a fairly regular basis, and he asked for my input into an annual seminar that he planned for the critical care nursing staff.

The supervisor for critical care was very supportive and actively assisted me in any way she could. She was also eager to have me help her problem solve; additionally, she freely discussed and asked for input into problems that affected the unit. These problems were related to specific staff nurses, relationships or problems with physicians, policies, interdepartmental issues, or issues related to nursing administration. Although I realized it was vital to approach the head nurse first with problems or concerns in the ICU, there were times I used the supervisor as a liaison if the head nurse's resistance was great and the issue was important.

I had sensed varying degrees of resistance and mistrust from the head nurse. It was difficult to deal with these feelings because they seemed to wax and wane. Sometimes she seemed very supportive and cooperative, and other times passively or actively resisted my efforts. For example, we spent considerable time discussing how to modify the change of shift report to reflect the nursing process, yet be time efficient. When I returned a week later, she had implemented a new method that met none of the objectives we had agreed were important. At other times she assisted me in attaining my goals with enthusiasm. Our relationship was always tenuous, however.

At the end of six months I was well established as the critical care clinical nurse specialist. The nursing staff seemed comfortable in approaching me to ask questions and to ask for assistance with their patients. Many were eager to learn about advanced education in nursing, as most of them had graduated from the local associate degree nursing program. Many asked for advice on how to deal with various professional issues involving physicians, peers, and nursing administration. I was surprised at the significance of my role as liaison between nursing management and the nursing staff. The nurses were open and eager, and I was impressed with their commitment to nursing and their patients.

RESEARCH IN PRACTICE

I made a point to share relevant nursing and medical articles with the nursing staff, emphasizing research that had significance for critical care nursing. Because of the part-time nature of my position, conducting research did not seem feasible, particularly the first year. Additionally, this community hospital was located in a rural area, and research was viewed by many as an esoteric activity carried out by university-affiliated academicians. I decided it was important to establish myself as a "real world" clinical nurse specialist, while easing into the idea of research.

SUMMARY

I have described my position as a part-time critical care specialist consultant in a medium-sized hospital. I work with the patient, patient's family, and nursing staff to resolve the complexities of clinical care as well as the communication difficulties. This kind of part-time consultative arrangement can be very effective. Success in this role can be enhanced by a variety of methods: working with selected complex patients, consulting with the nursing staff about the remaining patients, providing formal and informal educational programs, serving as a liaison with nursing management about critical care policies and procedures, and collaborating with physicians. As a consultant, success is reinforced by gaining nursing-staff support, dealing with resistance, role modeling professional practice, and communicating with the various health care team members.

SPECIFIC QUESTIONS

1. Both this chapter and chapter 5 discuss resistance from head nurses. Compare and contrast the strategies presented by both authors for dealing with it. What strategies would you use in such a situation?
2. What are the differences and the similarities between the role of the external consultant in a community hospital critical care setting described in this chapter and the role of the psychiatric external consultant in the non-acute setting described in chapter 8?
3. This author does not comment on whether or not she was re-

placed after her resignation. Do you think her evaluation methods were sufficient to support continuing the role? Why or why not?

4. How would you go about learning more about marketing the role of the clinical nurse specialist to small and medium-sized hospitals?

REFERENCES

Anderson, T., & Siden, A. (1982). A clinical study of the Guillain-Barre syndrome. *Acta Neurologica Scandinavica, 66,* 316–327.

Edlund, B., & Hodges, L. (1983). Preparing and using the clinical nurse specialist: A shared responsibility. *Nursing Clinics of North America, 18,* 499–507.

Gracey, D.R., McMichan, J.C., Divertie, M.B., & Howard, F.M. (1982). Respiratory failure in Guillain-Barre syndrome: A six-year experience. *Mayo Clinic Proceedings, 57,* 742–746.

Hamric, A.B., & Spross, J. (1983). *The clinical nurse specialist in theory and practice.* Orlando, FL: Grune & Stratton.

Morath, J. (1983). Putting leaders, consultants and teachers on the line. *Nursing Management, 14,* 50–52.

Padilla, G., & Padilla, G. (1979). Nursing roles to improve patient care. *Nursing Digest, 6,* 1–13.

Prydum, M. (1983). Guillain-Barre syndrome: Disease process. *Journal of Neurosurgical Nursing, 15,* 27–32.

Ropper, A.H., & Shahant, B.T. (1984). Pain in Guillain-Barre syndrome. *Archives of Neurology, 41,* 511–514.

chapter seven

The Pulmonary Rehabilitation Clinical Nurse Specialist in an Outpatient Setting

Janet D'Agostino Taylor

"My primary responsibility is to aid my clients in the reconstruction of their lives by providing highly individualized, personalized nursing care to mesh with their medical regimens" (Fanslow, 1976, p. 143). This quote by Fanslow probably best describes my role as a pulmonary rehabilitation clinical nurse specialist. I was hired 7 years ago to design and implement an outpatient pulmonary rehabilitation program for patients with chronic lung disease. An overview of the patient goals that I formulated for our pulmonary program are:

1. Optimize bronchodilatation
2. Provide patient education
3. Increase exercise tolerance
4. Alter smoking behavior
5. Instruct in diaphragm and respiratory muscle retraining
6. Improve psychological status
7. Provide vocational rehabilitation
8. Promote patient independence and prevent institutionalization by
   a. Improving the patient's ability to perform activities of daily living
   b. Mobilizing home care resources
9. Optimize nutritional status

Case Study

Mrs. B was a 52-year-old female with severe chronic obstructive pulmonary disease (COPD), a combination of both emphysema and chronic bronchitis. The patient was referred to the pulmonary rehabilitation program by her pulmonary physician. The patient stated that she first noticed shortness of breath with activities 2 to 3 years prior to referral to the program. She was diagnosed by her physician as having emphysema at that time. She said that her symptoms had gradually gotten worse over the past couple of years. She had bronchitis as a child but no other illnesses. Her medical history was significant for increasing weight loss over the past three years, the etiology of which was unclear. She also complained of paresthesia of her left leg and both hands. She had a thorough neurological workup one year ago and was found to have spinal stenosis. Her family history was significant, for a brother died at age 40 of lung cancer. Her medications included ventolin pills (bronchodilator), multivitamins, and Fiorinal as needed for headaches. She smoked two packs of cigarettes per day for 35 years, but quit (with the assistance of nicorette gum) one month prior to joining the pulmonary program. She was taking ten pieces of nicorette gum a day at the time. She denied occupational exposure to lung disease or any allergens. She formerly worked as a housecleaner, but was forced into retirement 2 years ago secondary to her lung problem. She was a widow with three grown children. She lived with her daughter, who was very supportive. Her other two children lived out of state. Financially, she was supported by social security disability and Medicaid. It was the assessment of the rehabilitation team members that she did not have vocational rehabilitation potential.

Functionally, she sometimes had dyspnea at rest; she experienced shortness of breath during her activities of daily living, walking one block on level surface, and climbing one flight of stairs. The patient was able to do light housekeeping, such as cooking, with her daughter performing the heavy chores. The patient and I both agreed that she did not need any home care resources such as a home health aide at that time. She had a chronic cough which improved since she quit smoking. She raised a small amount of clear sputum in the morning.

Her nutritional status was poor. She ate only one meal a day and "snacked" the rest of the day. She also had problems sleeping. She stated, "I'm up most of the night . . . I have my days mixed up with my nights." She had orthopnea and slept on three pillows. She denied nocturnal dyspnea.

On initial evaluation the patient was a cachectic looking female with obvious dyspnea on slight exertion. On auscultation her aeration was greatly reduced throughout without any adventitious sounds. Her resting respiratory rate was 22. She had a slight tachycardia, with a heart rate of 102. Her blood pressure was within normal range. Her breathing pattern was mostly upper chest with little movement of the diaphragm. During her initial 12-minute walk test, she walked 800 feet with two rest periods. The patient's blood gases showed hypoxia both at rest and with exercise. She also had slight cyanosis of the lips with walking. Her pulmonary function tests (PFT) showed severe obstruction without improvement after bronchodilators. Her chest x-ray showed no acute problem, but was consistent with COPD. Her weight was 85.5 pounds, and height was 61 inches. She correctly answered 15 out of 20 questions on the patient education test. Overall, the patient was very bright, motivated, and eager to learn, as assessed by the physical therapist and myself.

A summary of the mutual goals set with Mrs. B for the program were:

    1. To improve nutritional status and stabilize her weight
    2. To decrease airflow obstruction and mobilize secretions

3. To increase exercise tolerance, specifically to increase her ability to walk
4. To retrain breathing, altering from upper chest to diaphragmatic breathing
5. To educate Mrs. B. regarding her disease and treatment
6. To teach energy conservation techniques to increase her ability to perform activities of daily living
7. To support smoking cessation and weaning off nicorette

The patient was prescribed an exercise program, which she was to follow at home. This exercise program consisted of mobilization exercises to improve upper trunk mobility, warm-up exercises, walking program, and cool-down exercises. The patient was walking up to 15 minutes a day at home at the end of the program. She was taught self-monitoring of her heart rate and respiratory rate and guidelines to follow regarding her vital signs during exercise. The patient was taught stair climbing techniques and the importance of coordinating her breathing with stair climbing. Her home exercise diary was accurately completed and reflected that she understood her exercise guidelines.

The patient on occasion was acutely short of breath upon arrival at the clinic and was given a bronchodilator (Alupent) via a hand-held nebulizer. It was noted that the patient appeared much less dyspneic and subjectively improved after bronchodilator therapy, although there were no changes in her pulmonary function tests. The patient had been given a bronchodilator spray in the past, but was unable to activate the canister because of numbness in her hands. She also had difficulty coordinating her respiratory cycle with the activation of the canister. I consulted the pulmonary physician regarding another trial of bronchodilator spray and suggested that the patient use an inspirease device with the bronchodilator. The inspirease device eliminates the need for the patient to coordinate breathing with the activation of the canister. The patient initially had difficulty activating the canister with inspirease because of the numbness of her hands, but after some experimentation we found a position that allowed her to activate it. She was instructed to take Proventil spray with inspirease, two puffs four times a day. The patient reported less shortness of breath when taking a maintenance dose of Proventil.

Mrs. B was taught diaphragmatic breathing, and by the end of the program she was able to practice it with a 6-pound weight as resistance. Her breathing pattern at the end of the program was mostly diaphragmatic with slight upper chest movement. She was also placed on an inspiratory muscle training program to increase the endurance of her respiratory muscles.

Mrs. B was taught energy conservation and work simplification techniques. She was given some adaptive devices to use, such as long-handled reachers, since she experienced shortness of breath while reaching for objects. Mrs. B was able to incorporate these concepts into her daily activities and reported increased ability to perform activities of daily living by the end of the program.

Mrs. B attended the patient education program described in a later section and easily learned and retained concepts taught. I gave her a patient education booklet containing all concepts taught in the program, and she was able to answer correctly all twenty questions of the patient education test at the end of the program.

Although family members are encouraged to attend the program, Mrs. B's daughter worked and was unable to attend the program with her mother. The patient's daughter came into the program once to be informed about her mother's home program and to ask questions regarding her mother's condition. The patient's daughter was taught how to perform chest percussion on her mother at home. They were told to use this treatment during times of increased congestion or if she experienced a respiratory infection.

Mrs. B was prescribed continuous home oxygen because of her hypoxia and cyanosis with exertion. The patient was very receptive to having oxygen and wore it all the time, including when she went out of the house shopping. I felt that liquid oxygen would be the best system for this patient, since she wanted to be able to go out as much as possible. (With liquid oxygen, patients can fill their own portable tanks whenever they need to go out).

Mrs. B on initial assessment told me that she had difficulty relaxing and described herself as a "nervous" person. She was taught relaxation techniques and responded well to the relaxation tape. She was given a copy of a relaxation tape to use at home.

Mrs. B met with the nutritionist for intervention regarding weight loss. She was started on ensure feedings, one can three times a day. She was also given suggestions for food with high caloric and nutritional value. Her weight stabilized during the time she was in the program. She was told to continue weighing herself at home and to keep a diary.

The patient did not restart smoking and she was totally weaned off the nicorette gum.

The patient's sleeping pattern improved by coming to the program. She was unable to sleep during the day. She also used her relaxation tape to help her to get to sleep. To help improve her sleeping habits, she was told to try eliminating caffeine also, since she drank four cups of coffee plus several colas every day.

The patient was evaluated at the end of the program to determine if she met the outcome criteria established in the program. It was agreed by both the staff and the patient herself that she met all of the outcome criteria.

Mrs. B was asked to evaluate the results of the program. Overall, she felt that the program helped her, specifically to better understand her illness and treatment, increase her physical activity, be better able to do daily living chores, and better understand how to control her breathing when she was short of breath.

The patient met all of the goals set with her in the program. A summary of her goal attainment is as follows:

1. Increased exercise tolerance. Patient improved on her 12-minute walk test from 800 feet preprogram to 1000 feet post-program. The patient was walking up to 15 minutes a day at home
2. Improved breathing pattern from upper chest to diaphragmatic. Her abdominal excursion increased one inch on inspiration

3. Increased ability to perform activities of daily living as reported by the patient
4. Stabilized the patient's weight
5. Successful smoking cessation, and totally weaned off nicorette
6. Decrease in hypoxia using home oxygen
7. Decreased airflow obstruction using bronchodilators on a maintenance level
8. The patient's ability to learn and retain information was excellent. She was able to correctly answer all twenty questions in the patient education test postprogram

The patient was encouraged to continue all aspects of her home program after discharge from the rehabilitation program. At her one-month follow-up appointment, the patient was faithfully following all aspects of her home program and increased her walking up to 25 minutes a day. Her weight had stabilized at 85 pounds one month after the program.

CLINICAL NURSE SPECIALIST INTERVENTION

Method of Patient Selection

I have developed patient criteria for entry into the pulmonary rehabilitation program. The majority of my time and interventions are focused on the patients who meet these criteria and enter the program. It is my responsibility to screen and accept patients into the program. Patients are referred from a variety of sources including physicians, discharge planning nurses, visiting nurses, and staff nurses. The criteria for admission are:

1. *Diagnosis of chronic pulmonary disease; any stage is acceptable.* Individual goals are modified according to the severity of the patient's illness. The program is primarily focused on the patient with chronic obstructive pulmonary disease. Patients with other types of pulmonary diseases, however, such as pulmonary fibrosis, may also be candidates.
2. *Adults.* On rare occasions I am asked to help intervene with a child or teenager. In this case I would attempt to intervene on an individual basis with the patient, or refer the patient to the appropriate pediatric specialist.
3. *Absence of other acute medical problems,* such as recent myocardial infarction. Such diagnoses might interfere with the exercise program. Most of our patients, since they tend to be elderly, do have a combination of chronic diseases such as hypertension, old myocardial infarction, and cor pulmonale.
4. *Absence of any acute psychiatric problem, which could interfere with functioning in the program.* We have had several patients referred whose anxiety level was so high that it blocked their learning process. The behavior of these patients may also be disruptive to

the rest of the patients in the program. Such patients are not candidates for the program and are referred for psychological intervention. If their anxiety becomes better controlled, they would then be candidates for the program.

Criteria for Appropriateness of Method or Type of Intervention

My role as a pulmonary clinical nurse specialist includes job responsibilities in the following areas:

1. Outpatient pulmonary rehabilitation program
2. Outpatient services for other pulmonary patients not enrolled in the rehabilitation program
3. Inpatient consultation service
4. Respiratory home care program
5. Nursing education
6. Community nursing resource

A summary of my role in each of these areas follows.

Outpatient Pulmonary Rehabilitation Program. My primary job responsibility is to oversee the pulmonary rehabilitation program. I am responsible for coordinating the activities of the pulmonary rehabilitation team and patients. I am also responsible for screening and accepting patients into the program.

The major time commitment of my role in pulmonary rehabilitation involves providing patient education. I instruct patients on a variety of topics, such as medications, how to recover when they are short of breath, and how to eliminate irritants from the environment. The components of the patient education program are as follows:

1. Brief anatomy and physiology of the lungs
2. Overview of COPD
3. Medication
4. Energy conservation techniques
5. Breathing exercises
6. Dyspnea recovery techniques
7. Preventive care, such as signs of respiratory infection
8. Identification and elimination of potential irritants and allergens in the home and environment
9. Nutrition
10. Sexual activity and COPD
11. Traveling with COPD
12. Reduction of sleeping problems
13. Relaxation therapy

There is some overlap among team members providing patient education. For example, energy conservation techniques are taught and reinforced to patients by occupational therapists, physical therapists, and myself. There is also shared teaching of relaxation therapy; physical therapy instructs patients in relaxation exercises, whereas I use relaxation tapes with patients. The goal of providing uniform teaching and reinforcement of concepts by several team members is to increase patients' retention and incorporation of concepts into their lifestyle.

There are other job responsibilities that I have in the pulmonary rehabilitation program, including assessing the patient's need for home care services, such as the Visiting Nurses' Association (VNA) or having respiratory equipment, and corresponding with the various agencies concerning patient care needs.

The amount of time that I intervene with a patient depends on individual program needs. I see patients on a one-to-one basis, usually for one hour each unit. The rehabilitation team feels that the ideal time frame for patients to come is three times a week for a 5-week period. I do, however, individualize this time frame depending on the patient's needs. For example, if a patient is an appropriate candidate but is still working and unable to come three times a week, I would allow him to come once or twice a week for longer than a 5-week period. Of course, I also need to assess how quickly patients are able to assimilate and incorporate the components of the educational program. If a patient has been slower to incorporate concepts but is progressing toward individualized goals, it would be recommended that the patient come three times a week for longer than 5 weeks. Again, to summarize, the amount of my intervention is based on the patient's individual needs and progress in meeting his rehabilitation goals.

Outpatient Services for Patients Not Enrolled in Pulmonary Rehabilitation. This job responsibility is in providing nursing assessment and interventions to outpatients outside of the pulmonary rehabilitation program who are followed by the medical director of the pulmonary department in his practice. I would first perform a nursing assessment on these outpatients on a one-to-one basis, then my assessment and any suggestions are discussed with the medical director. The patient is then seen by both the medical director and myself. Whatever nursing interventions are needed are then provided. Patient education and assessment for the need for home care resources are my two main responsibilities in this setting.

The majority of my patients utilize me as a resource person in the home setting. Outpatients frequently call me if problems develop at home regarding their illness, home program, or in other areas. These phone calls need to be screened to determine which ones are appropriate for my intervention and which ones need to be referred to a pulmonary physician or other health care professional. This part of my role is reflected by Littell (1981), who stated, "Patients and families understood that I was available for reinforcement, questions, and support. This was one of my cherished roles" (p. 78).

Inpatient Consultation Service. Inpatient consultations are mostly related to three areas:

1. Assessment of the patient for eligibility for the pulmonary rehabilitation program
2. Smoking cessation
3. Problems related to home respiratory care

Respiratory Home Care Program. A new dimension recently added to my job description is respiratory home care. A continuing care agreement was signed between our hospital and a medical equipment supply company. The agreement is specific for respiratory home equipment. The company supplies the home equipment, and our respiratory department supplies the personnel to educate and follow up patients requiring home respiratory equipment. My role has recently been expanded to include coordination of this home care project. A respiratory therapist was hired to be responsible for most of the day-to-day operations of the program. My responsibilities are mostly administrative, but will also include making some home visits. This latest home care development gives us the opportunity to provide continuation of care in the patient's home. Our primary purpose in making a home visit is to determine whether the respiratory equipment is functioning properly and whether the patient is using it correctly. The home visit, however, provides the opportunity to clinically assess the patient and obtain intervention for detected problems. The home environment can also be assessed for pulmonary irritants and allergens that may adversely affect the patient's respiratory status. In addition it also provides an opportunity to increase patient education by answering questions the patient may have. For patients who have attended our pulmonary rehabilitation program, the home visit can help us to motivate the patient and reinforce the importance of following the prescribed home program. The home environment can be viewed as a critical area that needs to be included in the pulmonary rehabilitation of a patient.

Nursing Education. My role also encompasses several other educational activities, such as serving as a clinical preceptor for graduate and undergraduate students, providing nursing inservice lectures, and lecturing at schools of nursing.

Community Nursing Resource. Since our hospital has a community orientation, various community groups utilize me as a resource person.

"The Clinical Specialist also serves as a consultant in the community, when she has great responsibility to share her knowledge. She should be available for workshops, continuing education programs, district meetings, and lay organizations. She could also help organize such groups as emphysema clubs and be a resource for them" (McGann, 1975, p. 35). As part of my role, I have participated in a variety of community activities, such as co-sponsoring Better Breathing Clubs with the American Lung Association and participating in community health screening programs.

Support groups for individuals with chronic lung disease and their family members are sponsored by a social worker and myself on a monthly basis. These groups are open for all our patients, as well as anyone in the community interested in attending. A speaker or film on a topic related to lung disease is offered during the first part of the meeting, followed by time for patients to share ideas. We have had a favorable response from patients and families regarding this group.

Clinical Nurse Specialist and Patient Communication

As a pulmonary clinical nurse specialist, I am a primary provider of patient care. The majority of my time at work involves providing patient care, during which I communicate directly with the patient. Examples of my patient involvement include working with the patient to assess both functional and symptom management needs, mutually establishing goals, working with the patient to satisfactorily manipulate drug delivery mechanisms, directly teaching the patient and family, writing and distributing patient education materials, directing group education programs, and evaluating outcomes with the patient and family.

Clinical Nurse Specialist and Health Care
Team Communication

There are several members of the pulmonary rehabilitation team, including pulmonary physicians, physical therapists, occupational therapists, social workers, and nutritionists. Therefore, ongoing communication among the team members is essential. Since it was my job responsibility to develop the pulmonary rehabilitation program, I assumed the job of program coordinator once the program was established. As the program coordinator, it is my job to be sure that effective channels of communication remain open among rehabilitation team members.

I perform an initial nursing assessment on all patients admitted to the program. I then meet with other team members to discuss their assessments and goals. Mutual goals are set with the patient and an initial assessment note with goals and plans is written for each patient.

The role of the pulmonary physician is to assess patients during their initial evaluation, participate in the exercise testing and prescription, as well as in the patient's final evaluation. Otherwise, I usually function independently in the day-to-day operation of the program. I will request intervention from the pulmonary physician if a medical problem develops during the course of the program.

IMPACT OF CLINICAL NURSE SPECIALIST INTERVENTION

Method of Evaluation of Patient Outcomes

Although the role of different clinical nurse specialists may be similar, aspects of their jobs may vary. Clinical nurse specialists tend to impact on the health care system on several different levels. It is important to determine which level or levels of the health care system we impact on the most, since this is the focus for evaluating our effectiveness. Evaluation of my job effectiveness is related to the evaluation of the impact of the pulmonary rehabilitation program on patient care. In other words, program evaluation is closely linked to my job evaluation. Evaluation of the impact of the pulmonary rehabilitation program is made on each patient, so that any gains made or goals met can be documented. Each patient undergoes an extensive assessment both initially upon entering and later on completion of the program by a pulmonary physician, nurse coordinator, and physical therapist.

Pre-program and postprogram information is summarized on an outpatient evaluation form, which helps to document areas of improvement. We attempt to gather as much objective data as possible. For example, we have patients perform what is called a 12-minute walk test prior to entering the program. This is the distance the patient can walk in a 12-minute period. We repeat the test at the end of the program to see if the prescribed exercise program leads to an improvement. The data give us objective measurements of exercise tolerance. Objective data such as pulmonary function tests and arterial blood gases do not always tell us what a patient can do functionally. Preprogram patients are asked to fill out a functional assessment form that includes all activities of daily living. They are asked to fill out the same form postprogram to determine the patient's perception of functional improvement, if any.

Patient education is an important component of our pulmonary rehabilitation program. Patients are given an education test preprogram and postprogram. The questions focus on key principles that patients were taught during the program. This test helps to get some objective information regarding effectiveness of the patient education program.

Patient self-reporting diaries are also used to determine if patients are applying concepts learned in the teaching program (see Table 7–1). Patients are asked to fill out the diary on a daily basis. Much time is spent helping to teach the patient to identify and realize his exercise limits. Patients are taught to stop exercising if their heart rate reaches

TABLE 7–1. PATIENT DIARY

Date	Prewarmup Exercises	Postwarmup Exercises	Type of Exercises	After 5 min. Exercises	Symptoms/ Comments
	HR/RR	HR/RR	Bike/Walk	HR/RR	

peak or if certain symptoms such as chest pain occur. A diary helps us to determine if the patient understands his exercise guidelines. For example, if a patient continues exercising after he reaches his peak heart rate, then he needs more reinforcement in this area. Patients can also keep a diary about symptoms, treatment given, and medications taken to see if there is any change in the number and type of interventions utilized by a patient during and after the pulmonary rehabilitation program. This can be useful, for example, if one is trying to modify a patient's behavior such as using dyspnea control techniques rather than bronchodilator sprays to recover from shortness of breath.

Outcome criteria have also been developed for the pulmonary rehabilitation program. Both the clinical nurse specialist and the patient can evaluate whether or not the outcome criteria have been met. When many concepts have to be taught, a patient teaching record helps with organization and to ensure that all concepts are taught and documented. Our program uses program goals and outcome criteria based on a teaching plan by McCormick and Parkevich (1979).

Gallant and McLane (1979) developed an instrument for patients to rate whether or not they felt outcome criteria were met. This is particularly important since patients need to be viewed as consumers and hopefully will play an active role in their health care. Our perception of what a patient has learned may be different from his/her perception.

One can compare how the patient versus the clinical nurse specialist rate achievement of outcome criteria in terms of their agreement. The percent of patient and nurse agreement as to whether an outcome had been achieved could be viewed as a measure of the reliability of nurse judgment of patient outcome achievements.

At the end of the program, patients are given a questionnaire to evaluate the effectiveness of the pulmonary rehabilitation program. This questionnaire contains some open-ended questions that patients can answer, allowing them to give their suggestions or comments regarding the program.

Method of Evaluation of Cost Effectiveness

I do not have any data regarding my cost effectiveness, although this is an area that needs to be addressed by myself as well as by other clinical specialists. The pulmonary medicine department by whom I am employed also includes respiratory therapy. As a result, I can charge patients for some of my interventions, such as teaching patients breathing exercises and how to perform postural drainage at home. The respiratory home care program that I am involved in also generates some revenue for my department. However, I do not have any mechanism for charging for many other interventions, such as patient education and smoking cessation assistance.

Cost effectiveness of my role could hopefully be measured as a result of the impact made by the pulmonary rehabilitation program in providing care to patients with chronic lung disease. Patients with chronic lung disease often require frequent, prolonged hospitalizations. Interventions with both my pulmonary rehabilitation and other outpatients focus on increasing patients' understanding and compliance with their prescribed therapeutic regimens.

Preventive care is also emphasized with patients, such as early recognition and reporting of signs of respiratory infection by patients to their physicians. Patients are also taught how to recover from episodes of shortness of breath and to better "control" their respiratory symptoms themselves. As a result of the above interventions, one hopes that patients will have decreased hospital admissions and hospitalization days and increased compliance with prescribed therapeutic regimens. A decrease in lengthy hospitalizations in this patient population would be cost effective for the hospitals, especially with new cost-containment regulations.

The effectiveness of pulmonary rehabilitation programs has been studied previously. A review of the literature reveals that the following effects of pulmonary rehabilitation programs on patients have been reported: improved exercise tolerance, improved psychological status, improved ability for self-care, increase in gainful employment, fewer nursing home placements, decrease in patients' subjective symptoms, and decrease in hospitalization days.

ROLE OF THE CLINICAL NURSE SPECIALIST IN THE PRACTICE SETTING

There are a few factors that make my job different from other clinical nurse specialists. My job responsibilities focus primarily on an outpatient service, so that my role is isolated from most inpatient activities. This also minimizes my contact with staff nurses in the inpatient setting. Because of the nature of my job, if the impact of my practice on the nursing care on inpatient floors were measured, there would be little or no effect found. It was difficult for me to come to terms with the fact that, in my role, I do not have a great deal of interaction with staff nurses, since involvement with staff nurses was always what I viewed in graduate school as being a major component of the clinical nurse specialist role. However, one has to be realistic in terms of what one can accomplish. One needs to overcome the tendency to take on too many responsibilities and spread oneself so thin that effectiveness cannot be measured on any level. "The responsibilities of the clinical nurse specialist should be limited to a reasonably small area. It permits her to become a permanent and trusted member of the health care team" (Woodrow & Bell, 1971, p. 27).

My job is under the Department of Pulmonary Medicine rather than the Department of Nursing, and in some respects this tends to isolate me from the activities of the Department of Nursing. One may hear comments made by individuals in the nursing field that clinical nurse specialists working under medicine rather than nursing are "traitors," "handmaidens," or "looking for a 9 to 5 job." Clinical nurse specialists need to be open-minded about job opportunities in various settings, including those outside the traditional inpatient hospital setting. Actually, there is an interesting story behind how pulmonary medicine rather than nursing hired me. The personnel recruiter evidently did not know what a clinical nurse specialist was. The recruiter sent me on an interview for a pulmonary function technician's job in the respiratory department. However, during this "wrong interview" it was mentioned that the medical director of the department was interested in starting a pulmonary rehabilitation program, which was my area of interest. Subsequently, the medical director hired me to start the program. The medical director has given my role a lot of support and encouragement throughout the seven years of my employment in his department. One should keep in mind that some physicians hire clinical nurse specialists because they *do* value their knowledge and clinical expertise. One should try, however, to assess the motives or expectations of any potential employer hiring a clinical nurse specialist, whether it be nursing or medicine, before accepting a position. One should try to determine if the employer's expectations synchronize with yours.

One disadvantage of working in a department outside of nursing is that other staff in the hospital are not clear about your identity. Even though you identify yourself as a nurse, you are still probably viewed by nurses as somewhat of an outsider because you are not under the department of nursing. Even clinical nurse specialists employed by the department of nursing may experience some of these feelings. Woodrow and Bell (1971) asked the question, "Is the clinical specialist perceived as a nursing role model? It seemed to us that we were perceived as an oddity between nursing and other health related professions" (p. 26). Working outside the nursing department probably just accentuates the problem.

"There is often a tendency for the clinical specialist to feel isolated. In a small institution where there may be only one clinical specialist, the opportunities to attend professional meetings and workshops where she can discuss ideas with others in a similar position can be invaluable" (Castronovo, 1975, p. 51). There are several other clinical nurse specialists employed at the hospital where I work. However, my role is isolated from them, with little interaction, since my practice focuses on the outpatient setting. We have formed a clinical nurse specialist support group which meets on a regular basis. In addition to providing support for each other and a chance to share our feelings and concerns, we also work on projects related to the clinical nurse specialist area. This has really helped decrease my feelings of isolation and has broadened my support base. These meetings have also helped me to utilize the other clinical nurse specialists as resource persons more often.

Another source of support has been professional organizations such as the Massachusetts Thoracic Society Nursing Subsection, which offers an opportunity to interact with other nurses and clinical nurse specialists in my speciality area.

RESEARCH IN PRACTICE

I have not been involved in performing nursing research in my present role. I have dedicated more time and effort to writing for publication and lecturing professionally, and unfortunately have neglected nursing research. The main reasons I have not performed nursing research is lack of time, along with a conscious decision to give the other professional activities described above higher priority than nursing research. The main topic that I have interest in researching is patient compliance with a pulmonary rehabilitation program over various lengths of time. This study would supply more specific information as to which components of the home program patients are complying with and would help identify the problem areas.

I do feel that nursing research should, ideally, be an important component in the role of the clinical nurse specialist. However, the nursing research in my present role has been limited to incorporating current nursing research findings into my practice and helping graduate students that I precept with their research projects.

SUMMARY

Overall, I feel that my role as a pulmonary clinical nurse specialist in a nontraditional position the past seven years has been a very fulfilling and rewarding experience. My primary source of positive reinforcement and gratification on the job has been from patients (and their families) who verbalize that I have made a positive impact on their health care and status. Preparation at the master's degree level adequately provided me with the knowledge base needed to design the pulmonary rehabilitation program, function independently in providing in-depth patient assessment and nursing interventions, and then evaluate patient outcomes and the impact of the program on patient care. I feel that an area that I, as well as other clinical nurse specialists, need to address is the cost effectiveness of our role. The issue of cost effectiveness of the clinical nurse specialist has become increasingly important with the cost-containment restrictions affecting health care institutions. Because of these cost-containment restrictions imposed on hospitals and other health care institutions, I feel that there may be some shift in the clinical nurse specialist role to outside the traditional hospital setting. One can hope, however, there will be new job opportunities for expanded roles as clinical nurse specialists in the outpatient and community settings.

SPECIFIC QUESTIONS

1. This author maximized an unexpected opportunity and created a nontraditional role in the outpatient setting. Discuss how she maintained a clear nursing focus and identity and differentiated her role from the other health care providers.
2. How could this program design for patients with chronic lung disease be adapted to your specialty area? Identify the most important components.
3. Discuss the benefits of mutual goal-setting with clients.
4. Compare and contrast the criteria for patient selection in this chapter with chapter 13. What criteria would you use in your specialty area?
5. This author has not been involved in nursing research in her present role. Based on her description, identify possible research questions and suggest possible research designs for these questions. What support would she need to conduct research?

REFERENCES

Castronovo, F. (1975). The effective use of the clinical specialist. *Supervisor Nurse, 6* (5), 48–56.

Fanslow, C. (1976). Rehabilitation nursing. In R. Rockovitch (Ed.), *Quality patient care and the role of the clinical nursing specialist.* New York: John Wiley & Sons.

Gallant, B., & McLane, A. (1979). Outcome criteria: A process for validation at the unit level. *Journal of Nursing Administration, 9* (1) 14–21.

Littell, S. (1981). The clinical nurse specialist in a private medical practice. *Nursing Administration Quarterly, 6* (1) 77–85.

McCormick, R., & Parkevich, T. (1979). *Patient and family education: Tools, techniques and theory.* New York: John Wiley & Sons.

McGann, M. (1975). The clinical specialist: From hospital, to clinic, to community. *Journal of Nursing Administration, 5* (3) 33–37.
Woodrow, M., & Bell, J. (1971). Clinical specialization: Conflict between reality and theory. *Journal of Nursing Administration, 1* (6) 23–28.

chapter eight

The Psychiatric Clinical Nurse Specialist in the Non-acute Setting

Carrol A. Alvarez

The method of consultation used in the non-acute setting depends on the phase of the consultative relationship that has been developed between the clinical nurse specialist and the staff; the presenting problem also affects the method used, though to a lesser extent. The following case occurred in a setting in which my consultative relationship with the staff had existed for several years and was in an active working phase. Because the staff had received a great deal of previous training and consultation, and due to the complexity of the presenting problems, five consultation models were used.

Case Study

RM was a 31 year old man who, in July of the year prior to the referral, had been involved in a collision between his motorcycle and a pickup truck. The accident had occurred when the drunk driver of the truck made a left turn, without signaling, in front of RM's oncoming motorcycle. RM had received multiple fractures, a ruptured spleen, and multiple brain contusions with intracerebral bleeding; he was comatose for the first several weeks of his hospitalization. Also injured in the accident was RM's fiancée, who was comatose for 3 weeks and then died. Both were hospitalized in a university-affiliated county hospital, where RM remained for 8 months.

Following his hospitalization, RM was discharged to a long-term care facility that had a strong rehabilitation emphasis. This facility had 139 beds, all of which were filled by geriatric patients. The facility utilized consultants for speech therapy, physical therapy, mental health, nutrition, pharmacy, podiatry, social services, and occupational therapy. At the time of his admission, RM was wheelchair bound with poor muscle strength, poor motor control, and poor range of motion in his lower extremities; he had only 30° flexion in his right knee. RM also showed marked memory deficit: recent, remote, and short-term. A striking component of the memory loss was that RM had no memory of his fiancée nor of the 5 years that he had known her. Memories which this patient ascribed to the period just before his accident were, in fact, 5 years old.

Nineteen days after his admission to the facility, RM was referred to me, the psychiatric clinical nurse specialist. Staff had two primary concerns: episodes of anger, acted out verbally and physically by RM, which were frightening to staff members, and RM's loss of memory for and apparent lack of knowledge of his fiancée's death. Every staff member without exception was afraid that RM would at some point regain his memory of his fiancée and would ask one of them what had happened to her. Staff were unsure of the appropriate response in either problem situation, and several staff members were so uncomfortable that they avoided entering RM's room as much as possible.

The consultation focused on each of the presenting problems. My intervention with respect to RM's angry episodes focused on facilitating skills that, as a result of earlier consultation, were already within the staff's repertoire. This issue was resolved relatively quickly.

The issue of the memory loss was more complex, and intervention into this included direct service provided to RM by me. The memory loss did, to a large extent, become resolved. There was some evidence that a large portion of the memory loss was in fact functional, in that it helped RM to avoid the painful knowledge of his fiancée's death. In addition, once repression of these memories ended, RM made rapid progress in his physical rehabilitation; he moved quickly from wheelchair to walker to walkane, and discharge planning was begun 4 weeks after his memory had returned. Energy that had been required to repress painful memories, once released, seemed to work to RM's benefit in his physical progress.

My intervention then became necessary around a third issue, termination, which staff had not hitherto experienced so clearly. This intervention provided staff with knowledge and skill that enabled them to work through the termination with RM on their own. RM was discharged to a vocational setting, requiring no further nursing care, 14 months after his admission to the long-term care facility and 22 months after his accident.

CLINICAL NURSE SPECIALIST INTERVENTION

The form of the consultation I provided included five models, labeled according to Gallessich (1983). An inservice was held for all staff two days after my first interview with RM (education model). In conjunction with pertinent licensed staff and the social services person I developed a behavioral approach to the single most consistent precipitant to RM's angry outbursts (behavioral model). Concurrently, RM was involved in an anger management program that had been previously established in the facility by me in collaboration with the social services person in response to earlier referrals of patients with anger problems (program model). I worked in individual sessions with the patient to explore the function of and fears promoting the continued memory loss for the previous five years; the social services person and staff were kept informed of what occurred during these sessions and of the theoretical basis for interventions that were made (clinical model). Finally, at a certain point the social services person, who was also a skilled and intuitive licensed practical nurse (LPN), took over the individual sessions with the patient under my supervision (mental health model).

Before implementation of these approaches, however, an evaluation was done. Because of staff anxiety, I treated the situation as a crisis and saw RM the day after he was referred. RM was alert, cooperative, and generally pleasant; at times he was bewildered and at other times angry. The memory deficits, recent, remote, and short-term, were severe. For example, RM did not know the date, his birthdate, his age, the name of the president, the name of his hometown, nor that he had slept at that facility the previous night; he did not recall, after 5 minutes, my name or the names of three objects that he had been asked to remember. RM continued to have no memory of his fiancée nor of the previous five years. This patient did remember that someone had told him that he had been hit by a pickup truck while on his motorcycle; this was one focus of his anger (the other primary focus had to do with the rationing of his cigarettes by staff). No signs of depression were present, nor were signs of a psychotic thought process.

RM's family provided further history of his pre-accident functioning. The resulting picture was of a high-school graduate who had always been a loner, quick tempered and negative in outlook, rarely trusting of others. RM had known his fiancée for 5 years; they had planned to marry the summer of the accident. In addition, RM's mother mentioned that he had, on one occasion in the hospital, asked about his fiancée. RM's mother had been afraid to tell him of his fiancée's death and had changed the subject. This was the last time that the subject had come up between them.

Using this information, consultation around this patient focused on the two presenting problems, that of anger and of the memory loss for the previous 5 years. In fact, these two problems were seen as partially related. Based on his mother's report, I assumed that, at an unconscious level, RM was aware that his fiancée had been with him in the accident. The angry outbursts were seen as immediate and concrete forms of acting out the rage related to the fiancée's probable death. This formulation was based in part on the differences in the angry behavior exhibited by RM while in the hospital and that while in the long-term care facility. Although RM had been extremely angry in the hospital upon recovery from his coma, this had been a generalized rage consistent with the rage seen after major head injuries (Brigman, Dickey, & Zegeer, 1983; Coutant, 1982). Unlike the anger manifested in the hospital, the anger in the long-term care facility was always focused on a concrete event or object and had a specific precipitant; with one exception the precipitant was not predictable, and being angry was RM's most frequent emotional state. The hypothesized dynamic was not formally articulated to the staff. Rather, the focus of the consultation was to enable staff members to manage the resultant behaviors that they had identified.

In addition to the above formulation, the anger was seen as a response to the fact of the accident itself, with its resultant disruption of RM's life. In the consultation, responses were developed to the forms that the anger was taking within the facility; these were developed with and for the general staff. In the same way, a comfortable response was developed for staff to use should RM ever question one of them regarding the fate of his fiancée. The social services person and I then worked with RM on the issue of his memory loss.

The history and dynamic formulations were the basis for all my subsequent interventions. To provide immediate and practical assistance for staff members, an inservice was held which allowed them to discuss their fears and conflicting emotional responses to RM. Concrete responses were developed for those incidents which were most anxiety-provoking. For example, all staff members were afraid that RM would ask one of them what had happened to his fiancée. After discussion of whether it was possible to say "the wrong thing," it was decided that, should the event occur, the staff person could provide RM the opportunity to express his own fears; all were certain that they could be empathetic and honest with any response he might give.

I also shared with staff the history of RM as a private person and elicited empathy for his discomfort in the large facility where privacy was lacking; staff then developed specific times and places to provide him with time alone (a patio, the physical therapy room when it was not in use). This single inservice program, as well as continued availability of the social services person to staff members, kept their anxiety down and their interest up for the duration of the patient's stay in the facility.

In addition, a review was done of appropriate limit setting. Staff members were encouraged to remind RM that they had not yelled at him and that it was unfair for him to yell at them. The approach included leaving the room as soon as was possible, with a reminder to RM that yelling at people would not be tolerated.

Both staff and RM identified the rationing of his cigarettes as a frequent, specific precipitant to angry outbursts. Staff reported that, without rationing, RM would smoke two or more packs of cigarettes each day. This problem was complicated by the fact that RM did not remember when he had smoked his last cigarette, even if that had been within the previous 5 minutes. A behavioral approach was used. RM was consulted, and he agreed that twenty cigarettes each day was a reasonable limit. At the beginning of each day, RM was given twenty bills of play money, each representing one dollar. Throughout the day, RM traded one bill for one cigarette. Initially, when he asked for a cigarette, RM required a gentle reminder that he needed to trade a bill. Within 7 days, however, RM remembered this trade-off on his own, and counting the number of bills he had left would space his requests throughout the day. This plan effectively ended angry outbursts about the cigarette rationing.

Concurrently, to begin to deal with one of the two underlying issues and thereby to avoid simply a shift in the surface precipitant of the anger, I recommended that RM enter the anger management program at the facility. Three months earlier, I had identified the need for an anger management program in the facility in response to the needs of two angry residents, and I worked with the social services person to set it up. There are a multitude of emotions that are defended against with anger when a patient is admitted to a non-acute setting: hopelessness, loss of control, loss of identity, humiliation, and fear. Anger generated by these feelings is expressed variously, not always in a manner that would generate a referral for psychiatric consultation. The discomfort and defensiveness which is engendered by this emotion, however, can permanently alter the manner in which care is delivered to the patient; this affects both the efficiency of the nursing staff and the quality of patient care. I adapted the cognitive approach to anger management used for people with chronic anger (Novaco, 1976), to the long-term care setting and patients with moderate memory loss. This adaptation was in keeping with the role of the clinical nurse specialist in the use and development of theory.

In the program, using principles of anger management, RM was provided a safe time, place, and method of venting his anger (pounding on modeling clay in the small activities room when it was not in use). At the same time, some of the likely feelings underlying the anger were verbally identified and validated by the social services person. This intervention was based on the principle that anger is a secondary emotion which masks underlying, primary emotions (Beck, 1976; Moritz, 1978). Finally, non-angry responses to those primary emotions were provided verbally to RM as alternatives to his own anger-generating reflections (Novaco, 1976).

Eventually in these sessions RM was able to identify for himself, and to discuss specifically, his feelings of grief and pain at the many ways his life had been interrupted and disrupted by the accident. I did clarify that the focus of the feeling identification and validation should be the accident itself, with its immediate consequences, rather than the death of RM's fiancée.

The death of the fiancée was a more difficult issue. My decision to provide direct service to RM was based on my judgment that the repression of all memory related to the fiancée and the previous five years indicated in RM a powerful degree of anxiety and fear which required skilled intervention. In addition, at the time that this intervention occurred, RM was new to the facility; a safe and trusting relationship with staff members had not yet occurred. Later, when RM had developed strong relationships with the social services person and with other staff members, skilled interventions were made by them; I then acted as a resource.

I met weekly with RM for 1 hour. The focus of the intervention was safety. That is, within the therapeutic relationship, RM was allowed to discuss the accident and his reactions to it freely. Unlike staff and family, I was comfortable exploring with RM any feelings and concerns that came up. Initially, RM talked repeatedly of his anger at the person who had hit him and asked what the consequences had been for that person. RM described in detail the punishment he would like to mete out. Gradually the focus of the talk about the accident shifted to the physical consequences for RM, his dislike of being in the long-term care facility, his feelings of alienation from the other and much older residents, and his fears that he would not recover fully. Because of RM's continued short-term memory loss, he repeated a great deal from session to session. In each session, however, new material was discussed, and in this way RM gradually moved through the five stages of grief (Kübler-Ross, 1969) for the accident and its outcome for him.

As RM moved into acceptance of what had occurred, he began to talk about his continuing memory loss as one of the outcomes of the accident. After RM had been told that he was skipping 5 years of his memory he began to say such things as, "If I have to remember something sad, then I don't want to get my memory back." Gradually, still with the above disclaimer, RM began to speculate about what might have happened to him during the five years. Some of this speculation focused on probable girl friends, and eventually RM mentioned his fiancée's name as someone he had dated and had "probably" broken up with. The more this person was discussed, the more RM recalled events in their courtship, though without concurrent memory return for other events of that time. Finally RM spoke with sadness of his probable breakup with this woman and moved through the stages of grief for his loss of her. This process involved tears on RM's part, along with frustration at their appearance: "Men don't cry." At one point, RM hypothesized that his breakup with his fiancée had occurred because of his accident; when questioned about this, he stated that she might not have wanted to be burdened by someone as crippled as he was.

Following his acceptance of a breakup with his fiancée, RM made no further progress toward regaining his memory; he continued to state that he would prefer not to recall anything sad, saying that he had already had enough sadness. At this point it had been five months since RM had been referred to me. The relationship between this patient and the staff was positive. Staff members sometimes experienced RM as exasperating, but were no longer frightened of him. The social services person had continued to be RM's contact person whenever he was frustrated by something in the facility system; she was also the resource person sought by staff members with questions about RM's emotional needs.

I consistently informed the social services person and RM's mother of what occurred during my individual sessions with him. Because of the progress RM had made in his grieving, because of the skills of the social services person, and because of the relationship of trust and safety that had been established between RM, the social services person, and the staff, I terminated the individual sessions. At this point it was not clear whether RM would ever allow himself to remember that his fiancée had been in the accident with him. Everyone involved with his care, however, felt capable of dealing with that event should it occur.

One month later, while talking with the social services person, RM asked who had been in the accident with him. When his fiancée's name was mentioned, RM asked what had happened to her. RM was told that his fiancée had been badly injured and he then changed the subject. The evening of the same day, RM asked his mother what had happened to his fiancée in the accident. When told that she had been killed, RM became tearful and quiet; he began to remember portions of the accident itself and asked for pictures of his fiancée to be brought to his room. By the next day RM's memory of the accident and of the previous 5 years had returned.

Following the return of these memories, RM made rapid progress in his physical rehabilitation. Up to that point RM had remained wheelchair-bound, while walking a maximum of 400 feet with a walker in physical therapy. The day after he regained his memory of his fiancée's presence at the accident, RM walked 700 feet with the walker and 60 feet with the walkane; his endurance had greatly increased. Eight days later RM was out of the wheelchair permanently and showed a marked increase in his ability to manage his activities of daily living. Twenty four days later RM discarded the walker for the walkane. During this time RM began to talk about moving and began planning for the future; discharge plans were begun.

After RM regained his memory for the preceding 5 years, I was used as a resource person; most consultation occurred over the telephone. Telephone contact was on an as-needed basis, with more frequent contact being made during crisis periods. RM talked with the nursing staff and with the social services person about his fiancée; he reminisced and showed them pictures, and staff noted a continuing increase in his memory for and verbalization about the past. RM expressed relief at having his memory back. There were still occasional outbursts of anger, but staff members reponded to these appropriately and without assistance.

A major crisis ensued, however, when RM's discharge from the facility became imminent. RM began to spend most of his time in bed, was surly with staff, and began to talk of suicide. I then spoke with the social services person about the vicissitudes of termination. RM himself was able to verbalize that he felt trapped, no longer right for the facility and yet afraid to leave. The social services person then met regularly with RM to validate his fears and to help him leave the facility emotionally. The social services person also held an inservice for other staff members, to let them know the message behind RM's behavior and to help them plan interventions that they could make to ease the termination process. These interventions included such things as stopping in RM's room to let him know that they would miss him and to ask him to make return visits. Staff were useful in communicating to RM their expectations that he would continue to make progress outside the facility and that he would do well after discharge. The actual discharge was a successful though emotional event for everyone involved.

Criteria for Appropriateness of Method/Type of Intervention

In the case study, I used five models of consultation to intervene in the several aspects of the two presenting problems. One of these models (clinical model) involved direct service to the patient by the consultant rather than active consultation to staff. The criteria for using each model were products of the phase of the consultative relationship in that particular facility and the problems presented.

In my experience, consultative relationships in long-term care facilities typically follow a six-stage developmental process, as listed in Table 8–1. During the initial stages, the clinical nurse specialist uses the clinical and behavioral models almost exclusively. That is, the clinical nurse specialist is providing direct care (assessment, diagnosis, and treatment) and is working with staff members to set up a specific plan that they will implement. As the clinical nurse specialist gains credibility, additional staff members begin to support the use of the consultation; interest in inservice programs rises, and these programs in turn provide increasing visibility for the services of the clinical nurse specialist. This education, as well as the content of the consultations, sensitizes staff members to the emotional needs of patients while increasing staff skills;

TABLE 8–1. DEVELOPMENTAL STAGES OF CONSULTATIVE RELATIONSHIPS IN LONG-TERM CARE FACILITIES

Testing via crisis referrals
Referrals by a few psychologically-minded staff
Widening islands of staff support
Regular inservices and increasing visibility
Regular referrals and active working relationships
Skilled staff using consultant as a source of education and support
 for staff-generated interventions

this results in active working relationships with the clinical nurse specialist. Finally, as staff members become adept at assessing and intervening with patients, the consultant acts primarily as a resource for the planning of programs to meet needs that staff have identified and which staff will implement. The clinical nurse specialist also supports staff members and facilitates the use of their skills as they assess and intervene with patients (mental health model).

Clearly, the developmental phase of the relationship between the staff who were caring for RM and me allowed for the variety of models used in the consultation. In a facility in which the consultant was newer, the clinical model, the education model, and the behavioral model would all have been used more extensively. Each of these models relies more heavily on the intervention of the clinical nurse specialist into the presenting problems than does either the mental health model or the program model.

For example, only one inservice program was presented by me. Education that occurred during the inservice included venting of anxiety that had prevented staff from utilizing knowledge and skills that were already available to them. Information was presented, but a portion of this simply told more about the patient (i.e., the need for privacy) rather than providing formulations about patient dynamics or the presenting problems. A portion of the inservice was used for problem solving in which the staff participated. Following this inservice, staff members were generally able to manage their anxiety and to continue problem solving without my input; their ability to do so, and to use the inservice as effectively as they did, was a product of the active working phase of the consultative relationship. This type of inservice was not new to staff members and they had had previous successful experience with it.

Similarly, except for the instance with the cigarettes, a behavioral model was not used to manage the outbursts of RM's anger; staff sophistication in dealing with unpleasant expressions of emotion by residents precluded the need for such an approach. The inservice included a discussion of appropriate limit setting, another concept that was not new to staff members. Because of the staff's previous experience, this discussion was sufficient for the problem. In the absence of this earlier experience, I would have been more directly involved in supervising the management of the angry outbursts by setting up an approach using reinforcers and timeouts; this would have utilized strict operational definitions of the problem and of the consequences. I would also have directly intervened in individual sessions with RM to accomplish those things which in fact occurred in the facility's anger management program.

In the facility being described, at the time of RM's admission I used the mental health model primarily. Using this model, I was primarily a resource person for a staff that had become well-trained in intervening with most mental health problems encountered in the patients. As described above, I did intervene to provide direct service with RM; this occurred in an instance that I judged needed both time and skill not available to the staff.

A related criterion for direct intervention on my part involved the etiology of the presenting problem. In the case study, direct intervention occurred when the presenting problem was intrapsychic rather than being a function of the environment; that is, the problem was neither created nor exacerbated by the interaction of the patient's personality with the environment of the long-term care facility. With few exceptions, patients in a non-acute setting are long term. In addition, a non-acute setting automatically meets three of the four criteria for sensory deprivation (Suedfeld, 1969). Patients give up control in most aspects of their lives; arenas for decision making are greatly decreased. These aspects of being a patient create emotional crises and disturbances that are regularly referred to the psychiatric clinical nurse specialist.

These aspects of the non-acute institutional environment are best resolved through negotiation of institutional requirements, as perceived and carried out by staff, and patient requirements. Such negotiation precludes direct, clinical intervention with the patient by the clinical nurse specialist. In the case study, RM's anger about being in a long-term care facility was managed by interventions that staff were able to make. This increased the staff's sensitivity to RM's emotional needs and to his personality outside the role of patient. The interventions also altered the aspects of the environment that conflicted with RM's needs and provoked his frustration and anger. This alteration was more pertinent than my direct clinical intervention would have been. Furthermore, staff interventions were generalizable to similar episodes in future patients; the anger management program with the social services person is an example of learning that had been generalized from earlier consultation.

Operationally, use of the above criteria results in staff interventions that are behaviorally oriented, while I intervene directly when issues related to underlying psychodynamics of patient behavior must be addressed. Staff makes referrals to me based on behaviors that are causing practical problems in provision of nursing care; this can be as subtle as a referral for depression which seems to be preventing a patient from functioning at an expected level. Practical solutions are seen as more useful than information about psychodynamics, if the latter provides information without suggesting useful interventions (Lee, 1977). When the presenting problem represents, in part, a problem in the interaction of the environment with the patient's personality, a care plan that includes specific staff interventions with problem behaviors may be sufficient. In RM's case, the underlying dynamic of repression of the fiancée's death required intervention in order to resolve both presenting problems; this was the point at which I intervened directly.

Using the above criteria, the size of the clinical nurse specialist's caseload in any facility varies with the state of the consultative relationship and, to a lesser extent, with the etiology of the presenting problems. In the facility where RM resided, at the time of his admission I maintained a much smaller caseload than I had two years previously. The difference in the models of consultation required account for this change.

Several factors external to the relationship between the consultant and staff, however, can slow or alter the development of the consultative relationship. For example, staff turnover, with absence of a core staff, slows the development of the relationship. (Conversely, a strong consultative relationship that promotes skills and mastery can slow staff turnover.) At the time of the experience described in this chapter, I had been a consultant to another long-term care facility, of similar size, for the same length of time. Although the staff of this second facility were also in the active working phase of the consultative relationship, I carried a larger caseload and tended to utilize models of consultation requiring a large degree of direct intervention. This facility had recently undergone a change of ownership, with one year of subsequent constant change in management, policies, and the physical plant; staff energies had become divided. In this instance, I also provided consultation that was staff and systems oriented rather than simply patient oriented (organizational model).

IMPACT OF CLINICAL NURSE SPECIALIST INTERVENTION

Method of Evaluation of Patient Outcomes

I am a clinical nurse specialist in long-term care facilities where a mental health consultant is not required. Consequently, I am an external consultant working by contract for businessmen who look at cost effectiveness and concrete results. Insurance, Medicare, and public assistance do not pay for anything but direct intervention by me, and then only under certain conditions. Consequently, the facilities pay for the service from their operating budgets. My effectiveness is an important point in establishing and maintaining service contracts.

At present this effectiveness is shown empirically. My impact in the case of RM was clear to the administrator of the facility; he maintained a personal interest in the care of RM and spoke regularly with staff as well as the consultants involved in his care. When patients are referred for behaviors that are particularly dramatic or obvious, administrators often are aware of the referral. In addition, I provide narrative quarterly reports to administrators, summarizing work with staff and with patients. These reports include subjective reports on patient outcomes, changes in staff skill levels, and potential problems. Patient outcomes are defined in terms of the presenting problem and any underlying pathology. Such a regular reporting process helps the consultant maintain a clear sense of responsibility to the administrator as the actual client of clinical nurse specialist services.

Method of Evaluation of Cost Effectiveness

Cost effectiveness is also evaluated empirically. In the case of RM, several outcomes had implications for cost effectiveness. Staff overcame their fear of RM, stopped arguing with him (something that had originally occurred several times a day and required much staff time), and stopped avoiding his room and his care. The staff efficiency, as it related to RM's anger, was quickly improved because of the staff's ability to generalize from earlier consultation regarding angry patients. A later referral to me similarly demonstrated staff ability to increase efficiency by generalizing from a previous consultation experience; in that instance, staff utilized skills first discussed in the context of RM's termination from the facility.

In addition, staff from the rehabilitation unit of the hospital that had originally cared for RM remained aware of his progress and was impressed enough with his recovery to ask if the facility would be interested in receiving more trauma victims. A large rehabilitation center in the area similarly became aware of this facility and asked about referring patients. RM's improvement was a result of many people, such as myself, of different disciplines working together. However, to the extent that staff were able to provide prescribed care rather than avoid or argue with RM, and to the extent that his physical improvement was enhanced by the successful resolution of emotional problems, my intervention as a psychiatric clinical nurse specialist was cost effective. Certainly, the reputation of the facility was enhanced, leading to subsequent referrals from the community as well as expanding the number of facilities available to provide long-term care to similar patients.

As noted above, such evidence of impact on a setting is empirical and idiosyncratic; measurable, replicable evidence would be more useful. In long-term care settings, reduced length of stay has been less useful than in acute care settings for evaluating the effect of interventions. The focus of nursing care has been in providing care for people with chronic health problems and rehabilitating them to an unknown optimal level of function during their permanent residence at the facility. With the advent of diagnosis-related groupings (DRGs), however, many people are now being discharged from acute care facilities to complete their recovery in non-acute settings. In addition, increased community supports are available to maintain at home people who once would have resided permanently in a long-term care setting. Reduced length of stay is becoming an increasingly useful criterion for evaluation. Certainly, in the above case study, there is a suggestion that RM's length of stay in the facility was decreased by the return of his memory and subsequent physical improvement.

A more frequent criterion of the impact of the clinical nurse specialist has been that of staff turnover. This item is difficult to measure because of the many confounding variables. Again, empirical evidence predominates. In the facility described in this case study, I was asked to consult on an elderly woman who was bitter, complaining, insulting, and who had gotten a well-liked staff member fired because of accusations of abuse unsupported by physical evidence. Non-licensed staff refused to enter this patient's room, tried to avoid giving care to her, and even gave false names so that she could not complain about them. Since non-licensed staff were involved, not all facilities would have seen this woman as in need of referral. This facility, which does refer problems affecting staff at any level, has a low rate of staff turnover. The interventions I facilitated in this instance were useful in increasing staff's skill levels while decreasing patient-related sources of stress. Decreased staff stress and a low rate of staff turnover were also evidence of the general atmosphere of mutual support and community that has long been engendered by the administration. Thus this is a confounding variable in measuring the impact of clinical nurse specialist intervention on staff turnover.

Finally, in long-term care settings, clinical nurse specialists make a major impact on the quality of the nursing care when they improve the ability of staff to set appropriate priorities of care, which include the patient's emotional needs, and when they thereby improve the relationship between patients and staff. As noted previously, patients in non-acute settings are often present for the rest of their lives. Conflicting interactions that occur with staff can set up permanent negative cycles of behavior which are stressful for all. In the extreme, such conflicts can lead to patients being asked to leave the facility which leads to a sense of failure for staff, patients, and patients' families. Conversely, adequate support of patients' emotional needs can decrease symptoms of physical illness and can decrease the number and frequency of acute episodes of those illnesses; this is especially true for older adults, who are the predominant residents of non-acute care settings (Mumford, et al, 1984).

In summary, the impact of successful intervention by the psychiatric clinical nurse specialist is empirically shown through the following: positive change in the presenting problem; positive change in underlying pathology, as necessary to change the presenting problem or the provision of quality nursing care; increase in staff skill levels; increase in staff ability to generalize learning; increase in staff satisfaction, in part manifested by a decrease in staff turnover; and improved perceptions of the specific health care setting by the community. Recently, decreased length of stay has also been a useful criterion in evaluating the impact of the consultant. Finally, especially with older adults, impact of successful psychiatric consultation can be seen through the decreased incidence of acute illness and physical symptoms.

ROLE OF THE CLINICAL NURSE SPECIALIST IN THE NON-ACUTE SETTING

As described above, I am an external consultant working on contract in several long-term care facilities. As clinical nurse specialist, I rely on the definition of services to be offered as set out by the contract. That is, consultation is patient centered and is provided to nursing personnel on the pertinent unit. Each contract defines a minimum number of consultation hours per month as well as a minimum number of inservice hours per year. Additional amounts or types of consultation can be added as needed. My ability to affect nursing practice is influenced in several ways by this arrangement.

First, although I work closely with nursing staff, communication must be maintained with the administrator, who is usually a businessman. The danger in forgetting who is ultimately responsible for renewing the contract can mean termination of a clinical nurse specialist's services in the face of excellent consultative relationships with nursing staff. As mentioned previously, quarterly reports that summarize services and outcomes are useful in maintaining businesslike communication with the administrator.

Second, I am an external consultant, coming into the system from another agency. While this fact may enhance my expert and referent sources of power, it can also engender resistance. My impact is determined by the ability to: obtain formal and public sanction from the administrator; learn what is specific to the system, that is, the individual setting including norms, patterns of communication, and systems for eliciting follow-through; discern and remain neutral in system politics; work collaboratively with the internal consultant (in the case study, this was the LPN who was the social services person); provide information with practical applications; bring on changes slowly; and bring energy into the system.

Accomplishing these non-task components of the consultation is crucial in overcoming resistance and gaining credibility within the setting. Credibility is furthered by the quality of practical information that becomes available to staff in the context of patient behaviors that have been referred to me. This information is at the heart of the clinical nurse specialist role. I help staff members to increase their knowledge by providing educational opportunities and by facilitating staff utilization of knowledge available to them but not in use due to the stress of a given setting or situation (Fife & Lemler, 1983).

Both types of educational promotion occurred in the case study. RM's anger was so intimidating that staff were unable to utilize knowledge about limit setting which they had previously used with other patients. Similarly, staff had not referred RM to the previously established anger management program. In addition to facilitating the use of these resources, I provided new information about anger. I shared a theoretical understanding of anger as a secondary emotion that can be altered via a cognitive approach that was based on the literature on family violence.

This transfer of information, from a source not commonly used by staff at the long-term care facility, was important to the planning of interventions into one aspect of RM's angry episodes. As described in the case study, the interventions occurred at four levels, each based on a separate theoretical base or hypothesis. This planned intervention into a complex, multilayered patient response to illness and environment is another major component of the clinical nurse specialist role (Calkin, 1984).

This ability to respond with pertinent information to complex problems is what makes the role of the psychiatric (and geriatric) clinical nurse specialist important in the long-term care setting. Perhaps more than any other age group, the older adults who predominantly make up the population of such a setting have a multilayered, interwoven physiologic and psychologic response to illness. As many as 25 percent of all psychiatric symptoms in this age group have been found to be behavioral manifestations of physical illnesses (Mensh, 1979; Pfeiffer, 1977; Raskind, Alvarez, Pietrzyk, Westerlund, & Herlin, 1976). In addition, as mentioned earlier, research suggests that mental health counseling to older adults decreases the frequency and severity of physical symptoms and acute episodes of illness (Mumford et al., 1984). Patients in the setting who are not older adults are similar to RM; that is, they have complex physical disabilities, frequently with neurologic impairment. A consultant is necessary who can explain the complexity of the symptoms in such patients.

For these reasons, the clinical nurse specialist is preferable to a consultant in other professions. As in other settings, psychiatric consultation in long-term care facilities is provided by a variety of professions, including psychologists, social workers, and psychiatrists. Of these, the psychiatrist is best educated to the complexity of physical and emotional problems in older adults. The long-term care setting, however, is particularly a nursing setting. Although various consultants are available, nursing staff directly provide the majority of care: physical, rehabilitative, and emotional. Physicians, though directing that care, are seen much less frequently (30- to 90-day intervals) than in acute care settings. The nursing staff generally have a much longer time in which to develop a relationship with patients than in most acute care settings, and those relationships have implications for the stress levels of staff as well as the well-being of the patients. Independent nursing decisions abound.

The advantages of nurses consulting with nurses in any setting have been discussed elsewhere: the nurse consultant has a better understanding than other professionals of the limitations and stresses involved in providing patient care; the nurse consultant also has a unique vantage from which to discern individual and group strengths and possibilities on a nursing unit (Fife & Lemler, 1983). Because of the unique nursing environment that is the long-term care setting, however, these benefits are especially pertinent there. The nurse consultant is also likely to understand the demands and differences of the setting.

RESEARCH IN PRACTICE

As mentioned previously, I am a clinical nurse specialist consulting on contract from one agency to another. The contracting agency pays for patient-centered consultation that enhances staff skills. The provider agency, of necessity, emphasizes revenue generation. In this climate, nursing research is not emphasized. In addition, even within acute medical settings, no criteria have been established to evaluate the role of the psychiatric clinical nurse specialist (Fife & Lemler, 1983). For these reasons, I was unable to be involved in conducting research. From the case study and consultation experience in the long-term care setting, however, researchable clinical and management questions can be identified.

Researchable clinical questions include:

- What are the effects of psychiatric clinical nurse specialist consultation in long-term care facilities?
- What are the changes in recovery rates (or intensity/ frequency of symptoms) of physically ill patients who have been seen by the psychiatric clinical nurse specialist?
- What is the effectiveness of anger management techniques when modified for use with patients with moderate memory loss?

Regarding the latter question, in the case described and with other patients, there is much anecdotal evidence of the effectiveness of this adapted approach with this population. The next step is to objectively measure these effects.

Researchable questions that impact management can also be identified. With the advent of DRGs, cost effectiveness in every setting is being spotlighted. Psychiatric clinical nurse specialists provide a service that at times is difficult to quantify. Criteria for measurement and evaluation of these services must be developed and used. Empirically, I am aware that in long-term care settings in which a core staff has remained for more than two years, staff skills in dealing with problem behaviors have increased while referrals to the clinical nurse specialist have mark-edly decreased; this is a measure of success. Thus, questions suggested by anecdotal evidence include:

- What is the efficiency of nurses who have been taught anger management skills?
- What is the ability of staff to generalize the content of consulta-tion, as shown by frequency of patient responses that staff cannot manage, over time (Calkin, 1984)?

This knowledge must be quantified in a manner that can be shown to administrators, personnel departments, and legislators who determine health policy and funding.

SUMMARY

As a psychiatric clinical nurse specialist in a non-acute setting, I have demonstrated the integration of five consultative models in my relation-ships with the patient, family, and staff members. I have related the choice of model to six developmental stages that I identified in consulta-tive relationships in long-term care facilities. Throughout the case study, I illustrated the situations where direct involvement with the patient was indicated versus when I determined that it was appropriate to provide consultation to the internal provider, the social services person. Also, because I was a consultant in a business environment I have emphasized the importance of maintaining clear businesslike communication with facility administration including quarterly reports that summarize serv-ices, patient care outcomes, and referrals.

SPECIFIC QUESTIONS

1. What factors determine when direct care should be provided by the clinical nurse specialist? How is the boundary between the clinical nurse specialist and the internal care provider (in this case, the LPN) determined? Compare and contrast the cases de-scribed in this chapter and in chapters 6 and 12.
2. Discuss the adaptation and application of theory to the clinical problems presented in this chapter.
3. This author presented five consultation models and criteria for use of the models. How would you apply these to your own practice?
4. What are the similarities and differences in the business contracts described by the external consultants in this chapter and chapter 6? How is the impact of the clinical nurse specialist demon-strated?

5. This chapter generates a number of research questions. Select one and suggest a research design projecting both the time frame and cost required to undertake such a study.

REFERENCES

Beck, A. (1976). *Cognitive therapy and the emotional disorders.* New York: New American Library.

Brigman, C., Dickey C., & Zegeer, L.J. (1983). The agitated-aggressive patient. *American Journal of Nursing, 83* (10), 1408–1412.

Calkin, J. (1984). A model for advanced nursing practice. *The Journal of Nursing Administration, 14* (1), 24–30.

Coutant, N. (1982). Rage: Implied neurological correlates. *Journal of Neurosurgical Nursing, 14* (1), 28–33.

Fife, B., & Lemler, S. (1983). The psychiatric nurse specialist: A valuable asset in the general hospital. *Journal of Nursing Administration, 13* (4), 14–17.

Gallessich, J. (1983). *The profession and practice of consultation.* San Francisco: Jossey-Bass.

Kübler-Ross, E. (1969). *On death and dying.* New York: Macmillan.

Lee, A.R. (1977). Creating a mental health consultation package for community agencies. *Hospital and Community Psychiatry, 28* (10), 745–748.

Mensh, I. (1979). Acute, reversible, psychotic reactions in geriatric patients. In O.J. Kaplan (Ed.), *Psychopathology of aging.* New York: Academic Press.

Moritz, D.A. (1978). Understanding anger. *American Journal of Nursing, 78* (1), 81–83.

Mumford, E., Schlesinger, H.J., & Glass, G.V., et al., (1984). A new look at evidence about reduced cost of medical utilization following mental health treatment. *American Journal of Psychiatry, 141* (10), 1145–1158.

Novaco, R.W. (1976). The functions and regulation of the arousal of anger. *American Journal of Psychiatry, 133* (10), 1124–1128.

Pfeiffer, E. (1977). Psychopathology and social pathology. In J. Birren & K.W. Schaie (Eds.), *Handbook of the psychology of aging.* New York: Van Nostrand Reinhold.

Raskind, M., Alvarez, C., & Pietrzyk, M., et al. (1976). Helping the elderly psychiatric patient in crisis. *Geriatrics, 31,* 51–56.

Suedfeld, P. (1969). Introduction and historical background. In J.P. Zubeck (Ed.), *Sensory deprivation: 15 years of research.* New York: Appleton-Century-Crofts.

chapter nine

The Pediatric Surgical Clinical Nurse Specialist in a University Hospital Setting

Lori Howell

The clinical nurse specialist for pediatric surgery in a university setting sees patients referred for tertiary care, for example, those children requiring extremely specialized surgery. Due to the multiplicity of body systems requiring pediatric surgical intervention, the pediatric surgical clinical nurse specialist is a generalist, but should choose to become expert in a few and proficient in all areas.

Patients referred to a university hospital come from a wide referral radius, including the state, country and, occasionally, the world. Depending upon the urgency of care required, these children are frequently transported immediately after birth and often require prompt surgical attention. The infant born with VATER syndrome will be used to illustrate a case in which the pediatric surgical clinical nurse specialist typically would be involved. These infants may have all or a combination of the following anomalies: vertebral, vascular, anorectal, tracheo-esophageal atresia and/or fistula, radial, and renal; hence the acronym VATER (Barnes & Smith, 1978). The specific case presented is that of a child born with a tracheo-esophageal fistula, esophageal atresia, talipes equinovarus, and imperforate anus.

Case Study

LS was born with VATER syndrome and was transported from the county hospital shortly after he was born. His mother had immigrated from Mexico and spoke no English. She was a single parent; the father was not involved with the family. Her support system consisted of a brother and sister-in-law, whose child she also cared for. LS was admitted to our intensive care nursery (ICN) to begin a diagnostic workup of his anomalies. He immediately went to surgery where the pediatric surgeons ligated his tracheo-esophageal fistula and anastomosed the proximal and distal ends of his esophagus. A gastrostomy was performed to vent off air to relieve intragastric pressure; it would be used later for feedings while the esophageal anastomosis healed. A colostomy was created as a first stage in the

163

repair of his imperforate anus. In the following week LS had apneic episodes which were caused by a malacic segment of his trachea, necessitating a tracheostomy. He was also seen by the orthopedic surgeons for management of his talipes equinovarus. After discharge from the ICN, LS has been readmitted to the pediatric surgical floor to revise his colostomy and close his tracheostomy.

CLINICAL NURSE SPECIALIST INTERVENTION

Method of Patient Selection

As the clinical nurse specialist for a busy service which includes admissions to pediatric surgical, medical, and intensive care units as well as the intensive care nursery, I cannot routinely see every pediatric surgical patient. Prescheduled admissions to the surgical floor are checked regularly to assess which patients might require clinical nurse specialist services. If a particular diagnosis connotes a tremendous amount of discharge planning, such as tracheomalacia, or a poor prognosis, such as biliary atresia, the clinical nurse specialist would typically see these children and their parents on admission to complete a formal assessment of both.

Referrals from the staff nurse, head nurse, maternal–child divisional nursing director, and director of nursing are another method by which I select patients. The patients I am asked to see by the staff nurse and head nurse usually relate to the subspecialities I have developed, for example parenting, growth and development, intermittent catheterization, and skin care.

The divisional director of nursing usually requests my services when a quality of care issue is involved. A clinical assessment of a patient's status may be required to expedite admission to or from an intensive care unit. If an untoward incident occurs, the divisional director of nursing may ask for an evaluation of the care provided. Additionally, since the divisional director of nursing and I are colleagues, information must flow bi-directionally, that is, each is kept abreast of issues requiring clinical or administrative intervention. In general, the clinical nurse specialist should have a keen appreciation of the administrative structure of one's particular institution so that decisions can be made which promote the highest standards of care for the child and family.

Another potential patient referral source are physicians. The number of pediatric clinical nurse specialists continues to increase as physicians are witnessing the comprehensive care a clinical nurse specialist is able to provide. A physician may request the clinical nurse specialist's consultation in areas such as patient-family support, education, implementation of new procedures, and usage of new products.

Criteria for Patient Case Load

While patients with a variety of surgical clinical problems are cared for by the staff nurse, the clinical nurse specialist selects those patients with a higher complexity of care than the staff nurse may be able to provide. For example, the staff nurse caring for a child with an ileostomy is able to inspect skin, apply an appliance, and work with the family and child to educate them in the care of an ileostomy at home. When a school-age child with a recently created ileostomy has a poor body image, however, her parents cannot accept the ileostomy, and skin erosion has begun to occur, the higher level of expertise provided by the clinical nurse specialist is necessary.

In addition, since the nursing staff work 12-hour shifts and may only work 2 to 3 days per week, the continuity of care required during the child's hospitalization and follow-up care via phone contact and on return visits can often only be provided by the clinical nurse specialist. In institutions where nurses work 8-hour shifts, continuity of care by the clinical nurse specialist might not be as important during the child's hospitalization, but may be more so after the patient is discharged. An assessment of a particular setting's staffing pattern should be undertaken to determine how the clinical nurse specialist role can best be implemented.

The ICN nursing staff asked me to see LS because of their unfamiliarity with tracheostomies. When I was a novice clinical nurse specialist, I investigated areas of practice where the procedural incidence was low and the patient acuity was high, such as tracheostomies. My prior experience as a pediatric critical care nurse caring for a large number of children with tracheostomies furnished the necessary technical expertise to provide the staff with a needed service.

Well-developed clinical skills, however, are not all that is necessary to care for children with tracheostomies. A thorough understanding of the underlying anatomy and pathology and an awareness of the parental support and education necessary to provide home care are also essential (Aradine, 1980). With a well-developed home care program and team approach, the reported mortality rate in children less than one year of age with tracheostomies cared for at home has decreased from 25 to 50 percent (Tucker & Silberman, 1972) to 3 to 8 percent (Ruben et al., 1982; Wetmore, Handler, & Potsic, 1982). As the pediatric surgical clinical nurse specialist, I am in a position to provide not only the skills necessary to care for these children, but also the depth and breadth of knowledge necessary to identify and evaluate the discharge planning needs of the child, family, and nursing staff.

As I began to develop consultation services in the area of pediatric tracheostomies, I critically reviewed the current literature, observed surgical techniques for performing a tracheostomy in the operating room, assumed direct patient care postoperatively, and discussed postoperative care guidelines with the pediatric surgeons. Initial guidelines for tracheostomy care were developed and feedback was sought from the nursing staff and pediatric surgeons. From this input, instructions for the parents (Table 9–1 and Fig. 9–1) together with a discharge checklist (Table

---

TABLE 9–1. PARENT INSTRUCTIONS: TRACHEOSTOMY CARE OF INFANTS AND CHILDREN

I. **Cleaning tracheostomy site**
   A. Clean site at least twice a day and every 8 hours if any drainage or odor is present. Normally, tracheal secretions are clear/white with no odor. Odors and green/yellow drainage from the tracheostomy may indicate an infection and should be brought to the attention of your doctor.
   B. Roll applicators soaked in ½-strength hydrogen peroxide (equal parts water and hydrogen peroxide) over the tracheostomy site to remove any crusted areas. When through, rinse area with applicator dipped in clear water and dry.
   C. Do not use powder or lotion around tracheostomy.

II. **Changing tracheostomy ties**
   A. Clean neck area daily and change ties when soiled.
   B. Use two people if possible, or wrap your baby "mummy" style in a blanket to prevent wriggling.
   C. Slip the old ties up to the top of the holes on the tracheostomy tube.
   D. Tie new ties as shown in Figure 9–1.
   E. Secure with a knot. Prevent sores by changing the place of the knot each time you change the ties.
   F. Ties should be snug enough to let only the little finger slip underneath the ties.
   G. Check the neck daily for redness and sores.

III. **Suctioning**
   A. Use the bulb syringe at the tracheostomy tube opening if your baby coughs up secretions.
   B. For catheter suctioning:
      1. Wash hands well; this is the best way to prevent infections.
      2. Open the sterile glove and suction catheter package without touching the contents.
      3. Open sterile water container for rinsing catheter.
      4. Put on sterile glove by touching only the cuff. Remove the sterile catheter from the package with your gloved hand. Do not touch anything with your gloved hand holding the suction catheter.
      5. Attach catheter to suction tubing using nongloved hand.
      6. Wet the catheter in the container of sterile water.
      7. Turn on the suction machine.
      8. With the nongloved hand, put several drops of saline into the tracheostomy tube to loosen up secretions.
      9. Gently insert the catheter into the tracheostomy tube until resistance is met and then pull it back about ¼ inch. Withdraw the catheter by rotating it between your thumb and index finger and applying intermittent suction.
      10. Let the baby breathe again for a couple of minutes. If you can still hear secretions gurgling, suction again.
      11. Rinse the connecting tubing with water.
      12. Throw catheter, glove, and sterile water away.

TABLE 9–1. (Continued)

    C. Tips on suctioning:
1. Always suction before feedings and diaper changes.
2. Suction only as needed. Remember crying and too frequent suctioning will increase the amount of secretions.
3. Let your baby breathe after each pass of the suction catheter. Suctioning removes secretions and oxygen.
4. Blood-tinged secretions might mean too vigorous suctioning or that the suction machine is turned on too high.
5. Make sure you have enough supplies to get you through weekends and nights.

IV. Humidity
    A. The tracheostomy collar and nebulizer are used to moisten the air entering the trachea.
    B. Your baby may only need humidity during naps and during the night to keep secretions from plugging the tracheostomy tube. If secretions are thick, humidification is necessary.
    C. When travelling or during a power failure, one drop of saline put into the tracheostomy tube will keep the airway moist.
    D. Clean the nebulizer, tracheostomy collar, and suction bottle daily in hot, soapy water and rinse well.

V. Changing the tracheostomy tube
    A. Attach new ties to a clean tracheostomy tube and insert guide into the tube. Holding only the wings of the tube, put it back into the tray until ready to insert.
    B. Place a small blanket roll under your baby's shoulders to expose the tracheostomy site. Have another person help you if possible.
    C. Cut the old ties and remove the tube.
    D. Insert the new tube directing it to the back and then down; remove the guide.
    E. See that your baby is breathing easily and then fasten the ties.
    F. Throw the plastic tubes away after one use.

VI. Emergencies
    A. If the tracheostomy plugs, put saline into the tube and try suctioning. If you are unable to clear the tube, remove it and put in a new one.
    B. Keep a list of emergency numbers next to the phone.
    C. Always have a new tracheostomy tube with the ties attached at your baby's bedside.
    D. Keep a travel bag packed with all necessities for tracheostomy care.
    E. Enroll in a CPR class through the American Heart Association, Red Cross, or your local hospital.
    F. Notify the electric and phone companies that prompt service will be necessary.
    G. Talk to your local fire department and tell them about your baby.

VII. Taking care of your baby
A baby with a tracheostomy should be encouraged to grow and develop as normally as possible. He or she needs to be held, talked to, and loved as much as any child. A few things are different, though, in caring for a baby with a tracheostomy.
    A. Clothes should be open in the front so that they cannot plug the tracheostomy tube.
    B. Bathing or wading pools are fine. You may use the tracheostomy collar to prevent water from entering the tracheostomy. Just remember never to leave your baby alone.
    C. Quilted or smooth blankets are best. Blankets with a lot of nap should be washed several times before using.
    D. Small objects should be kept from the baby's playing area so that they won't accidentally get into the tracheostomy tube.

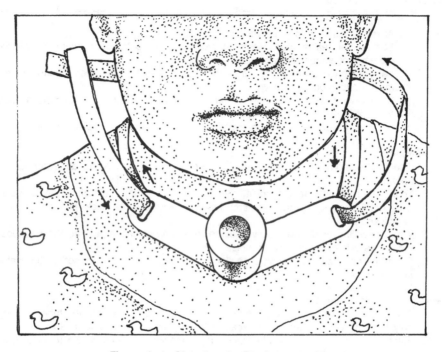

Figure 9–1. Changing the Tracheostomy Ties

9–2) and an equipment and supply list (Table 9–3) for the nurses caring for children with tracheostomies were written.

Involvement of staff nurses is critical to the success of the clinical nurse specialist role for many reasons. Staff nurses who possess advanced knowledge and expertise are better able to plan the care for complex patients. Also, the challenge presented by a higher acuity patient provides the staff nurses with a greater incentive to care for these patients and hopefully decreases staff turnover. Care should be taken by the clinical nurse specialist to positively recognize these superb clinical nurses and not to abuse them with overutilization. Finally, by increasing the expertise of the bedside nurse, theoretically the clinical nurse specialist would be able to devote more energy to other aspects of the role, such as research and consultation. In practice, with natural staff turnover, innovative treatments, surgeries, and the never-ending knowledge explosion, the reality is an increase in the complexity of referrals, but continued involvement in direct patient care. Currently, two clinical nurse IIIs (senior staff nurses) are participating in the revision of the initial tracheostomy guidelines and serve as additional expert resources to the staff in the area of tracheostomies.

TABLE 9–2. DISCHARGE CHECKLIST FOR PEDIATRIC TRACHEOSTOMY PATIENTS

	Date	RN	Parent
A. Persons involved in care are confident and have returned demonstrations of: 1. cleaning stoma 2. changing ties 3. changing tracheostomy tube 4. suctioning 5. vital signs 6. CPR 7. equipment care: monitor, nebulizer, suction machine, oxygen tank, and ambu bag			
B. Home care equipment obtained (see Table 9–3)			
C. Adequate supplies obtained for home and arrangements made for future needs (see Table 9–3)			
D. Home preparation completed 1. Formula and food supplies purchased 2. Room readied with 3-prong electrical outlets, good lighting, and adequate space for equipment 3. Intercom system discussed with parents			
E. Emergencies 1. Letters to telephone and electric companies and emergency services signed by physician and given to parents 2. Transportation arrangements 3. Emergency phone numbers posted by phone 4. When to call physician			
F. Caretakers are able to give well baby/child care related to bathing, clothing, activity, and childproofing needs			
G. Realistic feeding and suctioning schedule established			
H. Referrals 1. Chart copied or summary sent to referring physician 2. Parents aware of nearest hospital and community resources 3. Public health nurse referral			
I. Follow-up appointments made			

TABLE 9–3. DISCHARGE EQUIPMENT AND SUPPLY LIST

Equipment
Ordered from outside agency
_____ 1. Suction machine with connecting tubing
_____ 2. Cardiopulmonary monitor
_____ 3. Portable oxygen tank
_____ 4. Nebulizer with tracheostomy collar
_____ 5. Ambu bag

Supplies
Ordered from Materiel Services
_____ 1. 6 spare tracheostomy tubes (appropriate size and type for patient)
_____ 2. 1 roll 1/2 inch twill tape
_____ 3. Scissors
_____ 4. Suction catheters (appropriate size for tracheostomy tube)
_____ 5. Sterile gloves (appropriate size for caretaker)
_____ 6. 1 bulb syringe
_____ 7. DeLee suction catheters (appropriate size for tracheostomy tube)
_____ 8. Hydrogen peroxide
_____ 9. Sterile applicators
_____ 10. Normal saline pillows for suctioning
_____ 11. CPR Manual for Infants and Children
_____ 12. Cards for emergency phone numbers
_____ 13. Discharge Instructions for Children with Tracheostomies

Criteria for Appropriateness of Method/Type of Intervention

Children with tracheostomies require direct care of the tracheostomy, including critical care skills such as tracheal suctioning and changing tracheostomy tubes. Their care also necessitates a knowledge of home care required, anticipation of emergencies, and knowledge of which outside agencies to involve, for example, public health nursing, California Children's Services, infant development programs, speech therapy, and equipment vendors. A knowledge of adult learning theory to determine the parents' level of understanding, style of learning, and method of providing a supportive atmosphere are also essential.

As the proficiency of the staff improves, the amount of direct care provided by the clinical nurse specialist is reduced. If the incidence of a particular diagnosis is rare, such as infant tracheostomies in my setting, however, the nursing staff may not be able to maintain the skill level necessary to care for these children without receiving ongoing educational preparation as well as direct intervention by the clinical nurse specialist. LS required my interventions because the nursing staff were not familiar with infant tracheostomies, because they correctly anticipated a long-term care problem requiring continuity, and because I was an established resource in the care of children with tracheostomies.

To become an established resource in a particular area requires a success in one especially difficult case. In fact, the first time I developed plans for discharge for a 1-month-old infant with a tracheostomy, I worked with the neonatal clinical nurse specialist. She provided the necessary neonatal expertise while I provided the tracheostomy care expertise. Today, the patient we cared for is 7 years old, attends first grade, and no longer requires a tracheostomy. He still conjures up vivid memories of his frequent arrests, failure to thrive, and working parents who had limited English skills. While a success story is important, collaboration with other established resources, in this instance the neonatal clinical nurse specialist, can also be critical. Clinical nurse specialist colleagues can and should serve as advocates for clinical nurse specialist utilization within their primary unit.

In the case of LS, I arrived in the ICN at a prearranged time to meet with LS's nurse. After reading the chart, I discussed the infant's care with his nurse. The nurse told me that not only was she concerned about sending this baby home to a mother who did not visit very often, but she was not very familiar with tracheostomy care in particular, nor with the VATER syndrome in general. Based upon that information, I explained the VATER association, the rationale for surgical interventions, and which components were pertinent to LS. Further questioning revealed a lack of family coping abilities and the need for my continued involvement in LS's care. A nursing plan documenting the care required for his tracheostomy, gastrostomy, and colostomy, as well as the parent education necessary before he could be discharged was written with the staff nurse. My name was placed on the Kardex, to be called should any nursing problems arise. I also wrote a note in the medical progress section to keep the team informed of LS's nursing care.

The next day I ascertained if there were any problems encountered with the plan and provided the nursing staff with literature pertinent to the VATER association. The night-shift nurse had encountered difficulties with placement of the colostomy bag and, as a result, his peristomal skin had begun to break down. The nursing care plan was revised, based on discussion with the day nurse, to include suggestions to prevent further skin erosion.

For continuity, particularly where nurses work 12-hour shifts, communication with individual nurses is essential. This follow-up informs the nurses on night-shift that the clinical nurse specialist is concerned about the care being provided by them as well. It is also an excellent opportunity to market the clinical nurse specialist role and the ability to effect change so that consultations can continue. In a large teaching institution with a multiple array of health care providers, the staff nurse wants to know that the clinical nurse specialist can assist with and improve nursing care and is not just another person to call.

Once the staff nurse realizes that the clinical nurse specialist is readily available to help with nursing care problems, additional interventions can be made. For example, LS's mother also would require a great deal of education regarding LS's tracheostomy, gastrostomy, colostomy, nutrition, and feeding techniques, as well as the development of normal mothering skills. Procurement of resources, both financial and social, would also be necessary to facilitate parenting skills of LS's mother. I discussed the above proposed, necessary interventions with LS's nurse and suggested LS be assigned consistent nurses to further expedite discharge planning. The head nurse was approached about the problems this infant was likely to incur, and she readily agreed to rearrange the schedule to provide as much continuity of care as possible.

I communicate regularly with head nurses. I inform the head nurse if a serious or potentially serious incident occurs, for example, accidental dislodgement of a new tracheostomy tube. Since the head nurse possesses the line authority to resolve the issue, the clinical nurse specialist must work with the head nurse to achieve a satisfactory resolution for the benefit of patient care. I also involve the head nurse with "chronic" issues, where the gravity of the situation may be less but where my expertise might improve efficiency or patient care outcome. For example, after noting that chemical phlebitis occurred frequently, I developed a procedure based on the literature to reduce the sequelae of intravenous extravasations. When this protocol is followed, further care of the extravasation, such as dressing or ointments, is often not indicated.

Anticipation and planning for areas of concern improve the efficiency of nursing care because the staff nurse can practice defensive nursing rather than learn about problems after the fact. If untoward events do occur, however, the clinical nurse specialist can expedite learning by responding immediately, as in the case of LS. An unexpected malacic segment of trachea was found after LS experienced apneic episodes. I was able to provide a written plan of care and offer formal and informal classes to the nursing staff related to preoperative and postoperative care.

The clinical nurse specialist critically reviews the literature pertinent to the clinical problem at hand for its usefulness. With a strong clinical background and command of the current research in the area of pediatric tracheostomies, I was able to make recommendations to the health care team in planning the care of LS. The clinical nurse specialist walks a fine line, being careful not to assume the care from the staff nurse but rather to augment it. The clinical nurse specialist should also offer praise as well as constructive criticism. If high standards are expected, they will more likely be achieved.

Clinical Nurse Specialist/Patient Communication

As a clinical nurse specialist in a staff position, I am in an ideal role to coordinate the care the child and family receive. With advanced educational preparation, I am able to assess the patient from all perspectives within the context of the family and can thus provide nursing continuity over an extended period of time. The definition of the clinical nurse specialist role in a university setting includes a 24-hour responsibility for patients followed by a clinical nurse specialist. Therefore, if the nursing staff is also involved in the care of a child, the clinical nurse specialist will be notified of changes as they occur.

For the pediatric surgical patient, communication with the family is also essential while the child is in the operating room (Howell, 1980). Particularly if a case is unusually long, physicians may rely upon the clinical nurse specialist to support the family during this time and keep them informed of their child's progress. Because one then has access to this information, referrals to the chaplain or social worker can be made as appropriate. Once a child requires a number of services, or parents express anxiety over their child's condition, I will coordinate a multidisciplinary conference to clarify expectations and answer any questions. Prior to meeting with and providing clarifying information for a family, the health care providers meet to discuss potential concerns and reach consensus.

Parents need to be kept informed, have information clarified, and know that an attempt is being made to meet their needs. Because I do not do "shift" work, I am able to plan time to meet with families, assess their needs, and offer support. I can also assist the staff nurse in caring for the child by doing bedside care while simultaneously providing education. Confidence can be transmitted to the parents that the clinical nurse specialist is skilled in providing direct patient care and values the care given by the staff nurse.

In LS's case, my communication with the mother was hampered by the fact that I spoke no Spanish. An interpreter was obtained to help assess the situation. Even with an interpreter, difficulties arose in determining if the mother really knew what was being said. To find out why the mother visited so infrequently, the social worker was contacted to investigate the situation. She spoke fluent Spanish and learned that the mother was also caring for her brother's child in return for the rent payment, but that she desperately wanted to visit more often. Arrangements were made for her to use the clinic childcare services for her nephew so that she would be able to come to the hospital more frequently. Soon she began visiting regularly. The interactions she had with her infant boy were extremely loving and, even with all his ostomies, she assumed an *en face* position (mother and baby looking at each other), stroked him, and cooed to him. LS responded by maintaining eye contact with his mother whenever she spoke to him.

I began interactions with her by rewarding normal mothering activities, and I enabled her to come to the hospital with a minimum of distractions. Soon she began to bring clothes for her son and, later, teaching was begun related to caring for his ostomies and feeding him via his gastrostomy. Again, her efforts were encouraged. She began to return-demonstrate his care and later do his care without a prior demonstration. Finally, she would come for her visits and begin his care without being asked. Communication related to all of the above activities was carried out with interpreters, gestures, and smiles. Just when it seemed she would soon be ready to bring LS home, another problem presented itself. She was being asked to leave the home of her brother because she could not fulfill the responsibilities of caring for their child and hers as well. LS would require frequent clinic visits for cast changes, monitoring of his weight gain, follow-up of the surgical procedures, and normal pediatric visits. In order for LS to be discharged, it became necessary to find a home and help with transportation to and from clinic visits. With assistance from the public health department, she was established in her own apartment. She seemed excited about the prospect and came to take her son home. She brought a beautiful hand-knit blue outfit in which to bring him home, and when he was all dressed, pictures were taken. Everyone was thrilled he was going home after 2 months in the ICN!

Clinical Nurse Specialist/Health Care Team Communication

Involvement of the health care team in planning and coordinating care is necessary in every institution, but essential in a university hospital due to the multitude of people involved. Specialists of every body system, intensivists and their residents and interns, nurses, social workers, dieticians, chaplains, physical therapists, occupational therapists, and child life workers must be integrated into the child's plan of care. Families can become confused as to exactly who is in charge, and frequently this turmoil consumes their energy, particularly when their child has required a large number of consultations.

The clinical nurse specialist communicates on a variety of levels. First, the clinical nurse specialist role should be clearly defined (Colerick, Mason, & Proulx, 1980) and well-publicized. Visits to the head nurse and meeting with the nursing, medical, and other health professional staff to explain the clinical nurse specialist role are essential to good communication.

The clinical nurse specialist should document all the care delivered on the most appropriate forms. Proper placement of documentation is dependent upon hospital policy and the referral source; thus referrals from nursing indicate written communication should be placed in the nursing notes. Since the ICN nursing staff initiated the referral to see LS, his plan of care was placed in the nursing notes. Of course, if a modification in the medical plan of care was necessary, physician consultation would be sought. Later, when the physicians consulted me about discharge planning, pertinent information was then recorded in the medical progress section of the chart.

Communication is also greatly facilitated by visibility of the clinical nurse specialist (Blake, 1977). Posting a phone or beeper number where one can be reached, informing people when one will be away, and expressing appreciation in verbal or written form will enhance communication by conveying a message of approachability. The clinical nurse specialist should be friendly toward the staff and exhibit enthusiasm for nursing.

IMPACT OF CLINICAL NURSE SPECIALIST INTERVENTION

As the pediatric surgical clinical nurse specialist, I presented the teaching sessions to the mother, with the primary nurse in attendance, coordinated the plans for care, and anticipated discharge needs. In this case, I presented the teaching sessions for two reasons. First, there were no available tracheostomy resource nurses and, second, I used the teaching time to educate the staff nurse as well.

Following a patient for a period of time enables me to detect subtle changes. For example, when casts were put on LS's legs the first time and for several times thereafter, there was no alteration in skin integrity. With the next cast change, I noticed skin breakdown over his lateral malleolus. I requested that the orthopedic surgeon leave windows in the cast so that local wound care could be done. I was then able to follow the progress of his wound healing. Another example related to an order for a formula change. A formula which previously had caused diarrhea was suggested to increase his caloric intake. Having knowledge of previous problems with this formula, I suggested remaining with the current formula and adding polycose and medium chain triglyceride (MCT) oil to increase calories. If the formula change had been started, his stool frequency might have increased and the skin integrity at his colostomy site potentially would have been compromised.

As stated previously, the mortality rate of infants with tracheostomies cared for at home has been dramatically decreased by a comprehensive plan for care at home. Thus far I have been involved in the care of 52 infants with tracheostomies. Together with the health care team, I have coordinated the care of these children, written the educational material for parents, and provided the teaching for parents and nursing staff. Several parents have successfully resuscitated their children and changed the tracheostomy tubes on an emergency basis. I continue to follow these children, and three (including LS) have now been successfully decannulated. One child died from meningitis and one from sudden infant death syndrome. As a result of the team effort and extensive plan of care I have developed, however, none of the children has died or suffered morbidity as a result of their tracheostomy.

Evaluation and validation of the clinical nurse specialist role should occur through periodic examination and attainment of annual goals and objectives. In addition, the three phases of clinical nurse specialist role development—identification, transition, and confirmation—provide a useful reference point from which to qualitatively evaluate the progress of the clinical nurse specialist (Oda, 1977). Input should also be sought from patients and their families, staff nurses, administrative nurses, physicians, and peers as to their appraisal of the role performance.

The clinical nurse specialist can also measure effectiveness in a variety of other ways. For example, is the clinical nurse specialist called at all? Do requests for clinical nurse specialist services increase, decrease, or remain the same? Why? A log can be kept for documentation of these calls. How much of the clinical nurse specialist's recommendations are put into effect? If physician orders are required, in what period of time are they written? Are nurses recommending previous clinical nurse specialist suggestions to physicians in subsequent cases? Another gauge of effectiveness is how the nursing care plan developed by the clinical nurse specialist is followed, and if not, why not? Answers to the preceding questions can also help to evaluate the impact of the clinical nurse specialist.

The nursing staff recognized the expertise of the pediatric surgical clinical nurse specialist, as I was called immediately after LS's tracheostomy was placed. Additionally, the physicians sought my consultation regarding discharge planning. The suggestions of the clinical nurse specialist requiring physicians' orders were immediately put into effect.

Method of Evaluation of Cost Effectiveness

In light of these troubled economic times, the clinical nurse specialist should strive toward quantification of a qualitative role (Walker, 1983). There are inherent problems, however, in measuring cost effectiveness of the pediatric surgical clinical nurse specialist since patient outcomes are difficult to ascribe only to the clinical nurse specialist. For example, decreasing the length of hospitalization, which might be accredited to the clinical nurse specialist, may actually be increased when a language barrier exists necessitating detailed translator services, requests for home nursing services are denied and appeals are necessary, or the parents have special learning needs, such as being deaf, or live a long distance away.

Although evaluating cost effectiveness of the pediatric surgical clinical nurse specialist is difficult, I have undertaken several steps toward this process. Figure 9–2 represents one type of record I keep on every patient. These records are tabulated quarterly in an attempt to document particular unique services that I provide. Analyzing this information might later provide me with an opportunity to develop categories which would determine a fee-for-service scale. Since clinical nurse specialist roles are diverse, complex, and setting-dependent, I believe each clinical nurse specialist will have to share in the essential and immense responsibility for determining cost effectiveness.

PATIENT CONSULT RECORDS

Chart No _____

Service _____

Referral Source _____

Name _____ Birthdate _____

Diagnosis _____

Physician _____ Day of Surgery _____

Admission Date _____ Discharge Date _____

Parents _____

Siblings _____

Address _____ Phone _____

_____

_____

History _____

_____

_____

Date	Intervention	Notes	Time	Code

Code: A = Direct patient care   C = Consultation
      B = Education   D = Research

Figure 9–2. Patient Records

ROLE OF THE CLINICAL NURSE SPECIALIST IN THE PRACTICE SETTING

As the clinical nurse specialist in a staff position, quality of care issues must be discussed with the nursing staff, head nurse, and clinical director, as well as the immediate supervisor, in this instance the director of nursing. Comments should reflect not only the problem to be solved, but also convey a variety of approaches and a willingness to help in their resolution. The staff position allows the clinical nurse specialist to stay at the bedside to provide expert care with fewer administrative responsibilities. In a university setting, however, each clinical nurse specialist is frequently called upon to give expert testimony and participate on committees related to quality assurance, procedures, products, designing of new units, as well as educational planning. Administrative support from the director of nursing provides additional authority for the clinical nurse specialist role to function in an essential position within the university medical center. Fortunately, in this setting peer support is also available to share new ideas, discuss clinical issues which may have ramifications throughout the institution, and provide a forum for peer review, research, and publications.

RESEARCH IN PRACTICE

The selection of a particular area of nursing research should be practice-based according to the particular area of expertise a clinical nurse specialist possesses. As previously mentioned, I have critically reviewed all literature pertinent to infants and children with tracheostomies and discovered an alarmingly high mortality rate without a well-developed home care program. From these study results, I instituted a comprehensive training program for parents of children with tracheostomies. Therefore, by utilizing research findings and other available information, my practice has been enhanced.

Since my role is divided between direct patient care, education, consultation, and research, allocation of time to research often receives the lowest priority. I have many questions, however, and think that as the staff gain additional expertise in this particular area and less direct care interventions by me are necessary, additional time can be directed toward nursing research. Specifically, I would like to evaluate the usefulness of parent support groups with parents of children with tracheostomies, the incidence of granulation tissue developing as a result of suctioning techniques, speech development and training in infants with tracheostomies, and case reviews of infants with tracheal resections and cartilage grafting, to mention a few.

Currently, I am conducting case reviews for every child with a tracheostomy in whose care I participated. To date, because I am the primary person responsible for the program, the conclusion can be made that the intervention by a clinical nurse specialist is an important factor as evidenced by a near-zero mortality rate in children discharged home with a tracheostomy. Evaluation and refinement of the educational materials is being undertaken to make revisions based upon parent and staff input. As a result of these case reviews and parent surveys, patients and their families will receive the benefit of information shared by other parents of infants and children with tracheostomies.

SUMMARY

In this chapter, I have described my role as a pediatric clinical nurse specialist in a busy university medical center. By using the example of caring for a complexly ill infant with VATER syndrome, I have illustrated the critical involvement of the staff nurse in the success of the clinical nurse specialist role. I focused on methods for enhancing this relationship and effectively transferring knowledge to the nursing staff, thus leading to an increase in the overall quality of care provided.

SPECIFIC QUESTIONS

1. Compare and contrast the clinical nurse specialist role as a generalist in this chapter and the subspecialized role in Chapter 10.
2. This author describes the clinical nurse specialist as walking a fine line, being careful not to assume the care from the staff nurse but to augment it. Discuss the methods she uses for doing this and their applicability to your practice setting.
3. Discuss the effectiveness of the methods described in this chapter to transfer advanced knowledge and expertise to staff nurses.
4. Compare the Patient Consult Record with the Patient Information Card in Chapter 5. How would you design one for your own use?

REFERENCES

Aradine, C. (1980). Home care for young children with long-term tracheostomies. *Maternal Child Nursing (MCN)*, 5 (2), 121–125.

Barnes, J.C., & Smith, W.L. (1978). The VATER association. *Radiology, 126*, 445–450.

Blake, P. (1977). The clinical specialist as nurse consultant. *Journal of Nursing Administration, 7* (10), 33–66.

Colerick, E.J., Mason, P.B., & Proulx, J.R. (1980). Evaluation of the clinical nurse specialist role: Development and implementation of a dual purpose framework. *Nursing Leadership, 3* (3), 26–34.

Howell, L.J. (1980). *Preschool children after open heart surgery: Parental childrearing practices.* Master's thesis, University of California, San Francisco.

MacPhail, J. (1971). Reasonable expectations for the nurse clinician. *Journal of Nursing Administration, 1* (5), 16–18.

Oda, D.S. (1977). Specialized role development: A three-phase process. *Nursing Outlook, 25*, 374–377.

Ruben, R.J., Newton, L., Jornsay, D., et al. (1982). Home care of the pediatric patient with a tracheostomy. *Annals of Otology, Rhinology, and Laryngology, 91*, 633–640.

Tucker, J.A., & Silberman, H.D. (1972). Tracheotomy in pediatrics. *Annals of Otology, Rhinology, and Laryngology, 81*, 818–824.

Walker, D. (1983). Administrative utilization of the CNS. In A. Hamric & J. Spross (Eds.), *The CNS in theory and practice*. Orlando, FL: Grune & Stratton.

Wetmore, R.F., Handler, S.D., & Potsic, W.P. (1982). Pediatric tracheostomy experience during the past decade. *Annals of Otology Rhinology Larynogology 91*, 628–632.

chapter ten

The Surgical Clinical Nurse Specialist in a Tertiary Setting: Establishing a Subspecialty

Diane M. Cooper

Because of the diversity of conditions and level of illness of patients in tertiary care centers, specialization on the part of health care professionals in these settings has become a necessity. As a result, and in order to better meet the needs of patients, clinical nurse specialists employed in tertiary settings often develop and refine skills in subspecialties of the more generic speciality areas in which they were originally prepared. With this approach, increased numbers of clinical nurse specialists can focus on precise aspects of patient care and, combining their expertise, create an environment where the possibility of the patients' recovery and ongoing health are maximized.

The processes of role acquisition and role clarification take time; because of this the novice clinical nurse specialist is wise not to subspecialize. Frequently there is little need or desire for subspecialization until the clinical nurse specialist has been in the role for some time and has achieved some measure of success. As skills develop and a certain degree of comfort and acceptance in the role are experienced, the clinical nurse specialist is able to identify areas of particular interest or unmet patient care needs that can form the impetus for developing a subspecialty. At this juncture in role evolution, the climate for success in a subspecialty is enhanced.

Establishing oneself in the role of the clinical nurse specialist has been a topic of ongoing discussion (Hamric, 1983; Hamric & Spross, 1983; Henderson, 1981; Oda, 1977). Establishing oneself anew in a subspecialty, particularly one not assumed previously by nurses, creates a different set of challenges, some of which will be discussed in this chapter. Prior to role acquisition in either case, however, all clinical nurse specialists must be firmly grounded in the definition of the clinical nurse specialist as set forth in *Nursing: A Social Policy Statement* (American Nurses Association, 1980). It becomes apparent from reading the document that the clinical nurse specialist must function simultaneously as expert clinician, teacher, consultant, and researcher. A grasp of the synergy of these role components is essential to success in the role, whether the clinical nurse specialist functions in a broad area of practice or declares a subspeciality.

Besides incorporating the four role components into one's everyday efforts, the clinical nurse specialist must also be keenly aware of the metaparadigm concepts of nursing, namely that nursing's focus, its "rootedness" lies in attention to person, environment, health, and nursing (Fawcett, 1984a, 1984b). A clear grasp of and commitment to the meaning of these concepts insures that all clinical nurse specialists, but particularly those assuming subspecialties, will be perceived by nurses and other members of the health care team as being exquisitely clear about the focus of their work. A further enhancement, particularly in subspecialization, would be the selection of a nursing model by the clinical nurse specialist (Fawcett, 1984a). Careful attention to selection, testing, and translation of the model into one's everyday practice can serve both as a challenging guide and an underpinning to one's work with patients, as well as a means by which the clinical nurse specialist can assess effectiveness as an *advanced* nurse practitioner (Crawford-Gamble, 1986).

Although to some readers these introductory comments may seem obvious and to others academic, they are put forth to make the point that ambiguity about one's area of practice or perspective in approaching the patient has no part in the role of the clinical nurse specialist, particularly the clinical nurse specialist who chooses to subspecialize (Baker, 1973; Topham, 1987). Neither patients, nurses, nor other members of the health care team should be confused about what it is the clinical nurse specialist does, nor whether or not it is appropriate for a *nurse* to be doing it. The case study to be presented serves as a medium for examining one clinical nurse specialist's efforts at role refinement in the development of a subspecialty of surgical nursing.

Case Study

During nursing kardex rounds, the following patient was presented as "not progressing." His abdominal wound was described by the nurses as "worrisome," and it was evident that they were seeking assistance with assessment of his status, overall coordination of care, improved planning between nursing and medicine, and reclarification of the immediate and long-range goals of the patient's therapy.

JM was a 42-year-old white male who, though educated as a lawyer, had functioned for some years as the owner of a large corporation. At the time of the hospitalization under discussion, he had been divorced for a number of years. Two of his three teenaged children resided with their mother; his third child was away at college. JM lived the fast-paced life of the modern-day individual "on the move." He was affluent, extremely involved in his business ventures, and driven by self-defined goals of monetary and personal success. For a number of years prior to this admission he had suffered from ulcerative colitis and, after long-term treatment with steroids and other regimens, as well as repeated flare-ups, he had now chosen to undergo abdominal surgery. JM was well aware that the operation could result in the creation of either a temporary or permanent ileostomy. Both he and his surgeon hoped this procedure would reverse his chronically ill state and return him to a more normal existence. During the operation, however, JM's bowel was discovered to be so diseased that a more extensive surgical procedure, namely an abdominal-perineal resection, was performed. This resulted in removal of diseased portions of intestines, including removal of the rectum and creation of a permanent ileostomy. The postoperative course was troublesome; JM became severely septic twice, necessitating his return to the operating room on one occasion for exploration of an acute abdomen. Subsequently his original large abdominal incision (xiphoid to pubic bone) dehisced, and the wound was left open to heal by second intention. Because of the long-term steroid treatment JM had undergone in the initial treatment of his disease and the serious drain on his physical reserves as the result of a "bumpy" postoperative course, healing was severely retarded. Numerous setbacks occurred and JM's entire recuperative course was protracted. After approximately 3 months of diligent medical and nursing care, however, JM was discharged. To the delight of the staff, and the amazement of some, JM returned to his home where initially he was assisted in his daily care by his parents. Ultimately, and in fact as he had done with every milestone, ahead of schedule, JM returned to work and, as far as we know, to his previous way of life.

CLINICAL NURSE SPECIALIST INTERVENTION

Once it becomes apparent that the specific services I am able to offer are required by a patient, several factors determine the extent of my involvement. The following list enumerates the guidelines I use to determine the degree of my clinical nurse specialist involvement in direct patient care situations:

1. The acuity of the patient as assessed by the nurses through the use of the patient classification system
2. Whether the patient is on a unit where the nurses are specialized in the care of the problem for which they seek my intervention, or whether the patient is "boarding" on a unit where the nurses are skilled in the care of other patient populations
3. The level of collaboration in the relationship between the attending physician and the nursing staff
4. The general knowledge of the nursing staff of the method of treatment, or approach to care, being utilized

5. The amount of time and depth of previous interactions I have had with staff members on similar nursing care problems
6. The number of previous visits I had made to this particular patient
7. The degree of involvement, clinical knowledge, and accountability for follow-up on patient care issues evidenced by the administrative nurse (AN) and assistant administrative nurse (AAN)
8. Assessment of staff compliance with previous nursing care plans
9. The level of activity on the unit at this time
10. The staff-to-patient ratio as seen in nurse/patient assignments
11. The level of clinical expertise of the nurse caring for the patient (e.g. clinical nurse III, clinical nurse II, clinical nurse I, licensed practical nurse)
12. The degree of involvement of other clinical nurse specialists on this particular case, and the clarity with which it had been determined which specialist had assumed primary responsibility for coordination
13. The type of consultation being solicited by the nursing staff (i.e., expert, resource, etc.)
14. Assessment of current patient progress with the care plan as formulated
15. The specific patient problem for which my input is requested

Although staff on the units of patients undergoing major surgery had become increasingly clear about my capabilities in my area of subspecialization (i.e., wound healing) and thus were initiating appropriate referrals, as well as negotiating an appropriate degree of involvement, initially this was not the case elsewhere. As a result of the "word spreading" regarding successful interventions by me in the treatment of wounds, an increasing number of referrals were instituted from all over the hospital.

Initially I responded to all calls for wound care consultations. This deviation from the guidelines listed above was deliberate and occurred only in the early months of subspecialty acquisition. I responded to all calls because I strongly desired to increase my exposure to and demonstrate my availability for assistance with a broad range of wound care problems. Additionally, I noticed that a good number of nurses and physicians lacked knowledge of the theory underlying approaches to wound care and that they increasingly accepted the necessity for organized, theory-based, coordinated wound management. I also gained personal satisfaction from promoting healing and wholeness in patients with alterations in structural integrity.

Soon, however, responding to all calls for wound care consultations became overwhelming. Often the solution to the patient situation seemed obvious to me, and I felt myself stating the same approach to care so frequently that I became weary. In each case, though, I tried to remember that the nurse appropriately had sought my consultation.

It is easy for the consultant to forget the energy required by the individual requesting a consultation. In addition to the time involved in placing the call, the busy nurse also manifests vulnerability in seeking help from another, as well as revealing concern for quality care. At the same time, the nurse acknowledges varying levels of nursing expertise. Exposing one's values by seeking input from a clinical nurse specialist can involve risk. In responding to some requests for consultation, I had to remind myself of the influence I could have on patient care if I took the time to repeat, even if for the "thousandth time," the theory underlying various approaches to healing. Ultimately I knew a day would come when the nurses would request my services again and I could remind them of what they had already learned. In subsequent requests for consultation I could positively reinforce their selection of appropriate therapies. Finally, I could begin to build on the knowledge the nurses had already mastered. To this end, in the early stages of role subspecialization, I kept the names of the nurses who requested wound consultations. When these nurses consulted me appropriately on several occasions, or when I observed a high level of input on their part, I addressed a letter praising their initiative and clinical practice to their administrative nurse. I included a copy of this letter to the assistant director of nursing for that area as well as to the nurse being singled out. Utilizing this method of recognition served to reinforce the value I placed on quality nursing care and on utilization of nursing resources. Aware of the increased number of referrals in the initial stage of the assumption of my subspecialty, I also provided unit inservices when a new approach to wound care was being introduced. As a consequence, I was able to expect the same degree of accountability for the implementation of the suggested therapy from the staff in attendance as I had previously expected from the individual clinical nurses who had approached me. Thus many benefits were reaped from sharing knowledge and overextending myself in the early days of role refinement. In addition to insuring that more patients were treated with optimal therapies, multiple nurses could now implement treatments on their own.

The effect of the introduction of the subspecialty in wound healing was significant. Nurses were learning new theory and new interventions, and were responding positively to this change. Often I observed them manifesting a sense of pride and personal satisfaction in learning new approaches to care which, in turn, they were able to suggest to physicians and to other nurses. Additionally, educating staff in new approaches to patient care resulted in them challenging me and pushing me toward more complex patient situations. Consequently, as time progressed, I was freer to turn to the complex wound care situations because nurses all over the hospital were growing in their expertise.

Knowing that nurses on various units were increasingly competent in wound care assisted me in determining the degree of input I would need to have on specific units. Because I had kept records of the unit inservices, I could rapidly recall what knowledge base could be expected. Furthermore, I also was aware of nurses who had attended continuing education programs I had offered. Through review of my records I could identify clusters of nurses with strong, evolving backgrounds in wound care throughout the hospital. In a fashion similar to that already described, I took time to acknowledge excellence in wound care on a nursing unit in general. Here, however, I addressed the letter of praise to the assistant director of nursing and the director of nursing, but I still sent a copy to the nursing unit staff.

The majority of writings on the clinical nurse specialist conclude that the strength of the role lies embedded in the clinical nurse specialist's level of expertise as a clinician, coupled with the ability to transmit that expertise to others (Fenton, 1985; Steele & Fenton, 1988). Although clinical nurse specialists must always maintain their ability to act independently in patient care situations, their worth is measured by how well they "give away" their knowledge and skill, thereby elevating the overall quality of care. With this in mind, it has been my practice to always include the nurse(s) in every aspect of a patient's care, whatever the extent of my involvement. In all cases, the patient must be kept as the joint focus of the nursing staff and the clinical nurse specialist. Once I receive a referral, all patient assessments include the nurse(s) responsible for direct care. In most situations, the nurse accompanies me to the patient's bedside where she points out and describes the specific patient problem. This approach affords the nurse the opportunity to observe my assessment, seek clarification regarding uncertainties, and hear the patient/clinical nurse specialist interaction that occurs. For my part, seeing the patient jointly with the nurse allows me the opportunity to gain precise input from the nurse regarding the patient care problem. Underlying the exchange is a concern on my part that patients be introduced to the "outside" consultant by someone familiar to them. Successfully implemented, this initial assessment also serves to validate the skills of the clinical nurse (i.e., staff nurse) in the eyes of the patient and to convey to patients and their families the concern for patient care exhibited by the nursing staff. Regardless, all of this occurs with the patient's nurse clearly maintaining responsibility for the implementation of quality care, both in my eyes and, perhaps more importantly, in the eyes of the patient. Ideally, this approach also serves to teach the involved nurses skills they will utilize with future patients, thereby raising the quality of care on a long-term basis.

In JM's case, the nurses had assumed a great deal of initiative and responsibility for his total care. They looked to me for input as a resource and an expert. My initial interaction with JM occurred shortly after his return from the intensive care unit (ICU) following the episode of acute sepsis. At that time he was in full isolation and was receiving direct care from special duty registered nurses.

For several days staff nurses had observed JM's deteriorating state, manifested most graphically by an increasing number of episodes of altered mentation and the gaping, nonhealing, purulent abdominal wound. The nurses' level of concern regarding this patient evolved from their expertise and experience in caring for patients with his level of illness. It was imperative, then, that an outcome of their request for a consultation acknowledge their expertise and their readiness for learning new information. All staff involved with JM needed to feel included and important in each phase of the consultation.

The initial interaction with JM required a Class IV assessment (see Table 10–1). This involved a full review of his chart, including review of the surgical procedure performed, the medical orders, trends in lab values, and the overall progression of the plan as recorded in the nurses' notes. The medical progress notes were reviewed, as well as the written nursing care plan. Because JM's most apparent nursing problems, as assessed by the nurses and myself, were his deteriorating mental state and seriously compromised healing status, these became the prime foci of my attention.

Obviously, it was imperative early on that I be present at JM's dressing change. This tedious process, for both patient and nurse, revealed a wound with copious, purulent drainage, an adjacent ileostomy, and multiple drains. JM was in pain during the procedure, despite medication. He verbalized repulsion at his wound, his ileostomy, and his generalized dependent condition. Additionally, he appeared fearful of a situation over which he obviously lacked control. He sought guarantees regarding his future state of health.

The clinical nurse specialist is expected to act as a synthesizer and priority-setter of patient care needs. Furthermore, it is vital that the clinical nurse specialist bring to the patient situation a "bag of sound tricks" that, if carefully selected, will address the identified patient needs. Skill in selection of the most appropriate approach to the patient care problem, as well as conviction in the potential for positive outcome of the approach selected, are marks of the degree of expertise of one clinical nurse specialist over another.

Although JM was being supported maximally via total parenteral nutrition, antibiotics, and frequent respiratory treatments, the local care of his wound, on my initial consultation, was of an extremely traditional nature. Due to the volume of exudate, the treatment observed during my initial assessment required dressing changes every 2 to 4 hours. The tissue within JM's wound appeared greyish-pink and devoid of healthy, beefy-red granulation tissue. Moist, opaque exudate covered the walls of his wound and pooled in the base. Epithelial migration was nonapparent. Retention suture sites were purulent, taut, and encrusted with old secretions.

The patient was not receiving extra vitamins nor the 25,000 units of vitamin A suggested by some as beneficial during the steroid-dependent patients' initial postoperative period (Cooper, 1989; Ehrlich & Hunt, 1968; Hunt, 1976; Hunt, Ehrlich, Garcia, & Dunphy, 1969). At the conclusion of this first assessment, it was my recommendation to discontinue the current approach to wound care and to turn instead to treatment with Debrisan (dextranomer) twice daily. Not only is this therapy documented to be highly effective in wounds with moist exudate, but furthermore it is known to have chemotactic properties (Freeman, Carwell, & McCraw, 1981; Jacobsson et al., 1976; Oredsson, Gottrup, Beckmann, & Hohn, 1983). Among other things, increased migration of white blood cells into the wound was clearly needed in this immunosuppressed patient. In addition, reducing JM's dressing change schedule to once every 12 hours would afford him greater rest periods, hopefully less pain, and decreased stress over the thought of a painful and personally repulsive treatment.

The suggested change in approach to care was discussed with the resident following my initial observation. In addition, a lengthy note including an overall assessment of JM's status, suggestions for the alternative approach with Debrisan described above, and a statement describing my willingness to be integrally involved in the implementation of the plan was placed in the medical progress notes. I also referred to several pertinent articles on Debrisan (cited above), which I placed in the front of the chart, but not before I inscribed my name on them lest anyone be unaware of their source.

This meticulously formulated consultation went unheeded. Neither the resident, chief resident, nor the attending physician acknowledged it, either verbally or in subsequent written entries. It is important to point out that, up until this time, the attending surgeon had not utilized my services. Despite my meeting with him, during which time I described my role, his general approach to me appeared skeptical. Both the nurses and I found the rejection of our suggestions regarding JM disconcerting.

The situation described above is not without merit, however. Too often staff nurses feel that if only they had more "clout" they could accomplish great things. The lack of acceptance of the clinical nurse specialist's suggestions in JM's case clearly shows that advanced degrees and clinical expertise alone are not sufficient to result in immediate changes in behavior on the part of physicians. The fact that the orders suggested for JM went unheeded maximally tapped my creativity and professionalism, and demanded effective role modeling on my part. It is in circumstances such as these that clinical nurses observe the clinical nurse specialist's skill in areas beside mastery of physiological content.

The way the clinical nurse specialist handles rejection of suggestions can act as a basis for staff's future interactions with and reaction to the physicians involved. The clinical nurse specialist must assume responsibility for ensuring that the staff's subsequent behavior with physicians will be effective, constructive, and always oriented toward the good of the patient.

Despite the lack of acknowledgment of the suggested changes in the plan, it became my daily routine to be present at JM's morning dressing change, often assisting directly with the care. My strategy was not only to be able to observe progression or regression in healing, but to clearly demonstrate to the nurses, and the physicians, the level of involvement that I intended to maintain with this patient (Fenton, 1985). At the conclusion of each dressing change, I entered an evaluatory note in the chart, clearly writing my title and beeper number after my name. After several days of little progress, if not deterioration in the wound status, I again suggested the Debrisan approach to the resident. As before, it was heard but rejected as "unnecessary."

Fenton (1985) stated that one of the emerging characteristics of clinical nurse specialists which breeds success is "the ability to assert oneself in nurse–physician interactions with the expectation that the nurse is going to provide input" (p. 34). Even if as a result of such an interaction changes are not immediately apparent, confronting the situation directly often pays off in the long run. Knowing that the situation with JM was becoming serious, I approached the attending physician directly. Despite the interaction and although cordial, the petition for change in wound care management was again denied. It is only fair to point out that this rejection could have been based on several factors, one of which was the newness and unorthodox nature of the therapy I was suggesting. Not only was I an unknown to the attending surgeon as far as my capabilities in wound care management were concerned, but the treatment modality I was suggesting was unusual and not generally used on postsurgical wounds at that time.

Several days passed, and I continued to be present at the dressing change, as well as at the medical team discussions. Though quiet during these interactions, my presence was obvious. After approximately one and one-half weeks, the attending physician, seeing that wound healing was not progressing, sought me out and stated that he would write orders initiating the therapy I had suggested. It was clear from this interaction that the attending physician remained skeptical and that he initiated these orders on a temporary basis. Nevertheless, he had acknowledged me and was implicitly indicating that I might have something to offer his patient. Needless to say, the nurses and I felt that a great deal of coordinated effort and persistence had resulted in improved treatment for JM.

For the next week or so, this patient consumed a great deal of time;

besides formulating a detailed care plan which was copied and placed inside the patient's room, I also performed both dressing changes (assisted by the special duty registered nurse) on the first few days. Thereafter I attended only the morning change and gradually transferred the care to staff.

Among the other strategies I used to ensure JM's progress and the maximization of the plan was a request for continuity of the special duty nurses. The administrative nurse, who was aware of and involved in all aspects of this patient's plan, scheduled the nurses to provide the necessary continuity. The special duty nurses who assisted us in the early phase of this plan's implementation were excellent and I praised them frequently, not only privately but publicly in front of other nurses as well as the residents. Although the clinical nurse IIIs (senior staff nurses) on the unit had been involved all along, the administrative nurse and I selected several who were particularly concerned about JM and interested in learning more about wound care to oversee his daily needs.

A unit conference was arranged to discuss JM and the new approach to wound care. Likewise, and of extreme importance, the change in approach to wound care was described to the patient. He was shown Debrisan beads, and their mechanism of action was explained. He was also informed of the increased time between dressing changes that would ensue. It was important for him to realize that the longer time interval between dressing changes did not indicate staff were being less diligent or that less frequent dressing changes could result in further deterioration of his status. Although, initially, dressing changes were performed at times selected by me and the staff to facilitate observation of the wound by the physicians, JM was eventually approached regarding the times he would like the dressing changed. The goal of this latter action was to increase JM's control over his care, as well as to increase the likelihood of increased nutritional intake and rest on his part. Even early on, rest times were established. The special duty nurses were informed that these periods were to be observed as a part of care equally important as other aspects. Both physicians and nurses were informed of the schedule, which was posted on the door to JM's room. As a result, interruptions were reduced to a minimum.

Within 3 to 4 days of instituting Debrisan (dextranomer), marked improvement in the condition of the wound was apparent. At this point, I personally sought out the attending physician and scheduled a time with him to observe the wound. He was amazed at the progress. This is a day clearly etched in my mind; it signaled my "rite of passage" as a clinical nurse specialist in wound care with this skeptical surgeon. All the strategizing had been worth it. As the attending physician acknowledged the progress apparent in the wound, JM's face beamed, the nurses present stood taller as they took pride in what we had accomplished, and I felt the surgeon acknowledge me as a colleague instead of a foe.

Spurred on by the feedback they had received, and expert in the techniques in which I had instructed them, the staff assumed more and more involvement in JM's care, including promoting his independence in managing his ileostomy. Soon the extent of my involvement was reduced, although I continued to be present daily for at least one dressing change. These daily visits were important in many ways; besides allowing me an opportunity to assess the wound and decide whether or not changes in the care plan were required, they allowed me a predictable amount of time in which to communicate with JM. Although he was withdrawn and groggy in the early stage of his illness, we eventually established a significant relationship. On reflection, I became aware of the fact that I was the most continuous nursing figure in this man's recovery. The status he ascribed to me was evident when at one point he refused to allow modifications in the wound care regimen without my first being consulted. Though the attending physician and I were in constant communication regarding changes in orders, this behavior on the patient's part was significant to me.

As time progressed, JM and I discussed discharge plans, the events in his life he felt had contributed to his altered health status, as well as how he intended to modify his lifestyle posthospitalization. Although I continued to be the clinical nurse specialist primarily responsible for his care, the staff and I sought input from the psychiatric liaison clinical nurse specialist on an ongoing basis. There were times when JM would become extremely frustrated with his loss of strength, with the presence and permanence of the ileostomy, with the confines of his isolation room, with the protracted nature of his healing, and with the potential threat of altered sexual function as a result of his extensive surgical procedure.

Just before JM's discharge I visited him and, in the course of our discussion, he verbalized many of his frustrations; soon he became angry. The anger progressed, and in a matter of minutes his frustration was full blown and directed at me. I was stunned. I felt as if I had been kicked in the stomach and wanted to scream back at him, reminding him of all I had done for him. Instead, I retreated to the nurses' conference room where I tried to regain my composure and make some sense out of what had just occurred. I was hurt, and my initial reaction was to withdraw totally from JM. Suddenly, out of the distant past, I recalled the "Phases of the Nurse/Patient Relationship" suggested by Hildegard Peplau (1952). I remembered that often, in the phases of exploitation and termination, the patient must push the nurse away in order to move on and regain healthy independence. I was reminded that these were necessary occurrences in the total healing process and that they occurred most successfully in situations in which nurses had created a safe and trusting environment. Being accepted, supported, and allowed to evolve is one way the sick individual, restored of his structural integrity, moves on to restore his personal and social integrity (Levine, 1967, 1969a, 1969b, 1971, 1973).

At the time of the incident, several clinical nurses who were aware of the scenario described above came into the conference room to "console" me. They had overheard our interaction and were furious with JM. Although I accepted their consolation and acknowledged my hurt feelings, I was sustained by the writings of Peplau and Levine and discussed them with the nurses present. Though JM later apologized for his outburst, this final phase of our hospital relationship helped me to value anew my theory-based preparation. Technical skills alone, advanced physiological or psychological knowledge in itself, or excellent communication skills are insufficient of themselves to predict success as a clinical nurse specialist. It is the blending of all these factors, and an ongoing commitment to refining all of one's skills in caring for the total patient, that are the marks of a superior clinical nurse specialist (Steele & Fenton, 1988). JM had caused me to recognize the full impact of these realities and for that reason my experiences with him will long be remembered.

Method of Patient Selection

In addition to informing as many nursing staff as possible of my availability for wound care consultations, routine and systematic methods of identifying patients who might benefit from my services were also employed. Among the other means of identifying patients were nursing rounds and a close, supportive, trusting relationship with regular interaction between the various administrative nurses, assistant administrative nurses, and myself.

Nursing Kardex Rounds. Each week, on the same day and at the same time, nursing kardex rounds were held on the units with which I was involved. The day and hour had been established early in this process through joint agreement between the administrative nurse and nursing staff. The time selected for the rounds was one judged to allow the greatest number of staff to be present and not be interrupted. All attempts were made to meet at this time despite the tenor on the unit, in order to ensure the predictable nature and significance of this meeting. Furthermore, nursing kardex rounds were scheduled to occur prior to, and thus prepare for, another set of weekly rounds known as management rounds.

Management rounds were those meetings attended by the chief resident, the nursing staff, the nutritionist, and clinical nurse specialists involved in the care of specific patients on the unit. The focus of management rounds included clarification of the medical plan, discussion of the particular surgical procedure(s) undertaken on the patient(s), questions/suggestions regarding the patient's current status, clarification of approximate discharge date, and overall goals of therapy. Though management rounds frequently involved two-way discussion among the nursing staff and chief resident, they focused heavily on the *medical* aspects of patient management. Nursing kardex rounds, on the other hand, dealt with patients in a broader context. With the presence of the administrative nurse, assistant administrative nurse, primary nurse(s), the nutritionist, other clinical nurse specialists involved in particular cases, and myself, nursing kardex rounds provided a forum where multiple current and future concerns regarding an individual patient's care, as well as standards of nursing care regarding similar patients, could be addressed.

Format of Nursing Kardex Rounds. The format for nursing kardex rounds was as follows: the primary nurse, or nurse in charge of a cluster of patients, presented the patient to those in attendance. This included a short background on the patient, current status, and questions or concerns the nurse had identified regarding the patient's total care. Often these rounds afforded attendees the opportunity to teach; over time the level of information shared and expected advanced.

A positive aspect of nursing kardex rounds was the atmosphere created, which made it comfortable for anyone to ask any question that might arise and to receive feedback. Nurses did not have to "perform." They were not being graded or appraised by other non-nurse members of the health care team, so their genuine concern for the patients and the quality of nursing care issues could be raised in an unhindered manner. An additional service these rounds provided was preparation for management rounds. Because nursing kardex rounds were scheduled prior to management rounds, nurses, having assessed patient care issues on the previous day at nursing kardex rounds, could go to management rounds primed with salient questions regarding management. In this manner issues were addressed and patient care progressed expediently.

With regard to my role in particular, nursing kardex rounds served a number of purposes. First, because of my weekly attendance, staff came to know that this was a predictable time when they could pose questions easily about specific patients or request my involvement. Second, these rounds afforded me an opportunity to be seen as a knowledgeable resource, to be viewed as an integral part of the care of patients within my specialty, to serve as a somewhat objective "inquirer" who, because of relative distance from the moment-to-moment events on the unit, could raise issues or point out areas of concern that might not have been thought of by the nurses or physicians who were closer to the situation. Finally, nursing kardex rounds allowed me to identify specific patients with whom I should become directly involved, if staff had not already requested this. Suggesting the involvement of other clinical nurse specialists was an additional role I played in the early days of nursing kardex rounds. Not only did this last activity demonstrate support for my peers, but frequently the suggestion of a particular clinical nurse specialist provided an opportunity for clarification of their unique qualifications. In some cases, such clarification resulted in the clinical nurse specialist's ongoing interaction with the unit.

Although not directly related to patient selection, nursing kardex rounds also allowed me to act as a visible supporter of the standard of care set by the administrative nurse and her staff. Likewise, I assisted in actualizing the philosophy of the department of nursing, which addressed the ready availability of clinical resources aimed at improving patient care through the stimulation and growth of staff (UCSF, 1983). Nursing kardex rounds also served as a method of determining staff's inservice needs and acted as a gauge by which the general temperament of the staff could be evaluated. This latter assessment frequently afforded the administrative nurse and me an opportunity to provide input to the psychiatric liaison clinical nurse specialist about unit or patient issues that might require her discussion or resolution. Nurses who attended nursing kardex rounds on a regular basis, having listened to the series of questions asked by me on a repeated basis, eventually incorporated into their own practice assessment criteria for evaluating clusters of conditions.

It could be said that nursing kardex rounds afforded me the opportunity to offer input on *all* patients on the service. The amount of direct involvement in each case, however, was determined by criteria discussed previously. (see Clinical Nurse Specialist Intervention).

Attending Rounds. Prior to the appearance of clinical nurse specialists, the hierarchy in nursing had followed a more traditional pattern. Clinical nurse specialists signaled the implementation of a clinical ladder (Colavecchio, Tescher, & Scalzi, 1974) and the overt recognition of varying levels of nursing expertise (Hirsch et al. 1987). Until that time, medical management had been viewed as dominant. With the changes came the opportunity for increased collaboration between nurses and physicians.

With this in mind, before I had chosen a subspecialty, I decided it was necessary that, along with the pharmacist, pharmacy students, and nutritionist, I also be present at "attending rounds." This set of rounds consisted of interns presenting all the service's cases. Status reports on the patients were presented by the interns and residents, and the proposed operative procedures were discussed with the attending physician.

During the several years I sat in on these rounds, I was the only nurse present and, though the vast majority of cases focused on discussion of the optimal surgical approach, these rounds did provide me with cues regarding nursing care issues. Attending rounds also alerted me to particular patients with whom I should become involved and became another source of identifying patients.

With the exception of the first few weeks of my tenure in the role of clinical nurse specialist for major abdominal surgery and, later, wound care, however, it became unnecessary for me to actively seek out patients; I was never without a full case load. The major sources of patient referrals were nurses and physicians throughout the institution, although I also received requests from physical therapists and nutritionists. Nursing kardex rounds and attending rounds, however, remained steady checkpoints, reassuring me about patients with whom I was already involved and pointing out other patient situations requiring investigation. Although weekly attendance at several sets of rounds may seem tedious to some, these forums served this clinical nurse specialist well as sources for selecting patients.

Criteria for Appropriateness of Method and Amount of Intervention

In an attempt to objectively document my involvement with patients, I adapted an approach originally suggested by Welch-McCaffrey (Welch-McCaffrey & D'Agostino, 1984) and described in Chapter 5 of this book. Utilizing that format, I established a classification system for fre-

TABLE 10-1. ACUITY OF WOUND CARE CONSULTATIONS

Class	Example of Type of Intervention	Approximate Time
I	Re-evaluation of satisfactory ongoing treatment Brief progress note Short interaction with nurse assigned to the patient Brief interaction with patient regarding his/her assessment of the plan and progress	10 minutes
II	Observation of moderately complex dressing change on which I had already consulted and formulated a plan Re-application of polyurethene sheet More detailed progress note and brief discussion with nurse	20 minutes
III	Assistance with and re-evaluation of complex dressing change Updating of written plan Progress note with request to change medical orders Discussion and some informal teaching with RN(s) Brief clarification of plan changes with AN	30-45 minutes
IV	Complete evaluation of patient with a complex wound Assistance with direct wound care of a complex wound Initial formulation of a written nursing care plan, coupled with progress note and clearly delineated request for new orders Teaching of staff to ensure proper implementation of new plan for wound care	60-90 minutes

quently requested activities. To create the system, I reviewed individual patient cards—3 × 5 cards on which I kept the patient's name, diagnosis, referral source, consult requested, action taken, and time required to complete the call. The information noted revealed clusters of activities I performed repeatedly, as well as time frames by which I could begin to determine levels of interventions. With time, descriptions of my activities during consultations became increasingly refined. From year to year, the complexity of requested consultations increased. Yearly analysis of the evolving nature of consultations assisted me in evaluating whether or not my presence in the institution affected the quality of care. Additionally, information on these cards provided a source for inservice needs among staff, as well as potential areas for research. An example of a "roughly hewn" classification system formulated in the early phases of role reclarification is presented in Table 10–1.

Clinical Nurse Specialist Communication with the Patient and Health Care Team

Communication occurs on multiple levels and in many ways. Clinical nurse specialists are often assessed and evaluated by others on the basis of the manner of their communication. Whatever it is that is communicated forms the substance on which assessments by staff and others are made of the individual in the role. Even the clothing selected by a clinical nurse specialist has meaning (Beecroft & Papenhausen, 1988). For the surgical clinical nurse specialist in particular, lab coats make a statement, as do uniforms. In my experience, lab coats convey academia and distance from the physical care of the patient, while uniforms convey a readiness to be involved in direct care. Where, when, and what attire is selected by the clinical nurse specialist should be considered in relation to the message intended. Other nonverbal communicators, such as the time one arrives at work, the time one leaves work, the availability of the clinical nurse specialist to staff, all give messages about the availability, the enthusiasm, and the professionalism of the individual in the role.

The promptness with which the clinical nurse specialist responds to requests for help with patient care issues, the tone of voice used on the phone, the affect used in listening to a question or request, the compliment given or not given to staff involved in direct patient care all relay a message. The praise that is accepted solely for oneself, or that acknowledges the *joint* efforts of the clinical nurse specialist and staff, never falls on deaf ears. Role modeling for collaboration and vigilance concerning the maintenance of a patient-centered focus all serve to communicate and promote a constructive milieu. The support given peers and the ability to give honest, constructive feedback to individuals in need of it all are translated by those observing the actions of the clinical nurse specialist. The clinical nurse specialist, then, like anyone with additional expectations, needs to be acutely aware of the impact of nonverbal language. Whether verbal or nonverbal, the clinical nurse specialist's abilities in communication act as determinants of success in a way that is second only to skills as a clinician. Some of the methods of communication utilized in JM's case have been described already. For the sake of clarity, however, they will be reviewed.

Patient. Depending on the patient's physical status, it is my practice to ask the nurse who accompanies me to introduce me and explain who I am and my purpose for being called to see the patient. When initially observing JM's wound, I doubt he was aware of my presence. As he became more lucid, however, introduction and clarification regarding my involvement in his case was necessary. If the plan of care changed, this was discussed with the patient and his family. I make it a habit to indicate when I will return to both patient and nurses and, if appropriate, I leave my business card at the patient's bedside. Leaving this card helps to remind the patient who I am and what my credentials are. Often in the hospital setting, particularly the tertiary care setting, introductions are confusing. It can be comforting to the patient to clarify identities at a later date, as well as be aware of how I may be contacted.

In subsequent visits I ask the patient if there is any objection to discussing the wound with the nurses present. It has been my observation that gradually the patient not only looks forward to this discussion but also eventually enjoys becoming involved in it. In all, I attempt to communicate to the patient reassurance and the attitude that it is our purpose to provide the best care possible and that neither patient nor family should be disheartened (Benner, 1984). Before leaving, any patient inquiries are addressed.

Physician. Communication with the surgeon greatly determines the surgical clinical nurse specialist's latitude in direct patient care, particularly the clinical nurse specialist for wound care. Communication is best if it is direct and occurs at the lowest level possible. Keeping this dictum in mind in JM's case, I approached residents first. Attempts were made to provide them with adequate information to support the changes I was recommending in the plan. Even if the changes in JM's care plan had been accepted immediately, I still would have written a detailed note in the medical progress notes. My entry there always begins with the title "Nursing," and on completing the note my name, full title, and beeper number are recorded. Initially, I duplicated this entire note in the nursing notes section of the chart. This duplication was based on the rationale that I did not want to communicate to nurses that their notes were less important. Soon, however, this duplication became unmanageable and I modified the entry in the nurses' notes. As an alternative, I entered an abbreviated note in the nurses' notes describing an overview of my visit and referred the reader to the lengthier note in the progress section of the chart.

The format I use is that of problem-oriented charting. Under the section entitled "Objective," I include the name of the nurse, physician, physical therapist, or nutritionist who has asked me to see the patient. Under "Action Taken" I describe in some detail the plan I am suggesting. I divide the plan into nursing orders and physician orders and attempt to state each as succinctly as possible, numbering the orders as I go along. It is my observation that this facilitates medical orders being written accurately and in an expedient fashion. Often I have observed that physicians remove the sheet on which my entry is noted and copy each of the orders I have suggested, and in the exact manner I have suggested them. This format frequently reduces unnecessary calling for additional details or clarification. If I have discussed the suggested plan with a particular individual, I also include that person's name. Names are important. Including them in my note helps me not only to get to know individuals and acknowledge who has called me, but also increases accountability for follow through. When direct communication with the first line physician (i.e., usually the resident) is ineffective, I progress up the ladder. In the early days of role refinement, as my expertise was recognized, direct communication with attending physicians gradually became the norm, although I never stopped communicating at the levels already mentioned.

Written entries in the progress notes serve multiple purposes. In some cases I have noted nurses beginning to use the terminology only I had previously used. The notes also quietly speak to physicians and others of my continued presence, even if daily face-to-face encounters have not occurred. Additionally, these notes can serve as teaching tools for graduate students in nursing. Furthermore, my entries in the chart serve as a means of refreshing my own memory when my caseload is extensive. To this day, the notations remain in charts and could act as a source of data on the care and treatment of wounds for research purposes.

Nurses. Multiple methods of communication are used with nurses. Kardex rounds, unit conferences, daily discussions, and the written care plan all serve as avenues of interaction. Though it is not my usual routine to actually formulate the entire plan, in certain cases, as with JM, this becomes necessary. The newness of the procedure and the complexity of the technique in his particular case required it. The guidelines for determining the degree of CNS involvement in patient care situations (under Clinical Nurse Specialist Intervention) assist in deciding the degree of participation in formulating or updating the written plan.

When wound care is complex, or the patient is in isolation, a copy of the nursing care plan is placed in a strategic place in the patient's room. This copy is not removed unless the original is updated. A rough sketch of the wound is drawn on the plan, and if several wounds are apparent, each is numbered individually. This approach facilitates everyone having a common orientation when referring to the specific wound. All supplies necessary to accomplish the dressing change are listed, thus decreasing waste, variations in the plan, and ineffective use of nurses' time. I have already addressed my own nurses' notes, but whenever I read excellent nurses' notes, I make it a point to compliment the nurse.

Director of Nursing. Depending on one's accessibility to the Director of Nursing, it is important to establish a method of communication with the individual in that position. Because of the complexity of JM's case and my desire to successfully gain entre onto his case, I spoke to the director of nursing about the progress I was making. This method of keeping the director of nursing apprised of my activities on an ongoing basis is a strategy I have used over the years. Such information allows the director of nursing to be aware of the impact of the clinical nurse specialist. This and other information provides the data needed to support the role within the institution. After discharge, JM wrote to the hospital administrator, the director of nursing, the administrative nurse and the nursing staff, and myself, thanking us for the quality of care he had received. Although letters of appreciation are personally rewarding, it is my feeling that such letters are read with greater attention if individuals who are removed from the delivery of direct care are aware of the efforts that went into providing that care.

Other Clinical Nurse Specialists. The institution in which I practiced supported numerous clinical nurse specialists. At times, patients were discussed at our bimonthly meetings. Although this occurred less frequently than we all would have liked, it was an important means of support, particularly in complex cases. Certainly other clinical nurse specialists within the institution could understand the demands of a difficult patient care situation and, in some cases, suggest alternative approaches with more expertise than anyone else in the hospital. The psychiatric liaison clinical nurse specialist was an invaluable source of ongoing support and provided a safe haven for me to vent my frustrations in JM's case, and many others. Additionally, the psychiatric liaison clinical nurse specialist acted as a source of new insights which assisted in spurring me on when I felt drained.

Self. It was during my experience with JM that I realized the necessity of communicating with myself. In keeping patient cards, including the amount of time actually spent with patients and staff, as well as the strategies utilized in care situations, I came to see the progress I was making in role actualization. Without these concrete pieces of data, logged on a day-to-day basis, it could have been easy to become discouraged and miss seeing the progress actually being made. Prodding oneself to codify the information on these cards in an organized manner forces one to *see* what has happened in the role over the period of time evaluated. Furthermore, without diligent record keeping, it would have been easy to forget interventions with patients and staff that were effective or ineffective. Likewise, I could have assumed that effective behaviors were such only with specific patients. By logging them, I was able to analyze the significance of such interventions more objectively. I could selectively employ a broad range of interventions with future patients and thereby increase the number of nursing actions stored in my "bag of tricks."

IMPACT OF CLINICAL NURSE SPECIALIST INTERVENTION

No formal method of evaluation of patient outcomes was established at the time of my work with JM. In some ways, it is difficult to quantify an outcome measure in a patient for whom initially life itself was questionable. As time evolved, however, I did begin to tabulate (on the 3×5 patient cards mentioned earlier) the number of days between identification of a wound care problem, my involvement, and the patient's subsequent discharge. These ranges of time could have served as the basis of comparison in retrospective chart analysis regarding the length of stay of patients with similar wounds hospitalized before my tenure.

A nursing care problem that was particularly amenable to a time-sequencing format was the decubitus ulcer. In tabulating pertinent information on my initial visit, as well as the status of the patient and the wound at the time of discharge, I was beginning to compile a profile of the types of patients and patient care responses in individuals hospitalized in our institution. These data could have been compared with data on patients with decubitus ulcers in like institutions. Here again comparison would have afforded a measuring stick against which to analyze, among other things, the effect of having a clinical nurse specialist for wound care (Curtin, 1984). In reviewing data from several institutions I might have compared the presence or absence of formulated nursing care plans, the quality of charting regarding healing in nurses' notes, the use of theory-based versus less effective modalities in the care and treatment of pressure sores, and the criteria nurses used regarding patients' readiness for discharge.

Cognizant of the fact that decubitus ulcers are an ongoing problem in hospitalized patients, and realizing at the same time that pressure sores afforded a more concrete measure of the clinical nurse specialist's input regarding wound care, the nurse coordinator for quality assurance and I collected data on the number of pressure sores occurring within the hospital. The resultant data were classified as to whether the pressure sores were acquired during hospitalization or prior to admission. After formulating a model of practice (i.e., standard or protocol) describing recommended theory-based approaches to the care of the various stages of decubiti, we collected data on an ongoing basis, reassessing the incidence of decubiti. Through audits, carried out by nurses on the units, we were able to assess improving trends in care. Additionally, this approach to logging patient information acted as another check regarding the number of patients with whom I had interacted. These data also served to validate further the categories of nursing care problems I had established (see Table 10–1). Because of excessive costs incurred in the treatment of pressure sores, the data collected regarding them, if positive, could greatly support the position and effectiveness of a clinical nurse specialist for wound care.

Curtin (1984) said it best when, describing the contributions of a clinical nurse specialist for wound care, she stated:

> Medical and nursing research has increased knowledge, but the clinical expertise of the physician and nurse *improves* patient care which, in turn, shortens length of stay. Several years ago, administrators may not have found that exceptionally exciting, but today a few extra days in hospital are worth talking about: they may represent two or three thousand dollars the hospital will have to swallow. It is very difficult to measure cost saving for infections that did not occur, for wounds that did not burst open, for decubiti that failed to develop. You may not be able to track these savings neatly or place them in a ledger in a column, but they are "real gains" in the full economic sense of the word. The people who "produce" them are "profit makers" and no rational fiscal scheme sacrifices profit to reduce costs (p. 25).

Several other methods of assessing the impact of my interventions were: assessing the number and type of referrals within the institution, the source of referrals, the ongoing use of theory-based approaches to wound care by both physicians and nurses, and the number of interventions suggested by me that ultimately were written as medical orders. In evaluating this last indicator of acknowledgment of the impact of my interventions, I was pleased to observe that approximately 90 percent of the orders I suggested were transcribed into medical orders within 90 minutes of my having recommended them. This level of responsiveness by the nurses and physicians interested in promoting a therapeutic plan for their patients reinforced the importance of prompt response by me to referring sources, thorough assessment of the patient, organized charting of the patient's status and my suggestions, and open lines of communication with the nurses and physicians involved.

A final method of assessing the impact of my interventions was to document through photographs the appearance of extremely complex, open surgical wounds. Photographic documentation of the wound at the time of discharge supported our assessment that an organized nursing care plan, ongoing assessment and evaluation by me, frequent communication with the surgeon, and early incorporation of the patient and family into the overall plan of care facilitated early discharge—discharge that was definitely earlier than in other settings. Besides the sense of satisfaction experienced by the team in the realization that we had returned the patient to his family and community in an expeditious manner, Sovie (1984), in a more pragmatic vein, reminded us that "any reduction in LOS (length of stay) will contribute measurably to bringing the cost of care within prospective price, a necessity for fiscal solvency" (p. 90).

If problems arose postdischarge, patients were known to call me directly with questions or concerns about their wounds. Physicians also referred patients to me for follow-up once discharged. When a patient's wound was particularly complex, the visiting nurse who would care for the patient at home was invited into the institution prior to the patient's discharge. The wound care procedure was performed in the visiting nurse's presence and questions were answered. Such coordination also facilitated earlier discharge for the patient and reduced anxiety about what would occur after returning home.

Quoting Dr. David Knighton, a noted authority in the science of wound healing, Curtin (1984) stated: "A clinical nurse specialist in wound healing not only helps educate the staff, but also helps the patient with a healing wound. The clinical nurse specialist's clinical expertise helps get patients out of the hospital faster—helps control costs" (p. 37).

ROLE OF THE CLINICAL NURSE SPECIALIST IN THE PRACTICE SETTING

The role of the clinical nurse specialist in the practice setting in which I was employed has been described in some detail in several chapters in Part II of the text (see Chapters 9 and 12). Suffice it to say, however, that as a clinical nurse specialist in a staff position, it is paramount that one possess recognized expertise as both a clinician and consultant. Because the patient was my client and I was present to provide a service, it was mandatory that nurses perceive my services as beneficial. Although communication skills and clinical expertise greatly facilitated such utilization, reporting directly to the director of nursing and occupying the same level in the organizational structure as the assistant directors of nursing further enhanced appropriate utilization of clinical nurse specialists in care. Support from one's superior greatly facilitates any endeavor, and this is no more exquisitely evident than in the role of the clinical nurse specialist. Without overt support from the director of nursing and recognition of the clinical nurse specialist's expertise via strategic placement within the organizational chart, it is nearly impossible for even the most expert clinical nurse specialist to survive.

Role Refinement

It is imperative that anyone who uses the services of a clinical nurse specialist understand the particular scope of clinical practice for which the individual purports to be qualified. In my case, as the clinical nurse specialist for major abdominal surgery beginning to expand the focus to include wound care, this was especially true. Not only did the title and the focus of my nursing interventions present the possibility of territory issues between medicine and nursing but, additionally, because nurses have seldom identified themselves as specialists in the care of wounds, there was the potential that other care providers would ask what one does with a nurse who proposes to assist patients, nurses, and doctors with wound care. Because of the likelihood of some degree of confusion in my role title and the newness of the position, I found it necessary from the very beginning to explain the refinement of my speciality to all concerned. If these explanations were carried out effectively, they could provide clarity regarding my involvement in patient care situations and facilitate appropriate referrals.

Nurses. Aware of the issues described above, detailed discussions were held with the nurses involved most directly with patients undergoing major abdominal surgery. These nurses had used my services as clinical nurse specialist for major abdominal surgery patients for a number of years and needed to understand clearly the refinement of my practice focus. Through discussion sessions, both the nurses and I had the opportunity to clarify expectations and exchange ideas on the role as I envisioned it and as they saw it helping them with patient care. Issues such as examples of appropriate patient referrals, the degree of specialist versus assigned nursing staff involvement with patients, as well as the best methods of communicating with one another, availability, and so forth were addressed.

With time, the need for wound care consultations on similar types of patients on other units became evident. When consultations were requested on these other units, similar introductory sessions were arranged in a timely fashion, often during the unit's regularly scheduled nursing staff meetings.

Surgeons. Simultaneous with my meetings with the nursing staff on the primary units with which I would be involved, I met with the appropriate surgeons. Each of these meetings afforded me an opportunity to provide a clear explanation of the contributions I could make to the care of patients. Clear articulation of the scope of my practice, along with pertinent examples of some recent patient situations in which I had been involved, was the format used. Whenever possible, I met with the surgeons in their offices and provided each with a copy of my role description, explained what it was I could offer patients, and volunteered my services whenever I could be of assistance. Finally, I described the method by which I could be reached. These short meetings with the surgeons were vital. Without them it would have been difficult to become involved in selected aspects of patient care in a directive way, particularly as regards the care of surgical wounds.

New Staff. One additional and extremely useful method of "advertising" and clarifying my new role, thereby potentially increasing patient referrals, became available when it was decided that a clinical nurse specialist would explain to newly employed registered nurses how the CNS (clinical nurse specialist) role was implemented in the institution. Performing this task presented a wonderful opportunity for the presenting CNS. It afforded a face-to-face encounter with new nurses who received a first-hand description of the services of all clinical nurse specialists within the nursing department but, more precisely, an opportunity for the presenting CNS to provide a detailed role explanation. In the early stages of my role reclarification, these newly employed nurses became a frequent source of consultations, as well as acted as "ambassadors" by articulating to other nurses what new services I could provide patients. Likewise, even if clinical nurse specialists had not been used widely on specific units, these new nurses, unaware of the previous history, enthusiastically called upon me or my peers and sometimes were the impetus for a change in the unit's utilization of clinical nurse specialists.

RESEARCH IN PRACTICE

The myth that one will accomplish research projects as soon as everything else is done must be eliminated from nursing. In particular, if nurses are to succeed as clinical nurse specialists, research must be an integral part of their practice.

During the early stages of work with JM, dynamic changes in the tissue within his wound became apparent. Working with him and with other patients eventually led me to undertake ongoing research regarding the healing process. Because of time constraints inherent in the role, however, it was necessary to identify a project that could be conducted simultaneously with the delivery of patient care. Such a project was devised and carried out in collaboration with a faculty member from the school of nursing. Besides the personal satisfaction experienced when one actually sees a project come to fruition, such research efforts also serve other purposes: nurses are able to see the integration of research and practice and to experience the thrill of being part of the process, physicians and patients become aware of the types of concerns nurses have for patient care and the level of expertise present in nursing to carry out such efforts, and also, collaboration with faculty members greatly increases the alliance between education and practice so frequently spoken about. Ultimately, though, ongoing research serves to imbue the clinical nurse specialist's practice with a depth and means of growth difficult to attain in any other manner.

A research-supportive atmosphere was made evident in the institution in which I was employed. The value placed on research was clearly demonstrated by activities such as the director of nursing and the dean of the school of nursing making joint patient care rounds on the units, having the dean periodically attend both the clinical nurse specialist meetings and the executive nursing council meetings, having a clinical nurse specialist appointed as a member and later elected chairperson of the Committee on Human Research for the university, and the establishment of an active nursing research committee made up of faculty, clinical nurse specialists, and select clinical nurses.

In the early years of my employment in the institution referred to above, I was cognizant of my inability to bring all the prerequisite skills of an experienced researcher to any investigative undertaking. Realizing this fact, I was quick to establish affiliations with faculty members within the school of nursing.

Initially, my research interests were of a less focused and more general nature. Any problem that affected the general medical-surgical patient and had not been investigated previously was of interest to me. I was fortunate, then, to have faculty approach me and seek my assistance and participation in a study involving intravenous needle and tubing changes (Nichols, Barstow, & Cooper, 1983). This experience provided me the opportunity of observing the research process in action in the clinical setting and at a time when I was in a nonstudent position. Although data collection demanded time above and beyond "working hours," many benefits were reaped from interacting with faculty, demonstrating my commitment to nursing research to nurses and physicians and, perhaps most significantly, contributing to building nursing's body of knowledge.

As the focus of my expertise as a clinical nurse specialist became clearer, so did my research interests. From the start, I was committed to the fact that in order to assume the title of clinical nurse specialist one must demonstrate active participation in each of the four role components. Guided by this philosophy, and aware of the dearth of research-based guidelines for nurses regarding the care and evaluation of wounds, as well as being aware from my previous research experience of the time commitment involved in carrying out a research project, I set out to identify a project that could address relevant questions and yet be incorporated into my everyday practice with nurses and patients. A faculty member also interested in wound healing and I began systematically developing a series of research projects by which nurses could assess healing. Not only did these studies vitalize my activities as a clinical nurse specialist and move the research process into the everyday arena for the nurses who observed and participated in data collection, but for me these activities confirmed the necessity of my returning to school to obtain my doctorate. This decision, made after approximately 6 years in the role of clinical nurse specialist, validates to a degree the developmental stages articulated by this writer and others (Baker, 1987; Cooper, 1983; Holt, 1987). After acquiring the skills of a researcher and studying wound healing in depth, my ultimate goal is to return to the clinical setting as a doctorally-prepared clinical nurse specialist.

SUMMARY

An old adage states that "to live is to grow and to grow is to change." Though the sentiments expressed by the quote may sound obvious and somewhat trite, it speaks to the evolutionary experience of this clinical nurse specialist.

Each position I have held in nursing has afforded me opportunities to grow both as a nurse and a human being. In my interactions with nurses and patients I have been privileged to touch life in its most painful, most vulnerable and, at times, its most joyous moments. No position, though, has come close to the satisfaction I derived in being a clinical nurse specialist. As my area of specialization became clearer and my knowledge and experience with patients with wound healing problems increased, I found myself grinning inside. I realized that finally I had found my niche in nursing; I was like a round peg setting comfortably in the round hole. Arriving at this new place was not, however, synonymous with being unchallenged. On the contrary, I delight in knowing that I have a lifetime of practice ahead of me in an area of nursing I love and in a role that is open-ended, flexible, full of possibilities, and always able to be refined.

In my role as clinical nurse specialist for wound care I also learned that healing was far in excess of the prescriptions I proposed for local wound care. I came to realize that I contributed to the healing process far more, at times, by the way I supported the nurses' excellence in care, the assertiveness and manner in which I communicated with the physician, and the support I offered families. Most of all, though, I came to know that the patients with whom I interacted looked to me for knowledge, skill, understanding, encouragement, and caring. The patients, more than any textbook or teacher, taught me what it is *to heal.*

SPECIFIC QUESTIONS

1. This chapter describes many strategies for role reclarification. How can these strategies be used in your practice setting?
2. How does the role of the nurse differ from the role of the physician in the area of wound healing? Evaluate the strategies described in this chapter to develop working relationship with physicians. What if nurses and physicians disagree?
3. What research methods would be useful to test the effectiveness and outcomes of clinical nurse specialist participation in nursing kardex rounds, management rounds, and attending rounds?
4. This chapter discusses guidelines for responding to requests for consultation. How do you assess the client and the other health care providers to determine whether to become directly involved? What commitment are you making when you accept a referral?
5. Identify the strategies used by this author to develop accountability and commitment to quality nursing care among the staff. Give an example of how these strategies could be used in your practice.

REFERENCES

American Nurses' Association. (1980). *Nursing: A social policy statement.* Kansas City, MO: The American Nurses' Association.

Baker, P. (1987). Model activities for clinical nurse specialist role development. *Clinical Nurse Specialist, 1,* 119–123.

Baker, V. (1973). Retrospective explorations in role development. In J. Riehl and J. McVay (Eds.), *The clinical nurse specialist: Interpretations* New York: Appleton-Century-Crofts.

Beecroft, P., & Papenhausen, J. (1988). Editorial opinion. *Clinical Nurse Specialist, 2,* 1–2.

Benner, P. (1984). *From novice to expert.* Menlo Park, CA: Addison-Wesley.

Colavecchio, R., Tescher, B., & Scalzi, C. (1974). A clinical ladder for nursing practice. *The Journal of Nursing Administration, 4,* 54–58.

Cooper, D.M. (1983). A refined expert: The clinical nurse specialist after five years. *Momentum, 1,* 2.

Cooper, D.M. (1989). *Steroids, vitamin A, and soft tissue healing: What does it say for practice?* (Manuscript in process.)

Crawford-Gamble, T. (1986). An application of Levine's conceptual model. *Perioperative Nursing Quarterly, 2,* 63–70.

Curtin, L. (1984). Wound management: Care and cost—an overview. *Nursing Management, 15,* 34–37.

Ehrlich, H., & Hunt, T.K. (1968). Effect of cortisone and vitamin A on wound healing. *Annals of Surgery, 167,* 324–328.

Fawcett, J. (1984a). *Analysis and evaluation of conceptual models of nursing.* Philadelphia: F.A. Davis.

Fawcett, J. (1984b). The metaparadigm of nursing: Current status and future refinement. *Image. Journal of Nursing Scholarship, 16,* 84–87.

Fenton, M. (1985). Identifying competencies of clinical nurse specialists. *Journal of Nursing Administration, 15,* 31–37.

Freeman, B., Carwell, G., & McCraw, J. (1981). The quantitative study of the use of dextranomer in the management of infected wounds. *Surgery, Gynecology, & Obstetrics, 153,* 81–86.

Hamric, A. (1983). Role development and role function. In A. Hamric and J. Spross (Eds.), *The clinical nurse specialist in theory and practice.* Orlando, FL: Grune & Stratton, pp. 39–56.

Hamric, A., & Spross, J. (Eds.). (1983). *The clinical nurse specialist in theory and practice.* Orlando, FL: Grune & Stratton.

Henderson, V. (1981). Implementing the clinical nurse specialist role: A success story. *Nursing Management, 12,* 55–58.

Hirsch, J., Sparacino, P., & Doyle, M.B., et al. (1987). On the scene: Section II—University of California, San Francisco. *Nursing Administration Quarterly, 11,* 47–61.

Holt, F. (1987). Executive practice. *Clinical Nurse Specialist, 1,* 116–118.

Hunt, T.K. (1976). Control of wound healing with cortisone and vitamin A. In J.J. Longacre (Ed.), *The ultrastructure of collagen.* Springfield, IL: Thomas.

Hunt, T.K., Ehrlich, H.P., Garcia, J., & Dunphy, J.E. (1969). Effect of vitamin A on reversing the inhibitory effect of cortisone on healing of open wounds in animals and man. *Annals of Surgery, 170,* 633–641.

Jacobsson, S., Rothman, U., & Arturson, G., et al. (1976). A new principle for the cleansing of infected wounds. *Scandinavian Journal of Plastic and Reconstructive Surgery, 10,* 65–72.

Levine, M. (1967). The four conservation principles of nursing. *Nursing Forum, 6,* 45–59.

Levine, M. (1969a). *Introduction to clinical nursing.* Philadelphia: F.A. Davis.

Levine, M. (1969b). The pursuit of wholeness. *American Journal of Nursing, 69,* 93–98.

Levine, M. (1971). Holistic nursing. *Nursing Clinics of North America, 6,* 253–264.

Levine, M. (1973). *Introduction to clinical nursing,* 2nd ed. Philadelphia: F.A. Davis.

Nichols, E., Barstow, R., & Cooper, D. (1983). Relationship between the incidence of phlebitis and frequency of changing IV tubing and percutaneous site. *Nursing Research, 32,* 247–252.

Oda, D. (1977). Specialized role development: A three phase process. *Nursing Outlook, 25,* 374–377.

Oredsson, S., Gottrup, F., Beckmann, A., & Hohn, D. (1983). Activation of chemotactic factors in serum and wound fluid by dextranomer. *Surgery, 94,* 453–457.

Peplau H. (1952). *Interpersonal relations in nursing.* New York: G.P. Putnam's.

Sovie, M. (1984). The economics of magnetism. *Nursing Economics, 2,* 85–92.

Steele, S., & Fenton, M. (1988). Expert practice of clinical nurse specialists. *Clinical Nurse Specialist*, 2, 45–51.

Topham, D. (1987). Role theory in relation to role of the clinical nurse specialist. *Clinical Nurse Specialist*, 1, 81–84.

University of California, San Francisco. (1983). Philosophy: Department of Nursing. San Francisco: University of California, San Francisco.

Welch-McCaffrey, D., & D'Agostino, J. (1984). Documenting role effectiveness. Presented at conference on Progress, Promise, and Controversy. Good Samaritan Medical Center, Scottsdale, Arizona.

chapter eleven

The Medical-Gerontological Clinical Nurse Specialist in a Veterans Administration Medical Center

*Margaret K. Chang**

Distinctive characteristics of the clinical nurse specialist are flexibility and versatility. Whether the clinical nurse specialist changes focus over time in response to changing health care trends or to changing needs of an institution, the person in the role is in a pivotal position to respond to client needs and remain in the forefront of health care delivery. In this chapter I will describe my role as both a unit-based medical clinical nurse specialist, with a respiratory subspecialty, and a service-based gerontological clinical nurse specialist in a Veterans Administration Medical Center (VAMC).

Case Study

Mr. L was a 56-year-old white male who had had multiple sclerosis for 37 years. He was a paraplegic but active in a wheel chair. He was born in Detroit and moved to San Diego in 1979. Although he had not worked for the past 30 years, he received a bachelor's degree in economics and worked briefly as an accountant before being disabled by multiple sclerosis. He was married and had an attentive and caring wife but no children. As a veteran, he had a 100 percent service-connected disability for his multiple sclerosis. (Veterans Administration, 1984). This meant that Mr. L received all medical service free of charge, as well as a substantial monthly pension.

Mr. L's multiple sclerosis was minimally progressive and he remained reasonably functional until about 1980 when he developed tic Douloureux. In 1982 he required surgery for fifth-nerve ganglionic ablation. Following surgery, Mr. L had a respiratory arrest and a series of pneumonias that kept him in the medical intensive care unit for six weeks. A permanent

*The author wishes to express her appreciation to Susan Harris, RN, ACNSC of San Diego Veterans Administration Medical Center, and her clinical nurse specialist colleagues, Judy Haggie, RN, MS and Penny Schoenmehl, RN, MN, CS, for their input and support.

211

tracheostomy was placed during this time for airway protection. He was transferred to the medical ward for management of the permanent tracheostomy. After his wife learned to care for him with his permanent tracheostomy he was discharged home. During 1983, Mr. L did fairly well at home; he was able to go to church and maintained a limited social life.

In early 1984 Mr. L developed pneumonia and was hospitalized once again. He continued to have several episodes of pneumonia. During morning rounds one day the medical staff informed Mr. and Mrs. L that, due to the progression of multiple sclerosis and neuromuscular disorder of the larynx, Mr. L would have to stop eating by mouth to prevent recurrent aspiration pneumonia. Both Mr. and Mrs. L found this verdict difficult to accept. It was evident that an alternative to this verdict would be a critical factor in preserving those aspects of the lifestyle they treasured. Based on my review of the literature and discussions with other clinical nurse specialists in the medical center, I suggested an Ear, Nose, Throat (ENT) consultation to explore the alternative of a laryngotracheal separation.

In June 1984 the patient underwent a laryngotracheal separation, as recommended in the ENT consultation. After the operation Mr. L was allowed to consume food orally, and a speech therapist taught Mr. and Mrs. L to use the Cooper Rand Electrolarynx device to communicate. Eleven days after the procedure Mrs. L took her husband home.

Mr. L was readmitted again in February 1985 for nephrogenic diabetes insipidus syndrome secondary to medication. He had to be intubated for feeding. At this time, Mrs. L expressed that she was exhausted and could no longer manage to take care of the patient at home. A week later, Mr. L became more alert and was eating on his own. Mrs. L asked to take her husband home. After arranging various home support services, Mr. L was discharged home again. Mr. L remained at home approximately 10 months, at which time he was readmitted and ultimately died from urinary tract infection and upper respiratory tract infection.

CLINICAL NURSE SPECIALIST INTERVENTION

Method of Patient Selection

When Mr. L was transferred to the medical ward, he was referred to me by the ward intern and the ward nursing staff for management of the permanent tracheostomy. Patients are often referred to me in this manner, as well as by the head nurse or the social worker. Even patients' families and patients themselves have initiated referrals. I also self-select cases during discharge planning conferences and during change-of-shift nursing reports and morning medical rounds. For example, on one of Mr. L's subsequent admissions, during morning medical rounds I identified the need to readmit him to my case load due to the threat to their lifestyle which the proposed medical interventions suggested.

Mr. L met one of the informal criteria used for patients entering into my case load, that is, that the patient will be receiving complex nursing care involving the respiratory system. This includes patients who are chronically respirator-dependent, patients on the ward having difficulty adjusting to the presence of a permanent tracheostomy, and patients with COPD who require in-depth patient education. The tracheal-laryngeal separation resulting in a permanent tracheostomy was a relatively rare procedure that only once before had been attempted at this medical center.

A second criterion that is met by any patient/family in my case load is that they are experiencing difficulty coping with the hospitalization, the health problem or disease itself, or the medical or nursing plan of care. This coping difficulty is most often identified when the patient manifests behavior changes such as hostility and anger, high levels of anxiety, noncompliance, and/or attempts to leave the hospital against medical advice. The number of patients actually followed in the case load is limited at any given point in time, and there is no definite assigned case load.

While the above two parameters make up the boundaries of the typical case load, they do not set limits for the number of cases for which I provide consultation at any given time. The number of consultation visits varies depending on the day-to-day patient mix and needs on the ward, as well as my availability. Since the clinical nurse specialist role is divided into three other major components, in addition to the role of consultant in patient care, often a precarious balancing act is performed in order to meet the most critical demands. It is for this very reason that the actual case load and consultation visits often tend to be self-limiting in that the routine day-to-day nursing care needs of the average uncomplicated patient do not come to my attention. Rather, I focus on patients requiring complex nursing interventions due to multiple underlying problems. This may be the reason the staff responds in a positive manner to my intervention.

Criteria for Appropriateness of Type of Intervention

I used six major methods of intervention in managing Mr. L's case. The appropriateness of each method is discussed prior to listing the patient example with each intervention.

Intervention. Providing consultation

Rationale. This method of intervention was utilized both as a way of balancing the time of the one clinical nurse specialist assigned to the ward as well as a vehicle through which necessary education could be provided to both the nursing and medical staffs.

Case Examples. (1) As a consultant for planning the management of Mr. L's permanent tracheostomy, inservice sessions and direct bedside supervision of the nursing staff were provided to review the principles and psychomotor skills used in tracheostomy care. Assistance was also provided to the nursing staff in developing a nursing care plan to help the patient cope with the nursing diagnosis of impaired verbal commuication related to alteration in speech pattern. The patient's physical limitations and capabilities were assessed, and those findings were incorporated in designing appropriate nursing interventions. Mr. L first learned to talk by using his left hand to cover his tracheostomy. Other times he smacked his lips to make noises to get attention and then mouthed the words. Eventually he was able to tolerate talking with the tracheostomy button in place. Other nursing diagnoses identified that required my intervention were: (a) knowledge deficit of tracheostomy care, related to unfamiliarity with the procedure, and (b) ineffective coping, related to impending threatening procedure (permanent use of tube feeding).

(2) Based on data from the literature and my discussions with other clinical nurse specialists, I recommended to the medical staff to seek an ENT consultation for possible laryngotracheal separation. This surgical procedure would provide an alternate form of treatment more likely to maintain the quality of lifestyle to which the patient was accustomed.

Intervention. Providing patient teaching and offering solutions and alternatives.

Rationale. The tension in the staff, patient, and family interaction around teaching and learning tracheostomy care could be relieved if the concepts of adult learning and locus of control were utilized. The staff had not previously been exposed to these concepts and required clinical nurse specialist intervention.

Case Example. When the nursing staff taught Mrs. L how to care for Mr. L's tracheostomy, she would often modify the procedures without seeking advice, creating a frustrating situation for the staff. Principles of working with an adult learner and the concepts of educational diagnosis were reviewed with the staff and an effective teaching plan was developed. Mrs. L had demonstrated traits of a person with an internal locus of control; therefore she required guidelines and a clear delineation of the principles behind the caring of the tracheostomy so that she could understand them and adapt them to home care. Both the staff and I provided direct supervision for Mrs. L's learning process. When Mrs. L altered the techniques that were taught to her, the staff ascertained her reasons for the alteration and corrected her only when they violated the basic principles and interfered with the patient's safety. She learned quickly and was able to care for Mr. L's tracheostomy.

Intervention. Providing patient advocacy

Rationale. The clinical nurse specialist is in a pivotal position to understand the patient's perspective on the health problem as well as that of other health team members. In this case there was conflict among and between these varying views that needed to be resolved if the treatment plan was to be effective.

Case Example. Because of my continued association with the patient and his wife, I had a deeper insight into Mr. and Mrs. L's reactions to the verdict of "not allowed to eat by mouth again." Mrs. L was an excellent cook and enjoyed cooking. Inviting friends to their house for gourmet dinners was one of their few treasured joys in life. They seemed to enjoy the eating even more than the conversation. "Not allowed to eat" would take away from them one of the few opportunities for social interaction with the outside world. I arranged for Mrs. L to relate their feelings to the medical staff, which was a key to the subsequent willingness to change the suggested medical management of the patient's problems. For patients with repeated aspiration pneumonia, it is common practice to place the patient on tube feedings. Because of my knowledge and experience in caring for patients with aspiration pneumonia, and because of the success of my previous interventions, the medical staff responded to my request to seek consultation for an alternative method of treatment for the aspiration problem. After undergoing the laryngotracheal separation procedure, Mr. L was able to eat by mouth. Thus some quality of life was retained for this couple in a way that was meaningful to them.

Intervention. Coordinating discharge planning

Rationale. I often function as a case manager for case load patients with complex health care needs. My knowledge of clinical needs, as well as that of the broader system of the medical center itself, allows facilitation of a rapid and effective discharge through problem solving around obstacles that may occur that no one else on the health care team is as prepared to resolve.

Case Example. In recognizing the changing needs of the patient and his wife, I orchestrated the rather complex discharge planning by coordinating the efforts of the community health nurse, the social worker, the physician, and the respiratory therapist. For instance, I assisted the medical staff to use the appropriate assessment terminology to complete the complex request form required for Mr. L to receive funding for skilled home nursing care. Specialized medical equipment was identified by me, ordered, and delivered to the patient's home. Mr. L was able to go home again, avoiding permanent institutionalization.

Intervention. Providing continuity of care

Rationale. In a large teaching institution there is a rapid turnover of medical house staff and fragmentation of care can occur. Also, many patients, for example Mr. L, may be repeatedly readmitted for recurring or progressive health problems. These factors can be detrimental to the well-being of patients. For many of the patients, the nursing staff is the stabilizing force. In this situation, I serve as an advocate for continuous, comprehensive patient care and give the patient and family more control over their environment. As unique or complex patients are readmitted to different units, I extend my services beyond the medical unit and work with the nursing staff caring for that patient. Thus some sense of stability is created within the complex system when the clinical nurse specialist is involved.

Case Example. Whenever Mr. L was readmitted, it had been difficult for Mrs. L to relinquish her role as care provider to unfamiliar nursing and medical staff. I acted as a bridge during the traumatic periods by providing necessary instructions and information to the new staff or to the staff of the different units caring for Mr. L. Planned conferences were provided to solve the immediate issues. Since the staff nurses were ultimately responsible for the patient, they were encouraged to document the recommendations and results, and I also documented recommendations in the patient record to ensure continuity of care.

Intervention. Facilitating nursing student learning

Rationale. The Veterans Administration Medical Center (VAMC) is a teaching institution, and the goal is to provide experiences for students while maintaining quality patient care. Often a buffer is needed between students meeting their learning needs, patients receiving the care they require, and the nursing staff completing their daily routines. The clinical nurse specialist role involves not only providing patient care, but also facilitating the education of nursing students.

Case Example. Mrs. L also complicated the educational process of nursing students. When nursing students were assigned to take care of Mr. L, Mrs. L would critically observe the assigned students and sometimes would even suggest how to perform certain procedures. Through identification of specific learning objectives of the student and rearrangement of the time spent caring for the patient, with the cooperation of the instructor and nursing staff in charge, I facilitated a better learning situation. Mrs. L was permitted to assist the students in completing the morning care, thus allowing her to participate and at the same time providing an opportunity for the students to observe the interaction between the patient and his family. At other times, when students were learning to take care of the patient's tracheostomy, they did so without any confrontation with his wife.

Clinical Nurse Specialist/Patient and Family Communication

The special kind of communication with the patient and family that allows for an understanding of their predicament from their perspective is the driving force behind the unique contribution a clinical nurse specialist makes. The clinical nurse specialist takes the time to listen at times when others may be caught up in daily routines. The case study illustrates the importance of sensitive communication in the exploration of the intervention of patient advocacy. The case study also alludes to the healing relationship between the patient, his wife, and myself. Clinical nurse specialists create this healing type of climate through communication that allows for unconditional acceptance of the patient and family and their perspective.

Clinical Nurse Specialist/Health Care Team Communication

On the medical ward described herein, there was a weekly multidisciplinary health care team discharge planning conference. The health care team consisted of the staff nurse, head nurse, clinical nurse specialist, medical resident, social worker, dietitian, and the public health nurse. Discharge problems and needs of the patient were brought up and discussed during these conferences. Also facilitating the communication of the clinical nurse specialist and the health care team was the assignment of specific members of the team, such as social worker, dietitian, and pharmacist, to the specific ward. This increased the possibility of direct communication with them when there was a need. Communication with the nursing staff occurred through informal interactions and planned conferences. In the case study, I facilitated patient care conferences with the nursing staff and developed workable nursing strategies in the patient and family teaching plan. I acted as consultant to the staff nurses and demonstrated necessary clinical knowledge and skills to them. I also worked with individual nursing staff to provide guidance in applying the nursing process, enhancing patient assessment, identifying patient and family needs, selecting from among various nursing interventions, and evaluating the effectiveness of the care provided. I gave advice on the utilization of interdisciplinary resources and services available in the medical center. The level of consultation depended on the needs of the staff, that is, it varied from supervision of basic nursing care skills to assure quality care, to providing stimulation for growth to the more experienced nursing staff members. Communication with the medical staff was through direct individual contact and during daily morning rounds. The clinical nurse specialist is often in a position to recommend physician to physician consultation. In this case study, the recommendation was made to the intern following morning rounds. This was a face-saving strategy, as it avoided a potential power struggle with the resident physicians, which might have occurred had the suggestion for an alternative to the medical management been made openly in rounds.

IMPACT OF CLINICAL NURSE SPECIALIST INTERVENTION

One measure of the impact of the clinical nurse specialist interventions in this case study was the extended periods of time Mr. L was able to remain at home instead of in an acute care setting or extended care facility. Were it not for clinical nurse specialist interventions, this may not have been possible in this complex patient situation. My involvement made it easier for the patient and his wife to cope, thereby freeing up their energy to focus on learning how to care for problems in the home setting, rather than being frightened about day-to-day events in the hospital. This focus on coping may also have been a factor in preventing more frequent hospital readmissions.

An additional evaluation measure was the subjective patient and wife response to the care rendered by the clinical nurse specialist. They verbally indicated their appreciation frequently. Mrs. L would also contact me during each clinic visit to discuss how well they were getting along at home. Mrs. L wrote a letter of appreciation to me which detailed the more specific ways she felt they had been benefitted by the interaction. The following is a quote from the letter: "Without your love, caring, and support, I'm not sure I would have made it. Each time another crisis would arise (and, as you know, there were many) you were always there for me. And what's more, you rejoiced with us each time T was able to come home."

The patient's ability to maintain the quality of life he and his wife desired was perhaps the most impressive outcome facilitated by the clinical nurse specialist in this case. Other evidence of the clinical nurse specialist's impact was a decrease in the wife's anxiety with new staff. Through the teaching by the clinical nurse specialist, nursing staff were able to accept family participation in care, which also reduced the family's stress. While it cannot be claimed that this outcome was the direct result of the clinical nurse specialist interventions alone, it was significantly facilitated by the clinical nurse specialist.

In this case example, the impact of the clinical nurse specialist interventions have not been measured directly, either in terms of patient outcome or cost effectiveness. However, various approaches could be used to elicit this data in the future. These approaches include:

1. Length of stay and readmission data in complex cases where a clinical nurse specialist was involved could be compared to cases where there was no clinical nurse specialist.
2. The impact on quality patient care could be measured through various quality assurance monitors, such as monitoring patient falls, patient aspiration, etc.
3. Recruitment and retention data could be evaluated to see if there are differences in areas where there are clinical nurse specialists. Since the nursing staff in the medical ward function in a very hectic environment, with much interference and many tasks to be performed at specific times, frustration at times is high. Because of the broader perspective of the clinical nurse specialist, the staff can be assisted to avoid becoming overwhelmed by the stress of daily tasks, to begin to focus on the long-range goals of the patient, and to appreciate the progress that the patient has made (Blount et al., 1981). The staff members then derive some satisfaction from their efforts and feel better about the important contributions they are making.

ROLE OF THE CLINICAL NURSE SPECIALIST IN THE PRACTICE SETTING

The VAMC is a 577-bed acute care facility with an active ambulatory care department and a 62-bed nursing home unit. It is a teaching institution affiliated with a university school of medicine. My role as a clinical nurse specialist in a staff position at the VAMC has two distinct functions: I am unit-based on a 62-bed medical ward, and I am service-based for gerontology. My unit-based responsibilities are described in the previous case study. My service-based responsibility for gerontology was in response to both the growing needs of the patient population at the VAMC and to the Veterans Administration mandate that the nursing staff respond to the unique needs of gerontological patients.

Gerontology
The American population is growing older, but the veteran population is growing older even faster. In 1985 there were four million veterans over 65 years old, and there will be seven million by the year 1990. By the year 2000 two out of every three males over the age of 65 will be veterans and there will be over four million veterans over 75 years old (Mather, 1984, p. 37). Aging is characterized by an increased risk of acute illness complicated by chronic limitations and socioeconomic problems. Changing Medicare deductibles, co-insurance, and higher eligibility for Medicaid may result in large numbers of veterans unwilling or unable to pay for care in the non-Veterans Administration (VA) sector. Thus the demand on the VA may be even greater (Mather, 1984).

The clinical nurse specialist's functions and responsibilities in the area of gerontological nursing at the VAMC mostly involve consultation and education for the nursing staff and other health care providers. In the area of education, the clinical nurse specialist is responsible for the development and provision of activities which address gerontological nursing practice for all levels of the nursing staff on all shifts.

One of the earliest activities that addressed gerontological needs included a nursing audit on confused patients. Data on admission assessment for geriatric patients, including activities of daily living, sensory deficits, skin integrity, mobility, safety, and incontinence were reviewed. Learning needs identified from the audit were utilized to develop an educational program. The first class offered was "Introduction to Gerontological Nursing." The purpose of this 2-hour class was to sensitize the nursing staff to the needs of the older adult. The content of this program included demographic findings on the aging veteran and the aging population of America, the philosophy and standards of the VA nursing service on gerontological nursing practice, myths on aging, the examination of one's own values as well as society's biases, and a tour of the nursing home care unit. This class has been included in the orientation program for all nursing staff. It has been designed as an interactive class which focuses on attitudes. Many health care providers, including nursing staff, have preconceived myths about aging that could interfere with assessment and planning of care for aging patients. The tour of the nursing home care unit at the end of the class allows the participant to see concepts at work. It also provides an opportunity for the new employee to appreciate another alternative that the VA offers for the aging veterans. Teaching this class gives me a chance to meet every new nursing employee and familiarize them with the clinical nurse specialist role in gerontological nursing.

To increase the general knowledge base of the nursing staff, several other classes that relate to aging have been offered. Continuing education credit was offered for all classes. Some were 2-hour classes and others were all-day classes. Every one of the 2-hour classes was offered to all shifts and repeated several times to allow for optimal attendance. As a means of advertising, a green jacket was worn by the clinical nurse specialist on the days that a class on gerontology was held. The color green was chosen because it represented a sense of support, inspiration, and motivation, concepts that fit well with gerontological issues. At the request of the nursing staff, most of the nursing continuing education programs were offered as all-day classes. I coordinated a program on gerontological nursing entitled "Aging, an Individual Matter," in which other clinical nurse specialists participated in teaching gerontological nursing issues. In an effort to familiarize the nursing staff with current literature related to gerontological nursing, a gerontological nursing article was distributed monthly to each nursing unit. It was posted on a bulletin board with a green background. In keeping with the goals of the nursing service, concepts of competency-based education were utilized to develop several self-directed continuing nursing education programs. Every three months, through closed circuit television, programs on various issues, research findings, and educational opportunities in the community that related to aging were presented.

Additional responsibilities as a clinical nurse specialist in gerontological nursing include membership on the medical center's interdisciplinary committee on geriatrics and gerontology. As a member of the committee, I played a major role in the development and presentation of several hospital-wide educational programs on aging to all hospital employees. As an advocate of the aging patient, I participated in problem solving. One such problem identified was that of loss of patient dentures during hospitalization. By obtaining a dental marking kit and developing and implementing a protocol for its use, I found a means to protect patients' dentures. Due to the generosity of several veterans' groups, each ward in this VAMC now has a dental marking kit.

Another component of the clinical nurse specialist role in gerontological nursing is consultation. Nurses from various areas, especially the psychiatric unit, consult the clinical nurse specialist on problems associated with alteration in nutrition related to aging, self-care deficits related to cerebrovascular accident, and coping problems related to sensory deficit. Recently the psychiatric unit established a ward for the older mentally disturbed patients, and gerontological rounds were established. These rounds helped the staff to discuss some of the patients' behaviors related to physical problems and to identify whether they were normal physical changes associated with aging or associated with psychopathology. The nursing rounds decreased fragmentation of care for this particular patient population and increased the likelihood of care plans that incorporated the unique needs of the whole person. At the interdisciplinary conference, I was invited to make a presentation on how to work with the aging client experiencing sensory loss. Because of my dual focus in both medical-surgical and geriatric areas, the frequency of consultation for the psychiatric service increased. This occurred because it was easier for the staff to identify the medical-surgical problems of the geriatric patient than the aging problems alone.

Although the institution has identified the need to address the issues of aging, some of the health care providers in the acute care setting are not aware of their own attitudes nor do they realize the importance of the aging issue. I look for opportunities to introduce the facts and problems related to aging. For example, problems were identified and possible solutions were offered during medical and nursing rounds on the ward. Material related to aging was introduced in various educational programs, even when the program was not directly related to aging issues, such as 12-lead EKG classes. I further tried to enhance utilization of aging consultation services from the nursing leadership group by introducing aging issues during staff development meetings and other nursing leadership meetings.

Frequently social workers seek consultation of the clinical nurse specialist for evaluation of a patient's progress and status at discharge. On the unit, the social worker and I work closely to help the aging veterans and their families to cope with their problems.

The following case illustrated how I intervened on the patient's behalf and helped the staff to appreciate optimal function, not perfect health, of an aging patient.

Case Study

Mr. T was an 86-year-old retired sheriff. He was married, but his wife lived in a nursing home. He was admitted to the hospital with a 4-day history of syncopy and was placed in the medical intensive care unit (MICU) where a permanent pacemaker was inserted. After the patient was observed in the MICU for 24 hours, he was ready for discharge. The nurses in the unit, however, felt that Mr. T should not be discharged to his home because he lived alone and was not steady on his feet. Mr. T was transferred to our ward while waiting for placement, but he was very upset since he wanted to go home. I was called by the social worker to evaluate the patient's functional ability and self-care status. I identified that the patient had a severe hearing problem. With the proper approach, Mr. T understood what was said and followed directions well. He was able to get in and out of bed slowly but without assistance. Mr. T stated that he had been living alone for the past five years. He did his own cooking and he had a neighbor who took him shopping regularly. He did not want to spend his last penny on a nursing home. It was apparent that Mr. T could function in an independent living environment with the assistance of a supportive neighbor. I explained this to the staff. After arrangement with the neighbor, Mr. T was discharged home with instructions on pacemaker care and a referral to the hospital-based home care service for follow-up at home.

Many older persons entering acute care facilities live alone, and they must be prepared to meet their own needs when they are discharged from the hospital. Nurses and other health professionals tend to protect older adults from taking risks. Many of the older adults have taken many risks in their lives and are capable of weighing risks and benefits (Panicucci, 1983). The goal is to return the patient to his optimal function, not necessarily perfect health.

The hospital remains the primary point of contact for meeting the acute health needs of the elderly. The elderly are admitted three times more frequently, stay twice as long, and use five times more inpatient days than other adults (Bang, Morse, & Campion, 1984, p. 80). Despite the large numbers of elderly patients in acute care hospitals, few of these institutions have a comprehensive geriatric program geared to meet the long-term medical, rehabilitative, and social needs that are linked to acute illness (Bang et al., 1984, p. 82). These facts support the need for a clinical nurse specialist in gerontological nursing in an acute care VA setting.

Accountability

The clinical nurse specialist's accountability and responsibility is determined by service assignment. For example, mental health clinical nurse specialists are directly accountable to the supervisor of the psychiatric nursing service or the Associate Chief of Nursing Service Education (ACNSE) and the oncology clinical nurse specialist is directly accountable to the Assistant Chief of Nursing Service Ambulatory Care (SDVAMC, 1984). As one of the medical-surgical clinical nurse specialists, I am accountable to the ACNSE. Her administrative knowledge of resources allows her to advise the clinical nurse specialist of the most advantageous ways to implement new ideas. The focus of the functions and responsibilities differs from one clinical nurse specialist to another and is determined by the assignment. Most of the mental health clinical nurse specialists and the oncology clinical nurse specialists have primary responsibility for a selected patient case load. The medical-surgical clinical nurse specialists are assigned to a specific ward.

Clinical and Consultation Components

The clinical nurse specialist role on a ward emphasizes both the educational and clinical components. The head nurse works closely with the clinical nurse specialist in planning and implementing educational activities. The clinical nurse specialist does not have the administrative authority to enforce the implementation of planned changes, but does have recognized professional power based on the respect the staff have for the expertise offered. Both the head nurse and the clinical nurse specialist are ultimately responsible for and work together on the orientation of new nursing staff on the ward, staff development of nursing service personnel already assigned to the ward, and the quality of nursing care given to the patients. To ensure the quality and standards of care on our ward, both the head nurse and the clinical nurse specialist are responsible for direct supervision of new staff. The head nurse and clinical nurse specialist meet together with the new nursing personnel on a regular basis to evaluate their needs and progress and to establish goals for their practice. Although the head nurse is ultimately responsible for evaluating staff performance, she seeks the input of the clinical nurse specialist. The head nurse and I have developed a strong professional alliance and mutual respect, and the head nurse has provided specific feedback about the positive impact my role as clinical nurse specialist has had on staff performance and patient care.

Another area of my clinical emphasis is on chronic obstructive pulmonary disease (COPD) patients. I am a member of the multidisciplinary team teaching a program called "Living with COPD." I follow many of the patients with COPD throughout the inpatient/outpatient course. The medical ward to which I am assigned is the only ward in the hospital that provides care for patients on the mechanical ventilator outside the intensive care units. I evaluate all patients on the ventilator assigned to our ward and follow them closely; many of these patients remain in the hospital for long periods of time. I help the staff set long-term goals for these patients and appreciate the progress that each patient has made. Patients on ventilators sometimes present ethical problems. The head nurse and I work together to obtain resources to assist the staff to deal with these ethical dilemmas.

I act as a consultant to the nurses in the nursing process, and I am both a nursing advocate and a patient advocate. As nursing advocate I act on behalf of the nursing staff by interpreting policies and procedures that affect nursing practice. As patient advocate, I inform the patient and family about possible plans of care that can be expected from this facility. Because of my professional knowledge and interrelationship with other health disciplines I can improve cooperation and coordination with other departments. The clinical nurse specialist strives to facilitate excellent clinical practice in the environment by acting as an advocate for nursing staff and as a role model for successful practice within the bureaucracy (Blount et al., 1981).

The advantage of being both in a staff rather than a line position and unit-based rather than service-based is the opportunity to develop a strong relationship with the staff. I know each nurse as an individual in terms of abilities, interests, learning style, and self-perception. This relationship provides opportunities for staff members to use and develop their abilities, as well as get feedback about their contributions to the patients and the ward. Because of this relationship, experienced nurses often utilize me as a sounding board to verify their clinical assessment of patients and management decisions before communicating to a nursing supervisor or other professional health team members. In consultation, I validate the opinions of staff and provide guidance in considering other options. Because of the staff position, nurses often approach the clinical nurse specialist as a "safe" source for assistance in problem solving (Blount et al., 1981).

Because of the ward assignment, I am readily available for consultation. I am considered a trusted member of the health care team. Nursing staff and other health care team members feel comfortable in using my services. I have established gerontological rounds that allow me simultaneously to have an impact on patient care and staff development. The other advantage of a ward assignment is that it facilitates a broader understanding of the ward's assets and problems. This allows me to suggest workable nursing interventions that will be used by the staff.

Although assignment to a specific ward has many advantages, there are some disadvantages or inhibitions to the role. For example, I share an office with the head nurse. Role definition is thus sometimes made more difficult as nursing staff and personnel from other hospital services identify both the clinical nurse specialist and the head nurse as responsible for the total ward function and, therefore, expect the clinical nurse specialist to make decisions for administration of the ward. Yet the clinical nurse specialist is not in a line position to do so. Additionally, due to the various responsibilities the clinical nurse specialist has within the nursing service, conflicts over the amount of time spent on the ward must be negotiated. The staff sometimes rely on the clinical nurse specialist to function as "an extra pair of hands" rather than as a consultant. Clinical nurse specialists are expected to be a resource for broad system change. Using the clinical nurse specialist as "an extra pair of hands" can confuse and weaken the critical component of the role, which is to act as a change agent for the broader system (Everson, 1981).

Education Component

All the medical-surgical clinical nurse specialists are members of the staff development committee. As members of the staff development committee, the clinical nurse specialists participate in planning and developing central nursing educational activities. The medical-surgical clinical nurse specialists and the ward-based psychiatric clinical nurse specialist are also responsible for developing, supervising, and documenting the annual review activities that are required by the Joint Commission on Accreditation of Health Care Organizations and the VA for all nursing staff, such as the cardiopulmonary resuscitation review. The head nurse works closely with the clinical nurse specialist in planning staff orientation and inservice education. Weekly ward staff meetings and inservice sessions are scheduled and presented twice on one day to facilitate maximum attendance of all shifts. Since this ward provides care for patients with oncology problems, we also have monthly rounds with the oncology clinical nurse specialist. Utilization of other clinical nurse specialists is one effective way to assure that resources are being well utilized and allows one clinical nurse specialist to demonstrate to the staff that one need not be an expert in all things. This resource-seeking behavior enhances approachability of the clinical nurse specialist. Because of oncology rounds, our staff have gained new information and skills that enhance the quality of nursing care given to patients with oncologic problems.

This is one of the few hospitals in this community that still hires new graduate nurses. The clinical nurse specialist in this institute plays an important role in assisting the novice nurse to make the transition from student nurse to staff nurse. Benner (1984) states that new nurses are usually at the advanced beginner levels in most clinical areas, so clinical experts are needed on the patient care unit level to provide on-the-spot clinical training.

Administrative/Leadership Component

All of the clinical nurse specialists are members or chairpersons of major nursing committees, such as the quality assurance, policy and procedure, patient teaching, recruitment and retention, special projects, and standard patient care plan committees. Committee selection is made either by appointment or request and is based on the unique contributions a particular clinical nurse specialist may make in a particular realm.

Clinical nurse specialists historically have played key roles in the work and functioning of the special projects committee, serving as both committee members and chairpersons. The original purpose of this committee was to establish the policies and guidelines for implementing the nursing process hospital-wide. This was a natural fit with the focus of the clinical nurse specialists because they were assisting staff at the same time to learn how to write nursing care plans and to meet the JCAHO standards for care planning. After the nursing process policies were written, the purpose of the special projects committee shifted to that of implementing a nursing conceptual model as a way of advancing the science of nursing and reducing the gap between what is taught in academia and implemented in service. We felt that implementing a nursing conceptual model based on the nursing process would ultimately assist nurses in gathering nursing data on patient admission, which would be more likely to result in nursing diagnoses rather than medical diagnoses. The model selected by the special projects committee was Martha Rogers' Science of Unitary Human Beings. This model was most consistent with the staff's beliefs about nursing as reflected in a questionnaire and the already existing philosophy. Committee members were particularly impressed by the concept of holism and the future directions the model held for modern-day nursing practice. Clinical nurse specialists also played an important role in incorporating the Rogerian concepts in various educational activities for the staff.

The clinical nurse specialists have their own committee which meets once a month. The purpose of this committee is to increase the impact of specialty nursing practice on the kind and quality of health care services provided for patients at the VAMC and to work for the advancement and recognition of the clinical nurse specialist role. The chairperson of the clinical nurse specialists committee participates in the weekly meetings of the nursing executive committee, which directs and approves the activities of the whole nursing service. Clinical nurse specialists also serve as members of the nurse professional standard board, which reviews the records of registered nursing staff in this facility in relation to the VA qualification standards for hiring and promotion.

Other Activities

Other projects in which I have been involved are varied. Because of my background in critical care nursing, I assisted with the transition of the core curriculum for critical care nursing from didactic to auto-tutorial format. A basic electrocardiogram (EKG) course was initiated and presented by me several times to our nursing staff as a recruitment effort for the critical care units. Recently, the clinical nurse specialist from MICU and I taught a class on "12-Lead EKG" to the nurse practitioners. I was a member of the planning committee and a presentee of the VA-funded program for staff nurses, "Caring for the Chronically Ill Patients in the Acute Setting."

Professional Activities

The clinical nurse specialist's impact on the nursing profession is through participation in community activities, publications in various nursing journals, and membership in professional organizations. For example, in the community I gave a series of workshops on aging to a multidisciplinary team in a local psychiatric institute and was invited to teach a "Workshop on Aging" for the San Diego Nurse Practitioner Group. I also co-taught a course, "Advanced Acute Cardiovascular Nursing," at the Extension Service of the University of California, San Diego. I am a board member of the Chinese American Nursing Association and participated in teaching an RN State Board Review Course in both Chinese and English for Chinese-speaking nurses.

RESEARCH IN PRACTICE

The VA as an institution is strongly supportive of nurse involvement in research projects. In fact, research-related activity is a criteria for professional advancement. The research activities I am involved with currently are described below.

In conjunction with my clinical focus with COPD patients, I recently completed a research project on "The Effect of Diaphragmatic and Pursed Lip Breathing (DPLB) on Oral Temperatures." Many patients with COPD are instructed to utilize the DPLB technique to improve their breathing, and yet the effect of this breathing technique on the accuracy of oral temperature readings has been questioned. The research findings show that oral temperatures are indeed affected by the combined use of DPLB technique as well as by the use of PLB alone. Axillary temperatures were also found to be affected by this breathing technique. These findings have been incorporated into our teaching of patients with COPD. Patients with COPD are instructed to wait five minutes after use of DPLB or PLB before obtaining an oral temperature and to wait at least 10 minutes after use of DPLB before obtaining an axillary temperature (Chang, 1984, 1985). The above research study took 2 years to complete since, due to my other responsibilities, it is difficult to plan time for research. This is one of the inhibitors of the research component of the role. Yet nursing service does encourage nursing research and it is possible to negotiate for additional time in order to concentrate on a research project. At present, I am collecting data in the ambulatory care area with a staff nurse for phase II of the above study. We collect most of our data while working with patients in the pulmonary clinic or in the "Living with COPD" class. Also, I act as a consultant to a group of staff nurses who are doing a research study.

VA District 26 has established a yearly Nursing Research Conference, and many of the clinical nurse specialists from this VAMC have participated. Several of the clinical nurse specialists from this VAMC have been awarded the Research Nurse of the Year, and I received this honor in 1984.

SUMMARY

The clinical nurse specialist in this VAMC setting affects patient care by facilitating clinical competence of the nursing staff through consultation, education, role modeling, research, and administration. Since each VAMC chief nurse has a unique nursing management style, and since each VAMC Nursing Service has its own philosophy, the clinical nurse specialist needs to be innovative and flexible in capturing opportunities that exist in that particular VAMC setting. The VA health care delivery system is keenly affected by the current economic forces on the health care industry in general. The role of the clinical nurse specialist will need to continuously evolve in response to the changes in nursing and health care needs of society.

SPECIFIC QUESTIONS

1. Compare the advantages and disadvantages of unit-based and service-based clinical nurse specialist roles.
2. How could you incorporate the educational approaches used by this author in your practice?
3. This chapter describes the intervention of patient advocacy. When is this part of the nurse generalist role and when is it appropriately referred to the clinical nurse specialist?
4. How can the strategies described by this author for working with physicians be utilized in your practice?

REFERENCES

Bang, A., Morse, J., & Campion, E. (1984). Transition of VA acute care hospital into acute and long-term care. In T. Wetle & J. Rowe (Eds.), *Older veterans: Linking VA and community resources.* Cambridge, MA: Harvard University Press, pp. 68–69.

Benner, P. (1984). *From novice to expert.* Menlo Park, CA: Addison-Wesley.

Blount, M., Burges, S., Crigler, L, et al. (1981). Extending the influence of the clinical nurse specialist. *Nursing Administration Quarterly, 6* (1), 53–63.

Chang, M. (1984). The effect of diaphragmatic and pursed lip breathing on oral temperature. *Proceedings of Octoberquest '84: Nursing Research Conference.*

Chang, M. (1985). Temperature changes with breathing effort. *American Journal of Nursing, 85* (7), 775.

Everson, S. (1981). Integration of the role of clinical nurse specialist. *The Journal of Continuing Education in Nursing, 12* (2), 16–19.

Mather, J. (1984). An overview of the Veterans Administration and its services for older veterans. In T. Wetle & J. Rowe (Eds.), *Older veterans: Linking VA and community resources.* Cambridge, MA: Harvard University Press, pp. 35–48.

Panicucci, C. (1983). Functional assessment of the older adult in the acute care setting. *The Nursing Clinics of North America, 18* (2), 355–363.

San Diego Veterans Administration Medical Center. (1984). *Functions and responsibilities of the clinical nurse specialist.* San Diego: San Diego Veterans Administration Medical Center Nursing Service.

Veterans Administration. (1984). *A summary of veterans administration benefits.* VA Pamphlet 27-82-2. Department of Veterans Benefits.

chapter twelve

Clinical Nurse Specialist Collaboration in a University Medical Center

Pamela A. Minarik
Patricia S.A. Sparacino

The benefits of a clinical nurse specialist in a tertiary care setting multiply when clinical nurse specialists in different specialties successfully collaborate. This is dramatically demonstrated when such a collaboration positively influences the outcome of a complex patient care situation and addresses the nursing system issues associated with it. Collaboration has been defined as interactions between professionals that enable the knowledge and skills of both to influence synergistically the patient care being provided (Weiss & Davis, 1985). Weiss and Davis emphasize that collaborative problem solving has a high degree of both assertiveness and cooperation. Collaboration merges the insights of persons with differing perspectives and involves attempts to develop integrated solutions where both parties' concerns are recognized and important concerns are not compromised (Weiss & Davis, 1985).

The following case occurred in a university medical center. It describes the collaboration of a clinical nurse specialist in cardiovascular surgery and a psychiatric liaison clinical nurse specialist. The clinical nurse specialists collaborated in the development of effective nursing care approaches for the care of a complex acutely ill adult patient and in support and education for the staff. Due to the complexity of the presenting problems and the preexisting consultative relationships with the staff, both direct and indirect approaches were used by the clinical nurse specialists as a team. The needs of the staff as well as the needs of the patient were addressed.

Case Study

Admission

At the time of transfer to a large university medical center, JS was a 58-year-old white man who was separated from his wife and children. His medical history included several major procedures. He had sustained an above-the-knee amputation (AKA) of the right leg, performed several years previously because of severe gangrene that developed as a result of peripheral vascular disease. Six months prior to transfer he had had an aortofemoral bypass graft on the left and an aorto-common iliac bypass graft on the right. Two months prior to transfer he sought medical attention for a draining left groin wound, which was treated by his hometown physician with antibiotics, partial removal of some graft material, and a new bypass graft. One week prior to transfer, JS noted the onset of a cool, mottled, and painful leg. He had positive blood cultures for *Pseudomonas aeruginosa*.

At the time of admission to the university medical center, JS was critically ill with gangrene of the left leg to above the knee and a purulent draining sinus in the left groin. Because of the urgency of eliminating the source of JS's septicemia, emergency surgery was performed the evening of admission, with removal of all bypass graft material, oversewing of the aorta just distal to the renal arteries, and a guillotine amputation above the left knee. His postoperative course was very unstable, complicated by the following:

1. Multiple revisions of the amputations of both lower extremities, eventually resulting in bilateral hip disarticulations
2. Compromised peripheral perfusion and altered skin integrity due to extensive third-spacing of fluid and reliance on collateral circulation
3. Numerous septic episodes
4. Multiple surgeries for drainage of abscesses
5. An exploratory laparotomy for peritoneal adhesiolysis
6. Impaired mobility due to bilateral above-the-knee amputations
7. Impaired tissue oxygenation due to a long smoking history and chronic obstructive pulmonary disease
8. Anemia
9. Persistent urinary tract infections, incontinence, and contamination of surgical wounds, resulting in a temporary cystostomy
10. Numerous split thickness skin grafts
11. Nutritional requirements greater than voluntary caloric intake, resulting in prolonged nutritional support
12. Pain management problems caused by his recent surgery and aggravated by chronic low back pain from an old war injury
13. Impaired cognitive functioning due to numerous septic episodes and the unfamiliarity of the hospital environment
14. Depressed mood and withdrawal due to being hospitalized a significant distance from his home, extreme physical losses and body image changes, and the lack of an effective social support system

JS's physiological problems presented an enormous challenge to all members of the health care team, and thus the cardiovascular surgery clinical nurse specialist was involved in his care from the day of admission to the hospital. The problems encountered with his impaired cognitive functioning and depression created significant long-term obstacles to his care as well. This prompted the cardiovascular surgery clinical nurse specialist to request for collaboration with the psychiatric liaison clinical nurse specialist. The psychiatric liaison clinical nurse specialist was asked to provide a cognitive and psychological appraisal of the situation and to make recommendations for JS's care. It was anticipated that JS would move frequently between the intensive care unit, the intermediate care unit, and the cardiovascular surgery unit. Therefore, frequent collaboration was required between the two clinical nurse specialists. Additionally, JS's care necessitated the establishment of a framework of caregiver continuity.

The First Month

During the first month of hospitalization, nursing care was intensely focused on physiological care and ensuring JS's survival. By the third week, in conversation with the cardiovascular surgery clinical nurse specialist, the head nurse of the cardiovascular surgery unit enumerated several problems related to JS's care: (1) an anticipated prolonged hospitalization, (2) a family that was perceived to be severely disjointed and therefore unsupportive to JS, (3) difficulty in providing continuity of nursing care, and (4) lack of a comprehensive patient management approach that was consistently followed by all staff. During the same week, a senior staff nurse who frequently cared for JS consulted the psychiatric liaison clinical nurse specialist to discuss treatment approaches for behavior management, which were then added to the nursing care plan. The psychiatric liaison clinical nurse specialist suggested an indirect approach in which she would provide support to the nursing staff as they cared for the patient. With reassurance of the psychiatric liaison clinical nurse specialist's availability and willingness to be directly involved with JS if indicated, the staff nurse felt that an indirect approach was workable. The primary factors leading to a choice of indirect care at that time were the following:

1. The clinical problems presented by JS had been previously managed effectively by this predominantly experienced staff.
2. The most immediate need was for a consistently followed nursing approach.
3. The psychiatric liaison clinical nurse specialist carried an unusually high direct care case load of patients at the time, including another amputee on the same unit with similar complications and evidence of significant depression.
4. Most important, the unit census included an unusually high number of amputees with serious complications, extended hospitalizations, and depressive behaviors, resulting in strain on the nursing staff as a whole. An indirect approach with one patient under these circumstances would have the potential for positively affecting the nursing care of other patients on the unit.

The assistant head nurse, effective and experienced with psychological issues and stress among the staff, recognized that the problem was larger than one patient and one nurse and requested assistance from the psychiatric liaison clinical nurse specialist for the staff as a group. Therefore, in addition to the cardiovascular surgery unit's weekly patient care conferences, which were useful for evaluation and change of care approaches, a series of staff groups were initiated to provide support for staff and assist them in coping with their feelings. The predominant feelings that surfaced were frustration, hopelessness, sadness, compassion, helplessness, and sense of failure because of the number of amputees with prolonged hospitalizations.

During the fourth week, JS was presented at the weekly patient care conference to review and evaluate his nursing care plan. The chaplain, who was working on the cardiovascular surgery unit as part of her internship on the hospital's chaplain's service, said she was seeing JS on a daily basis. The chaplain was known to be highly competent in dealing with interpersonal problems and had developed excellent rapport with JS. All present agreed that the chaplain's regular visits in combination with a consistent approach from staff appeared sufficient to meet JS's needs for social and emotional support. Soon after, another conference provided an opportunity for shared planning, staff support, and ventilation of frustrated feelings.

The Sixth to the Twenty-third Weeks

By the sixth week JS was again presented at the weekly patient care conference, at which time the nursing staff reported he was disoriented and increasingly irritable, and questioned whether he was experiencing visual hallucinations. The nursing staff were eager to intervene assertively rather than let JS lapse into a worsening state. A preliminary evaluation by the psychiatric liaison clinical nurse specialist determined that a psychiatric assessment was necessary for evaluation of a possible acute confusional state. Because of the high probability that medication changes would be necessary and to prevent duplication of work, the psychiatric liaison clinical nurse specialist strongly suggested consultation with one of her medical colleagues from the psychiatric consultation liaison service.

The psychiatrist's assessment was that JS was not hallucinating and did not have a major depressive disorder. His confusion was assessed to be the result of unfamiliar surroundings, with decreased sensory stimulation, psychological stress, alteration in sensory perceptions because of prolonged supine positioning on a flotation bed, frequently interrupted sleep, infection, and multiple medications used for pain control. The psychiatrist's recommendations included medication changes and the continuation of nursing and environmental measures to decrease confusion. (For a thorough discussion of nursing management of confusion, refer to Wolanin & Phillips [1981] and Luna-Raines [1989].) JS's physiological status subsequently became critical once again. Not until the fourteenth week did he become more than monosyllabic and able to converse coherently even part of the time.

In the interim, the psychiatric liaison clinical nurse specialist facilitated multidisciplinary staff groups, which included nurses, the social worker, the physical therapist, and the chaplain, to deal with the discouragement and hopelessness everyone experienced while caring for the greater than usual number of amputees making slow progress. As staff in an acute care setting, they identified themselves as less accustomed to the slow changes more often seen in long-term care. Staff comments included: "Our mindset is 'up and out' with surgical repair . . . our mindset is not chronicity." "Is this a new trend? Who would want to live like this? Why are we doing this?

What are we doing?" Implicit in some of the comments was a wish to let JS die and end his suffering.

The psychiatric liaison clinical nurse specialist acknowledged the nurses' difficult role, which helped them to continue caring and to tolerate a seemingly intolerable situation. By maintaining the focus on constructive problem solving, the psychiatric liaison clinical nurse specialist assisted the staff in group meetings to develop a "sense of trying to work together as a group" and "turned feelings into professional action." In addition, the group served to identify the needs of individual staff members and to identify those staff members best suited to serve as primary nurses. The group shared the development of nursing care plans and facilitated communication of observations, information, and ideas.

By the 15th week, JS was becoming discouraged by his continuing medical complications and said, "I wish I could go to sleep and never wake up." Despite daily chaplain visits and fairly consistent nursing care providers, by the seventeenth week JS had developed further medical complications and as a result had again regressed to monosyllabic requests and answers with intermittent moaning. Several days later he was disoriented to person, time, and place. By the nineteenth week he was more often coherent, with variable appropriateness, and could usually be reoriented.

‧The Twenty-third Week

The cardiovascular surgery clinical nurse specialist was on leave of absence from the 8th to 23rd week of JS's hospitalization. Upon her return she was, quite frankly, amazed to find him still alive. A patient care conference, facilitated by both clinical nurse specialists, was convened to involve all care providers, including two attending physicians. This particular conference was prompted by extreme hopelessness and helplessness among the nursing staff, most of whom had grown to know and care for JS and were afraid he would never be well enough for discharge. A major problem with JS's behavior was revealed in one nurse's discouraged comment: "He's so dependent. We have to feed him." By this time, JS was making significant physical improvement, but his interpersonal behavior was abusive and demanding. He refused to feed himself or drink a necessary quantity of fluid, use the urinal or bedpan, assist with bathing, or leave his room, even on a guerney. The nursing staff, feeling angry and frustrated with lack of progress but also feeling sorry for JS, wanted to do everything they could for him. A possible interpretation of this overdoing behavior on the part of the nursing staff could be related to guilt because of their angry, frustrated feelings; this was not explicitly addressed by the psychiatric liaison clinical nurse specialist. The reasons were twofold: (1) the interpretation could result in defensiveness, and (2) the effect of the behavior was the key area that needed to be identified. The psychiatric liaison clinical nurse specialist instead pointed out that this compassionate approach resulted in increased dependency on the part of the patient and increased hopelessness on the part of the staff.

The psychiatric liaison clinical nurse specialist diagnosed the problem in
- terms of self-care deficit theory (Orem, 1985) and suggested a change in management; she recommended the staff stop reinforcing JS's dependent behaviors and instead provide a contingency relationship between compe-

tent independent behavior and positive reinforcement that would alter his behavior and subsequently influence his thoughts and feelings. The psychiatric liaison clinical nurse specialist suggested that daily self-care goals be developed with JS to influence his sense of competence and self-efficacy and to increase his sense of control. She also proposed that a chart be posted in his room to monitor daily progress with gold stars as reinforcement. The gold stars and the chart would also secure more meaningful reinforcement for JS by generating the praise and attention of numerous others. In addition, the chart and stars would give JS's care providers increased opportunities for positive interactions with him which would gratify them. The psychiatric liaison clinical nurse specialist recognized the level of psychosocial skill involved in implementing such an intervention. Because of her skill, consistency on the unit, and supportive relationship with JS, the cardiovascular surgery clinical nurse specialist was selected to develop the goals with JS Several days after the multidisciplinary conference, the cardiovascular surgery clinical nurse specialist met with JS to negotiate self-care activities he felt he could complete. The use of the chart proved to be a turning point in JS's care and came to be called the gold star intervention.

The first chart (Table 12–1) was developed by JS and the cardiovascular surgery clinical nurse specialist on a Thursday, and was posted in the patient's room. He was given a supply of gold stars and, for each task completed each day, a gold star was glued to the appropriate box by the nurse.

The following Monday, the cardiovascular surgery clinical nurse specialist returned to discuss with JS how his gold star chart was working and how he felt about it. One thing was immediately apparent; JS was quite angry that he had run out of gold stars. The nursing staff reported a significant improvement in his alertness, participation in self-care, and inquiries about staff and other patients. JS stated, "I really feel better about things. A while ago I never thought that I could get this far." By the following day, JS was inquiring about rehabilitation possibilities and placement.

McLean (1982) reported that Burgess recommended graded task assign-

TABLE 12–1. INITIAL GOLD STAR DAILY PROGRESS CHART

Goals	Sat	Sun	Mon	Tues	Wed	Thurs	Fri
Assists with meals							
Holds own cup							
Drinks: Morning: 1300 cc Evening: 1000 cc							
Brushes teeth							
Out of bed: total 20 minutes/day							
Turn flotation bed off 10 minutes every 4 hours[a]							

[a]In order to prepare JS for placement in a rehabilitation facility, it was necessary to wean him from the flotation bed so that he could return to a regular bed.

TABLE 12–2. UPGRADED GOLD STAR DAILY PROGRESS CHART

Goals	Sat	Sun	Mon	Tues	Wed	Thurs	Fri
Feeds self							
Holds own cup							
Drinks: Morning: 1300 cc Evening: 1000 cc							
Brushes teeth							
Brushes hair							
Washes face							
Assists with bath							
Out of bed: total 40 minutes/day							
Goes to solarium once a day							
Turn flotation bed off 20 minutes every 2 hours							

ment in order to encourage increasing opportunities for positive reinforcement and goal attainment. Therefore, 11 days after the first chart was posted the goals were up-graded (Table 12–2).

The Twenty-sixth Week

Because of his continuing physical improvement and, more importantly, because of his renewed interest in self-care, attempts at placement in a rehabilitation facility were initiated. Three weeks after initiating the gold star chart, the nursing staff reported that JS demanded that the goal charts be removed, that they were "stupid" and "baby stuff." When the cardiovascular surgery clinical nurse specialist entered JS's room to take down the gold-star-studded charts, he insisted that they in fact be left as is "because it helps the nurses remember what I'm supposed to do each day." A week later he decided that the charts cluttered his walls and could be taken down. Although placement efforts were begun on his 26th week of hospitalization, because of complex insurance problems JS was not transferred to a rehabilitation facility until 5 weeks later.

Readmission

Two and one-half months after transfer to the rehabilitation facility, JS was returned to the university medical center because of a draining tract from his hip disarticulations. The nursing staff greeted him with mixed feelings; they were elated to see his marked physical improvement and independence in self-care, but they were apprehensive about the significance and consequences of the purulent drainage. Shortly after readmission a psychiatric consultation was requested by a vascular surgeon because JS was having angry outbursts that were perceived to have a paranoid flavor. When the consulting psychiatrist and the cardiovascular surgery clinical nurse specialist spoke with JS, he stated that he was "scared and upset that it is going to start all over again and that I'll lose everything I've worked so hard for." The psychiatrist and the cardiovascular surgery clinical nurse specialist concurred that JS handled severe psychosocial stressors with bravado and denial and that he had assumed that the nursing staff who had previously cared for him for almost 8 months would provide a tolerant atmosphere in which he could express his anger, fears, and sadness. The cardiovascular surgery clinical nurse specialist and JS agreed to meet daily so that the cardiovascular surgery clinical nurse specialist could regularly assess JS's vascular status and JS could direct his frustrations to one person. This arrangement worked well; the nursing staff were generally spared JS's outbursts, which decreased in frequency, and the cardiovascular surgery clinical nurse specialist was singularly accountable to JS for any questions or concerns.

Discharge

After 2 weeks of diagnostic tests and wound care, JS returned to the rehabilitation facility for another 3 months and was then discharged to care for himself in an architecturally adapted apartment. The cardiovascular surgery clinical nurse specialist has phoned JS regularly to follow his progress and, 18 months after returning home, he still is able to live alone, despite persistent physical and social problems.

Summary of Clinical Nurse Specialist Interventions in Case Study

The key elements that made the significant difference in JS's positive outcome were the direct behavioral interventions as well as continuity of care coordinated by the cardiovascular surgery clinical nurse specialist, and the collaboration and indirect care of the psychiatric liaison clinical nurse specialist, as well as the level of care provided by the nursing staff. While the nursing staff of the cardiovascular surgery unit, who cared for JS for the majority of his 8-month stay, were highly capable of providing complex physical care and truly cared for him, certain obstacles observed by the two clinical nurse specialists restricted the staff's impact: lack of staff continuity and consistency because of many part-time staff and 12-hour shifts, lack of objectivity, lack of a theoretical framework or psychiatric clinical experience from which to view the problem and derive workable interventions, and an overwhelming intensity of feelings.

The psychiatric liaison clinical nurse specialist had primary responsibility for overseeing the nursing care issues related to self-care deficit, alteration in thought processes, ineffective individual coping, powerlessness, alteration in comfort (pain), disturbance in self-concept, and alteration in family process. The staff groups and patient care conferences provided the opportunity for the staff to gain an objective perspective on these problems and served as a release valve for intense feelings. The psychiatric liaison clinical nurse specialist selected theories appropriate for organizing the clinical data. She utilized the conferences for informal teaching of nursing care approaches and more useful frameworks for understanding the patient's dependent, depressive behaviors.

Theoretical Framework

Her input was based on Orem's self-care concepts (Calley, Dirksen, Engalla, & Hennrich, 1980; Coleman, 1980; Dickson & Lee-Villasenor, 1982; Joseph, 1980; Mullin, 1980; Underwood, 1980) and behavioral therapies for depression (Lewinsohn, Sullivan, & Grosscup, 1982; McLean, 1982). According to Orem's self-care theory (Orem, 1985), the purpose of nursing is to help individuals engage in and accomplish self-care activities to the extent of their abilities; the nurse's role is to facilitate, promote and, when possible, increase the self-care abilities, leading to the most independent level of functioning possible for the patient. The behavioral approaches for depression provide a means for accomplishing this goal. From the perspective of operant learning theory, there exists a contingency relationship between behavior and reinforcement. Thus, if there is no contingency between adaptive behavior and positive reinforcement, or if depressive behavior itself (e.g., inactivity, avoidance, complaints) is inadvertently reinforced by a sympathetic interpersonal environment for an extended period of time (as in the case of JS), the necessary conditions for the experience of depression are present. The gold-star intervention designed for JS included the four common denominators of behavioral treatments of depression: (1) systematic application of the principle of reinforcement, (2) self-monitoring of predetermined events to permit an on-going performance review, (3) focus on goal attainment, and (4) preparation for adaptive coping in the future (McLean, 1982). *gold*

The cardiovascular surgery clinical nurse specialist had primary responsibility for coordinating the nursing care issues related to alteration in tissue perfusion, impairment of skin integrity, alteration in nutrition, alteration in urinary elimination, and impaired physical mobility. Direct patient interventions occurred according to patient need or nurse or physician request, and with follow-up visits on a regular basis. Education as to why wounds did not heal or were slow to heal secondary to JS's complex and altered vascular anatomy generally took place in patient care conferences, with clarification of specific points often discussed in hallway consultations. The periodic patient care conferences were an opportunity to review total care for JS and discuss whether all possible nursing modalities had been considered or were being used. The cardiovascular surgery clinical nurse specialist collaborated with the vascular surgeons to evaluate the various stages of wound healing and to plan wound care that was not only most appropriate at a particular stage but was least painful and allowed the longest possible intervals of rest between dressing changes. Of no less importance was the continuity the cardiovascular surgery clinical nurse specialist provided in JS's care; JS was hospitalized for 8 months, with many interunit transfers, junior house staff monthly rotations, and senior house staff changes after JS's fourth month.

What both clinical nurse specialists felt was unique was the way in which each of the clinical nurse specialist roles complemented the other, providing a balance to each other's skills and utilizing the best each had to offer to make a difference in JS's outcome. At no time was competition for primary involvement even a consideration, and only in a retrospective case review did it become obvious that, in some situations, it could have been a major issue leading to interference with the patient's progress toward recovery. Competition between clinical nurse specialists can occur when each feels so advanced in theoretical knowledge and clinical practice skills that there is no longer a need to call upon colleagues for consultation, assistance, or utilization of knowledge or skills that another has to offer. Competition can also occur when one is unclear about one's specialty or feels inadequate and prefers that no one recognize this. Collaboration develops from a recognition and respect of one's own expertise, respect for the expertise of others, and a strong interest in the consideration of differing viewpoints (Johnson, 1985). Both the cardiovascular surgery clinical nurse specialist and the psychiatric liaison clinical nurse specialist share the attitude essential for collaboration. From collaboration comes a complete picture, an expanded perspective on problems, issues, and solutions. Collaboration results in quality patient care beyond what one individual could provide. When it is the positive outcome for the patient that is at stake, then the elements of collaboration become not only essential but should be an integral part of a clinical nurse specialist's practice.

CLINICAL NURSE SPECIALIST INTERVENTION

To further develop and explain the elements of collaboration between specialists, this section will describe the roles of the cardiovascular surgery clinical nurse specialist and the psychiatric liaison clinical nurse specialist. Methods of patient selection and criteria for patient case load will be included, as well as criteria for appropriateness of the type of intervention. Summaries will delineate the similarities and differences.

Cardiovascular Surgery Clinical Nurse Specialist

The philosophy of the cardiovascular surgery clinical nurse specialist about the clinical nurse specialist role encompasses two basic tenets:

1. While each of the four basic components (patient care, consultation, education, and research) must be incorporated into one's role, patient care must always remain one's primary priority.
2. The purpose of one's role is not to attain omnipotence to the exclusion of professional development of colleagues, nursing staff, and other members of the health care team, but to share one's knowledge and skills to the theoretical point of working oneself out of a job.

Method of Patient Selection and Criteria for Patient Caseload. The patient case load of the cardiovascular surgery clinical nurse specialist is a result of referrals by staff nurses, head nurses, other clinical nurse specialists, and/or physicians or by patient request, or by self-selection based on anticipated or actual patient acuity. Because the nursing staff on the cardiovascular surgery unit are known for their longevity of employment and thus well-developed skill level, the patients of the cardiovascular surgery clinical nurse specialist tend to be those who, by mutual agreement between the referring person and the clinical nurse specialist, require continuity because they are long-term patients or patients who transfer frequently between critical care units and the surgical floor, those who have a pathophysiological problem or surgical approach with which the staff is unfamiliar, those who have a treatment intervention that is new or infrequently performed, or those who have ineffective coping behaviors and who require consistency and continuity.

Criteria for Appropriateness of Type and Amount of Intervention. The amount of the cardiovascular surgery clinical nurse specialist's involvement is one that undergoes continual reassessment and negotiation with the staff nurses; there is no standard degree of involvement, as it remains flexible according to the needs of the patient and the staff. In any single patient care situation, the involvement of the cardiovascular surgery clinical nurse specialist may be indirect at times and direct at others, depending on the presenting problems and the ability of the staff to manage them. Theoretical content is presented at patient care conferences or staff meetings, classes through the nursing service's department of education, individual nursing consultations, and collaboration in the development or revision of nursing care plans. Likewise, when it is determined that involvement of the cardiovascular surgery clinical nurse specialist in a patient care situation is unique because of the knowledge or expertise needed to deliver a particular aspect of care, then the cardiovascular surgery clinical nurse specialist's patient involvement will remain direct and continuous, although it is still necessary to consistently communicate with the staff nurses and health care team as well as in the patient's chart.

Clinical Nurse Specialist/Health Care Team Communication. It is communication that makes or breaks the continuity of a patient's care. Effective communication becomes a challenge when: nursing staff work 12-hour shifts and therefore may work only fourteen shifts per month as well as rotate between days and nights; house staff rotate every 1 to 2 months; attending physicians are often out of town; surgical schedules and office and clinic appointments remove the physician from direct patient involvement for a major portion of each day; a significant number of health care team members and consultants are involved in some aspect of the patient's care; and the patient may predictably be on three or four nursing units during the course of hospitalization.

Communication, then, must be both verbal and written. Every attempt is made to verbally communicate the cardiovascular surgery clinical nurse specialist's assessments, interventions, and results of interactions with the staff nurse caring for the patient if, in fact, the cardiovascular surgery clinical nurse specialist and the staff nurse have not worked simultaneously with the patient for the purpose of role-modeling. Verbal communication, whenever possible, must be a part of the collaboration with the charge nurse or the head nurse and with all health care team members, whether by phone, on rounds, by chance encounter, or during a patient care conference. Whereas verbal communication encounters the risk of being variously interpreted as it is transmitted from one person to the next, written communication is not as easily misinterpreted. Our institution still separates nurses' notes from other health care professionals' progress notes; where the cardiovascular surgery clinical nurse specialist's notes are written depends on who the primary audience is for the specific purpose. If, for example, the cardiovascular surgery clinical nurse specialist's assessment or intervention has implications for the patient's medical care or overall management, the cardiovascular surgery clinical nurse specialist's note is written in the medical record section where the physicians enter their notes; an entry is made in the nurses' notes to refer to the progress notes. If, however, the cardiovascular surgery clinical nurse specialist's assessment or intervention has greater implications for the continuity and measurement of the outcomes of nursing care, then the findings are written in the nurses' notes, with an entry in the physician notes to refer to the nurses' notes.

Clinical Nurse Specialist/Patient Communication. The cardiovascular surgery clinical nurse specialist's method of communication with patients and families varies considerably according to the situation or intent. When it is a preoperative visit, after the initial introduction, the questions are phrased so that the patient's or family's questions are answered first. The purpose of this approach is to assess how much the patient, family, or both already knows, the level of comprehension, the degree to which the patient/family is ready or willing to learn, and the level of anxiety. In answering questions, sensory and cognitive content is intentionally incorporated that is anticipated to be beneficial for the patient/family to know, and subjective and objective anticipatory information is provided after answering the initial questions (Johnson, 1972; Johnson, Fuller, Endress, & Rice, 1978). In subsequent visits with the patient/family, the cardiovascular surgery clinical nurse specialist's interactions may appear social in nature when, in fact, they are intended to assess family functioning, patient/family coping, accuracy of patient/family interpretation of hospital course of events, problems encountered, and progression of the patient/family toward self-care. Interactions may take on a more formal instructional approach as discharge planning and teaching occurs, but the usual pattern is to gradually incorporate information into the patient's daily hospital activities, so that new content or new behaviors have functional meaning. When it becomes apparent that there is a complex patient/family situation where communication or behaviors are out of the ordinary, then the psychiatric liaison clinical nurse specialist is readily consulted for advice, direction, or perhaps direct involvement.

The Psychiatric Liaison Clinical Nurse Specialist

The emphasis of the multifaceted psychiatric liaison clinical nurse specialist's role is on consultation to nursing staff, aimed not only at the solution of immediate patient problems, but at the improvement of the observational, assessment, and intervention skills of staff nurses (Nelson & Schilke, 1976). An important aspect is support activities for the nursing staff, both individually and in groups. As consultant, the psychiatric liaison clinical nurse specialist serves as expert and as facilitator. Formal classes, patient care conferences, and consultation with individual nurses provide the framework for teaching. With expertise in psychiatric illnesses and in the range of normal as well as pathological responses to chronic and acute physical illness, the psychiatric liaison clinical nurse specialist may serve as a role model for staff in the provision of direct, specialized care to patients and their families. A selection of patient and family care activities includes psychosocial or psychiatric assessment, or both, brief supportive therapy, crisis intervention, grief counseling, mental health referral, teaching relaxation and imagery techniques for pain management and anxiety reduction, and teaching self-care strategies for managing illness, disability, or pain. Because the psychiatric liaison clinical nurse specialist provides services to thirteen nursing units in the medical center, a smaller proportion of time is spent in direct care activities; greater emphasis is placed on consultation and teaching.

Within a consultation-liaison model of clinical practice, characterized by an educative, collaborative alliance with nursing and medical colleagues, the primary responsibility for the patient and the recommended interventions remains with the consultee. In nurse-to-nurse consultation, three intervention models are considered: (1) direct care relationship with the patient or family members, (2) a patient-centered relationship with nurses, and (3) a consultee-centered relationship with nurses.

Method of Patient Selection

In the university medical center, referrals may come from nursing staff, other clinical nurse specialists, attending physicians, residents, students, social workers, chaplains, administrators, physical therapists, friends or family of the patient, or patients may refer themselves. Therefore, because of the size of the potential case load on thirteen units, patient selection rarely results from case finding by the psychiatric liaison clinical nurse specialist.

Criteria for Appropriateness of Type and Amount of Intervention

Once a consultation is requested, the psychiatric liaison clinical nurse specialist will make an initial assessment of the situation in terms of the appropriateness of the consultation for the psychiatric liaison clinical nurse specialist. Problem identification begins or continues, and the need for direct or indirect service is determined in discussion with the consultee. Making this determination involves "diagnosing the total consultation" (Lewis & Levy, 1982, p. 98). The evaluation is extended beyond the patient to include the nature of the request, the nurse, the physician, the family, the chart, the medical illness, and the ward culture. Whether the problem involves the nursing or the medical domain must also be considered. Some of the questions to be addressed are:

- Who is making the request and how is it expressed?
- How complex is the problem?
- Is continuity over time a factor in the request?
- What is the relationship of the psychiatric liaison clinical nurse specialist with the consultee?
- What is the consultee's level of experience, skill, knowledge, and anxiety about the problem?
- How does the physician view the problem?
- What knowledge does the psychiatric liaison clinical nurse specialist have of the unit and of the people involved in the problematic situation?
- What does the family contribute to the situation?
- How might the problem be related to the medical illness?
- What information is provided by the chart?

The decision about direct or indirect service is also influenced by pragmatic factors, some of them related to the simultaneous demands in such a varied role. Pragmatic factors include time available, acuity and number of current patient (direct care) case load (currently 4-11 per month), extent of other responsibilities (such as support groups, patient care conferences, teaching, committees), institutional expectations, areas of expertise of the psychiatric liaison clinical nurse specialist, and the needs or interests of the consultation–liaison psychiatry service in the institution. In other words, what is feasible in the time available and in this setting, from a practical as well as a therapeutic point of view?

A direct care relationship may be indicated if psychiatric nursing care is required or if there is inadequate time, opportunity, knowledge, or motivation for the consultee to develop the required skills. In general, an attempt is made to limit the numbers of new people introduced into a situation and, if possible, to assist someone already involved to develop the skills or knowledge necessary to intervene effectively.

Clinical Nurse Specialist Communication with Patients and Health Care Team

Successful intervention in a direct care relationship depends on open and frequent communication. Counseling or teaching with the patient and family members is infrequently fully observed by the nursing staff due to the time involved; therefore discussions with the assigned nurse or primary nurse for the purposes of continuity and teaching occur before and after each visit. Any other health team members involved in the case are included in the discussions. Written documentation of each visit using the problem-oriented format is done in the physician's progress notes with a notation in the separate nurse's notes to see the progress notes. The responsibility for developing and writing the nursing care plan normally is retained by the nursing staff with the guidance of the psychiatric liaison clinical nurse specialist. This method augments the teaching value of the verbal communication and ensures that the feasibility of the recommended interventions is jointly determined.

When indirect care is indicated, interventions are implemented through a patient-centered or consultee-centered relationship with nurses (Minarik, 1984). Support for the staff, as well as expressed willingness to be involved directly with the patient, is provided. In general, the least complex interventions are utilized first and may become more complex as necessary (Lewis & Levy, 1982). Flexibility, open and frequent communication, and continued negotiation with nursing staff regarding direct versus indirect care, as described in JS's first month of hospitalization, is necessary.

In a patient-centered indirect care relationship, the clinical nurse specialist assists the nurse-consultee(s) in the development of nursing care strategies based on the presenting needs of the patient and his family. These are then documented in the care plan, the nursing notes, and communicated in report by the nurse. The appointment calendar of the psychiatric liaison clinical nurse specialist serves as a personal record of indirect care. Frequent verbal communication with the nurses involved with the patient and the leadership of the unit over a 5-day work week provides follow-up and aids in continuity of care. In contrast to the patient-centered relationship, a consultee-centered relationship focuses on the nurse-consultee's need for knowledge or skills or the resolution of "interfering themes" such as personal biases, value judgments, or anxiety.

When consultation is expanded to a liaison approach, the psychiatric liaison clinical nurse specialist intervenes by working continuously with the total environment to facilitate the interrelationships among patient, family, staff, and the hospital unit milieu and to raise the awareness of psychological needs and issues (Lewis & Levy, 1982). The focus is on indirect care activities with nursing staff, such as informal and formal teaching, preventive management, patient care planning with individual staff, participation in ward rounds and patient care conferences, and facilitation of nurses' groups or team-building activities.

Due to the complexity and interaction of multiple relationships in the liaison approach, impact is difficult to measure and must be viewed in terms of increased knowledge, skills, problem-solving ability, self-awareness, and clinical judgment in the nursing staff. This is demonstrated when the questions addressed to the clinical nurse specialist become more complex because nursing staff's skills are more refined and they become resources for each other. Currently, perceived impact of the psychiatric liaison clinical nurse specialist is measured using two methods. One is the use of a clinical nurse specialist services contract

TABLE 12–3. CONTRACT FORM FOR CNS SERVICES

CNS Provider: _____

Administrative Nurse: _____
Date of Agreement: _____
Time Period Covered: _____

SERVICES	EVALUATION METHOD
1. _____	_____
_____	_____
_____	_____
2. _____	_____
_____	_____
_____	_____
3. _____	_____
_____	_____
_____	_____
4. _____	_____
_____	_____
_____	_____
	_____
	Signature of CNS
	_____
	Signature of Administrative Nurse

TABLE 12-4. CONTRACT FOR CNS SERVICES (Sample)

CNS Provider: Pamela Minarik

Administrative Nurse:	HN, Medicine
Date of Agreement:	6/86
Time Period Covered:	6 months

SERVICES	EVALUATION METHOD
1. Consultant to nursing rounds	• Increased use of care plan for psychosocial issues • Increased use of cognitive testing tools and appropriate nursing approaches for management and prevention of confusional states • Increased knowledge of methods of utilizing psychiatric resources
2. Consultation on individual clinical problems (direct and indirect care)	• Document type, number, and specific consultees, and specific requests for consultation • Increased appropriateness of referrals • Administrative nurses to follow up on problem identification and assessment
3. Consultant to administrative nurses on behavior modification of crisis mode of problem-solving in staff group	• Monthly staff group with core group attendance and participation • Increased identification of own difficulties • Observable improvement in preventive problem-solving among core group
4. Relaxation/imagery training for staff	• Participation in seminar by interested staff • Fewer requests to CNS for relaxation tape • Increased use of relaxation/imagery techniques by involved staff • Increased use of trained staff for consultation by other nursing staff
5. Available for individual staff support, crisis intervention on personal work-related issues	• Appropriate use • Staff self-report of effectiveness and follow-through on discussed plan

Signature of CNS
_____

Signature of Administrative Nurse
_____

(see Tables 12-3 through 12-5) which is reviewed and renegotiated with the head nurse once or twice a year. The second method is the clinical nurse specialist evaluation (see Table 12-6), completed by selected members of the multidisciplinary health care team as part of the annual performance appraisal.

TABLE 12–5. CONTRACT FOR CNS SERVICES (Sample)

CNS Provider: Pamela Minarik

Administrative Nurse:	HN, Surgery
Date of Agreement:	6/86
Time Period Covered:	6 months

SERVICES	EVALUATION METHOD
1. Patient consultations—involve staff more, especially primary nurses	• Document types, numbers, reasons for referral, staff who refer, level of knowledge and problem-solving demonstrated in request • Review/assess needs
2. Patient care conferences—increase the number of conferences called to prevent problems or communicate with increased number of staff vs. "fire-fighting"	• Document staff member who called conference, patient problem, reason, outcome • Review/assess needs
3. Personal counseling/crisis intervention with staff—availability PRN	• Feedback from staff • Staff member follow-through on self-defined plan
4. Work with administrative nurse to assess level of functioning of staff group and develop intervention strategies	• Level identified • Strategies implemented • Level increase in problem areas/growth

Signature of CNS

Signature of Administrative Nurse

TABLE 12–6. CLINICAL NURSE SPECIALIST EVALUATION

Date: _____

My position is: _____

The CNS with whom I have worked: _____
                                                Name

Instructions

Please indicate the degree to which the CNS engages in the behaviors described. If you do not feel qualified to comment, please check Not Applicable.

Please place your check marks in the middle of the space, not on the boundaries.

                                (this)   (not this)
                                  x   x

_____ :_____ :_____ :_____ :_____ :_____

    never   always   n/a

Please place only one check mark on each item.

1. Overall evaluation of performance.

_____ :_____ :_____ :_____ :_____ :_____

    not   very   n/a
effective   effective

TABLE 12–6. (Continued)

2. The CNS responds to requests for consultation in a timely and professional manner.

———————:——————:——————:——————:——————:——————

   never   always   n/a

3. The CNS effectively participates in health-care decisions.

———————:——————:——————:——————:——————:——————

   never   always   n/a

4. The CNS demonstrates a high level of interpersonal skill and is overtly helpful in interactions with other members of the health care team.

———————:——————:——————:——————:——————:——————

   never   always   n/a

5. The CNS demonstrates a high quality of clinical knowledge, contributing useful suggestions for patient problem management.

———————:——————:——————:——————:——————:——————

   never   always   n/a

6. The CNS brings appropriate patient problems to your attention and assists in their resolution.

———————:——————:——————:——————:——————:——————

   never   always   n/a

7. The CNS, when appropriate, renders skillful care directly to patients and/or their families.

———————:——————:——————:——————:——————:——————

   never   always   n/a

8. The CNS involvement has a positive impact on patient and family outcomes.

———————:——————:——————:——————:——————:——————

   never   always   n/a

9. The CNS teaching to patients/families is accurately and skillfully accomplished.

———————:——————:——————:——————:——————:——————

   never   always   n/a

10. The CNS teaching to staff is accurately and skillfully accomplished.

———————:——————:——————:——————:——————:——————

   never   always   n/a

11. The CNS provides appropriate feedback to the nursing staff.

———————:——————:——————:——————:——————:——————

   never   always   n/a

12. The CNS facilitates quality nursing care and serves as a role model.

———————:——————:——————:——————:——————:——————

   never   always   n/a

13. The CNS involvement facilitates patient and family readiness for early discharge.

———————:——————:——————:——————:——————:——————

   never   always   n/a

14. The CNS facilitates and contributes to research projects.

———————:——————:——————:——————:——————:——————

   never   always   n/a

15. The CNS acts as role model for house and telephone standards.

———————:——————:——————:——————:——————:——————

   never   always   n/a

Your comments amplifying your ratings are most appreciated.

(Continued)

TABLE 12–6. (Continued)

Positive Comments: _____

_____

_____

_____

_____

_____

_____

Any Constructive Criticism? _____

_____

_____

_____

_____

_____

From The Clinical Nurse Specialists at the Medical Center at the University of California, San Francisco, copyright 1986. Reprinted with permission.

Similarities and Differences

Similarities and differences in role implementation influence the quality of collaborative problem solving. Similarities and differences in the roles of the cardiovascular surgery clinical nurse specialist and psychiatric liaison clinical nurse specialist will be summarized here. Both clinical nurse specialists receive referrals from multiple sources. Due to her continuing presence on the three units caring for adult cardiovascular surgery patients, the cardiovascular surgery clinical nurse specialist is more likely to identify and self-select patients, as in the case of JS, for direct care. The psychiatric liaison clinical nurse specialist may self-select patients when attending nursing rounds, but is more likely to focus on consultation and teaching to the nursing staff. Both clinical nurse specialists select patients for direct care based on similar factors. Both assess the complexity of the patient's situation as well as the individual nurse's or staff's level of knowledge, skill, and anxiety. Either clinical nurse specialist may become directly involved if a relationship is already developed with the patient/family, if the complexity and acuity of the patient exceed the present skills of the staff, in cases where patient continuity may be compromised (e.g., when the patient is transferred to a variety of units), or when a procedure that is unfamiliar to the staff nurse needs to be done. Both clinical nurse specialists expect that nurses caring for patients will accompany them to see the patient, if time permits, to learn necessary skills, assist with the plan of care, verbalize questions concerning unfamiliar aspects of care and, in the process, increase problem-solving skills. If, after clarification, validation, or reassurance from the clinical nurse specialist, the nurse involved feels capable of handling the patient problem, the clinical nurse specialist may eliminate direct involvment.

The cardiovascular surgery clinical nurse specialist has a more focused area of concern and therefore a smaller potential case load but a larger proportion of direct care activities. Much of the work of the psychiatric liaison clinical nurse specialist is focused on the systems around the patient and therefore on indirect care. The cardiovascular surgery clinical nurse specialist works primarily with nursing staff in the same speciality, while the psychiatric liaison clinical nurse specialist, as the "nurse's nurse", works with nursing staff in non-psychiatric specialties.

Because both clinical nurse specialists are first and foremost nurses, both share a common language, a concern for the whole patient, and an agreement about nursing diagnosis and treatment of the response to illness. In this context of shared discipline and role, their different specialty areas enhance collaboration by offering distinct expertise and knowledge; this provides different vantage points for evaluating a situation. Clinical nurse specialists working in collaboration can transfer knowledge to each other. The constant spreading of clinical knowledge from specialist to specialist and specialist to staff is an enrichment process of great importance to nursing care. The expertise of clinical nurse specialists eventually spreads to benefit patients throughout the institution, patients whom these nurses might never see (Poole, 1986).

IMPACT OF CLINICAL NURSE SPECIALIST INTERVENTION

Method of Evaluation of Patient Outcomes

The one area of practice that creates the greatest degree of frustration is developing an objective method of evaluation of patient care outcomes. Methods which the clinical nurse specialist peer group at the University of California, San Francisco (UCSF) have developed have been for patient case documentation only—a feat in itself to have eighteen clinical nurse specialists with diverse specialties come to a consensus. The dilemma of evaluating patient care outcomes is that many of the patient outcomes are not exclusively dependent on the expertise of clinical nurse specialist interventions even though the outcome is influenced highly by them. Clinical nurse specialists may believe that a patient's length of hospital stay was significantly shorter because of clinical nurse specialist interventions, but ultimately it is the attending physician who determines the day of discharge. One would also presume that one's influence has significantly improved the patient's ability to provide self-care and to utilize resources of health care providers, thus notably reducing recidivism. Various professional groups are attempting to study this problem, but the progress has been extremely slow. In this age of cost containment, clinical nurse specialists feel increased pressure to develop an objective method of documenting the value of clinical nurse specialist positions to save current positions and to open new ones.

The psychiatric liaison clinical nurse specialist and the cardiovascular surgery clinical nurse specialist have not yet developed a formal method of documenting patient care outcomes beyond the clinical nurse specialist's quantification of patients to whom care is provided directly. When direct care is provided, clear documentation in the patient record is essential, not only as a legal record but also as a method of communicating one's interventions and their effects to other members of the health care team, thereby building a positive image. The clinical nurse specialists have relied on subjective data based on a variety of feedback mechanisms including letters from patients, families, other health team members, and the clinical nurse specialist evaluation tool (Table 12–6). Changes in patient care trends are monitored through the nursing audits of the department of nursing's unit-based quality assurance program, although these improvements may not be directly tied to the intervention of a particular clinical nurse specialist. Other components of the evaluation process include self-evaluation and administrative review using the job description as a base for the measurement of effective performance. The clinical nurse specialists at UCSF also use a form of peer review in which, on a rotating basis, individual clinical nurse specialists present their role, including areas of difficulty in implementation. As a group, the clinical nurse specialists prepare an annual report for the director of nursing and the director of the medical center.

If it is impact the clinical nurse specialist is hoping to demonstrate, the search for quantitative methods may not be the only useful approach at this time. Many of the outcomes of clinical nurse specialist intervention are affected by a complex of other variables as well as other members of the health care team, as in hospital discharge times. Persuading colleagues in the health care community of the clinical nurse specialist's value might be accomplished through effective story-telling and description, in addition to formal research or program evaluation. Media persuades powerfully. It does so by telling stories and anecdotes about people, full of rich detail, creating pictures that excite the imagination and engender new possibilities. Leah Curtain (1987), in the editorial "About Nurses: Perceptions and Misperceptions," makes the point that nurses should be building a media campaign that builds on preexisting positive perceptions, is emotive rather than cognitive, and offers something to the public. She suggests building on the "Nightingale" image of the nurse as competent clinician, decision maker, social activist, researcher, educator, administrator, and reformer. The clinical nurse specialist is ideal to represent this image to the public, and in promulgating a dynamic, committed profession, clinical nurse specialists will also demonstrate their own impact.

Within the last few years, with the support and often at the initiation of the director of nursing, clinical nurse specialists have been featured in high quality UCSF publications (Callister, 1985; Poole, 1986; *The Science of Caring*, 1985, 1986). Successfully weaving anecdotes with more formal description, the articles attest not only to the specialized clinical contributions of clinical nurse specialists, but also to the breadth of the role.

Positive benefits have resulted from these publications which are distributed locally, nationally, and internationally. One publication led to a feature article about one of the clinical nurse specialists in a San Francisco newspaper. Since the publication of the article by William Poole (a pediatric nurse who is also a professional writer), various physicians joined together to request the development of additional clinical nurse specialist positions to support their patient populations. Many nursing staff have also been requesting new positions in particular areas. Because of these requests and other factors, four additional clinical nurse specialist positions were funded; this is in stark contrast to reports of clinical nurse specialist positions being eliminated elsewhere. In the Northern California Clinical Nurse Specialist Group, discussions are periodically held to track unpublished and in-house reports of projects that formally document the clinical nurse specialists' impact on patient care outcomes.

In a complex tertiary care setting, cost effectiveness of a particular care provider is difficult to measure. If one is the primary clinical nurse specialist working with a nursing staff, it may be possible to measure one's clinical nurse specialist impact on the efficiency of nursing care provided as the staff learn new skills and work toward improving the quality of nursing care. Decreased readmissions can certainly be measured; JS is an example.

ROLE OF THE CLINICAL NURSE SPECIALIST IN THE PRACTICE SETTING

At the Medical Center of the University of California, San Francisco, the majority of clinical nurse specialists involved with the hospitalized patients are hired by nursing service, hold a staff position, and report directly to the director of nursing; several other clinical nurse specialists are funded by physicians and report dually to the physician and to the director of nursing. None of the clinical nurse specialists is unit-based; all are service-based in order to be more flexible and available for patient care needs. The clinical nurse specialists are direct caregivers, consultants, educators, and researchers, with primary responsibility to the patients in a particular specialty area and to the staff nurses caring for them. Free from formal administrative responsibility, the clinical nurse specialists also act as leaders, innovators, and change agents.

A staff position for the clinical nurse specialist, as opposed to a line position with managerial responsibilities, does allow greater time to attend to clinical issues and allows staff to be more open about their vulnerabilities or needs. The autonomy of a staff position allows the clinical nurse specialist to be free to make decisions about priorities and to be responsible for these decisions. The other side of the coin is that ambiguity may result and lead to confusion on the part of others about how to use the skills of the clinical nurse specialist.

A possible disadvantage of the staff position is that without the authority of being part of the administrative hierarchy, the clinical nurse specialist does not carry the responsibility for the overall patient care and may be seen as an outsider. Thus expert and referent power must be combined with excellent interpersonal skills to achieve clinical goals. Working in a staff position in a large institution, it is necessary to develop solid, respectful working relationships with administrative nurses and the clinical leadership on each unit to increase the follow-through and effectiveness of recommendations, as well as to promote continued learning.

RESEARCH IN PRACTICE

The aspect of the clinical nurse specialist role that is most often neglected is that of research. As expressed in Chapter 4, the clinical nurse specialist has the unique opportunity to significantly influence the direction in which the scientific basis for nursing is to be expanded. It is expected that any nurse in advanced practice will identify researchable questions and will share and implement research findings in patient care situations; however, the clinical nurse specialist must be actively involved in practice-based research. In spite of the yearly increase in the total time devoted to research endeavors, the smallest proportion of the cardiovascular surgery clinical nurse specialist's and psychiatric liaison clinical nurse specialist's time is spent in research (for both, less than 5 percent). A university medical center, by definition, supports research, education, and patient care, in that order. The department of nursing also supports research with an active research committee providing some monetary and enthusiastic people support. In addition, one of the members of the clinical nurse specialist group is currently the chair of the university's three-site committee on human research. However, because the primary focus of the clinical nurse specialist role in the institution is quality patient care, research is necessarily a lower priority. Therefore, linking research to the area of clinical practice in which one is already involved increases the possibility of doing research.

Because most clinical nurse specialists have clinical expertise but lack sophistication in research methodology, and likewise because nurse researchers who are expert in research methodology often lack access to patient populations or recent clinical experience, there is the prime opportunity, but more often unused possibility, for collaboration (Jacox, 1980). Once the commitment to collaborative research has been made, there are certain guidelines that may be used by the clinical nurse specialist to promote a successful research endeavor:

1. Select a research topic whose results will, presumably, make a difference in patient care outcomes.
2. Investigate a clinical area which will hopefully expand the scientific basis for nursing practice.
3. Clarify with your co-investigator(s) the responsibilities of participation and extent of time allocation.
4. Take care to fulfill the agreed-upon percentage of participation but, on the other hand, do not jeopardize your primary responsibility for patient care needs.

Research activities of the two clinical nurse specialists will be reviewed briefly. The cardiovascular surgery clinical nurse specialist and the psychiatric liaison clinical nurse specialist, with two other investigators, completed data collection on a survey of clinical nurse specialists at the annual UCSF Clinical Nurse Specialist Conference, and have been working with statisticians at the UCSF School of Nursing to analyze the data.

For more than 7 years the cardiovascular surgery clinical nurse specialist has been a co-investigator in a series of research projects investigating the impact of cardiac surgery on patient recovery and family functioning (Gilliss, Sparacino, Gortner, & Kenneth, 1985; Gortner, et al. 1985). The participation has been invaluable for many reasons, the greatest of which have been the validation of the value of clinical research, the impact on personal practice, and the ability to teach and counsel patients based on research outcomes. The series of research studies have also illustrated the interaction of human biology and social behavior, or the interface of social and biological sciences with illness and health.

Participation in clinical research has highlighted the several advantages and the one disadvantage of the clinical nurse specialist's research role component. The advantages are that the clinical nurse specialist can rapidly translate the findings into personal practice (Barnard, 1980), the diffusion time for new findings to reach the practice level is eliminated at least for the clinician involved (King, Barnard, & Hoehn, 1981), and there is the satisfaction derived from implementing new content into nursing interventions and observing the impact on patient welfare and outcomes. The one disadvantage identified by the cardiovascular surgery clinical nurse specialist has been the difficulty in remaining objective during data collection phases and avoiding premature translation of subjective results into clinical practice, thereby potentially contaminating the research and minimizing the hoped-for effect in the experimental group.

The cardiovascular surgery clinical nurse specialist's involvement with the Family Heart Study project also illustrated the many advantages, and few disadvantages, of collaborative research. The research team for the Family Heart Study was composed of several experienced nurse researchers and two expert nurse clinicians, each of whom had unique, separate, and yet complementary roles. The clinicians provided access to patients and guidance on what relevance the study outcomes might have for improving patient care delivery, and the nurse researchers provided the expert knowledge on theoretical frameworks, methodology, and statistical analysis. Such collegiality demonstrated that the perceived, if not real, gap between the roles of clinicians and researchers can be bridged and that collaboration between nurses in the practice setting and nurses in the academic setting is not only feasible, but is productive and mutually satisfying.

The cardiovascular surgery clinical nurse specialist identified two disadvantages of collaborative research: one is specific to the difference between clinical and academic responsibilities and the other is a hazard of any collaborative project. Inherent in any collaborative endeavor is the issue of ownership. While original intent is based on trust and good will, commitment and accountability may change and conflict may arise when seniority of authorship needs to be decided. A potential problem specific to the differences between the clinical and academic roles is one of time allocation. While neither type of role has more time than the other, the academician tends to have more predictable time and a research priority, while the clinician's available research time must necessarily be whatever can be squeezed between priority patient needs.

The cardiovascular surgery clinical nurse specialist has gained personally and professionally from continued involvement in collaborative nursing research. The professional gains have been the opportunity to be integrally involved in generating new knowledge that will hopefully improve nursing care and reduce costs, and the continued learning of research methodologies. The personal gain has been the colleagueship and the opportunity to participate in presenting the findings at the local, national, and international levels.

The psychiatric liaison clinical nurse specialist and three co-investigators are currently involved in an exciting project that developed as a part of activities in the Department of Nursing's Quality Assurance Committee, of which the psychiatric liaison clinical nurse specialist is a member. Within the Quality Assurance program, the project is called Positive Case Review, and it was developed to enlarge the focus from problem-monitoring and standard-setting to identification of factors that produce positive outcomes in patient care. The Positive Case Reviews have proven gratifying and energizing for the nursing staff. They have also aided in the identification of nursing attitudes, behaviors, and interventions related to positive patient outcomes. The investigators are currently writing a proposal for an exploratory study to determine the factors antecedent to positive outcomes in patient care. Multiple study sites will be utilized. The focus on positive situations is expected to produce data that are descriptive of more or less ideal circumstances, identify what a positive outcome is, and suggest personal, interpersonal, and social variables that people associate with positive outcomes.

Contributions to the development of nursing science may also be made by participating as a research subject. Both clinical nurse specialists have served as subjects in a number of studies of the clinical nurse specialist role. In addition, the psychiatric liaison clinical nurse specialist was selected as a subject in Benner and Tanner's (1987) study of expert nursing practice, thereby contributing to the understanding of the role of intuition in expert nursing practice. From participation as a subject, other collaborative activities have developed, including writing for publication and giving presentations in school of nursing programs as well as at international conferences.

If clinical nurse specialists broaden the definition of research to include a variety of contributions to the scientific base of nursing practice, the research component of the role may not appear neglected. The advantages significantly outweigh the disadvantages.

SUMMARY

While differences are evident between the implementation of the roles of cardiovascular surgery clinical nurse specialist and psychiatric liaison clinical nurse specialist, significant similarities exist. Both differences and similarities enhance collaboration and lend to integrative solutions to complex patient care problems. Positive impact on patient care outcomes is the result, although it may be difficult to single out and measure the impact of the clinical nurse specialist alone.

SPECIFIC QUESTIONS

1. Compare and contrast clinical nurse specialist behaviors that enhance collaboration and behaviors that may lead to territorial competition between clinical nurse specialists.
2. How do the types of consultation identified in this chapter complement each other? Which of these types of consultation do you use most often and why?
3. Based on descriptions in this chapter, identify the factors you

consider most important when making a decision regarding direct versus indirect care.
4. Describe a situation in which you have applied theory to practice to design an intervention. What was the outcome? Compare your answer to the case study in the chapter.

REFERENCES

Barnard, K. (1980). Knowledge for practice: Directions for the future. *Nursing Research, 29* (4), 208–212.

Benner, P., & Tanner, C. (1987). Clinical judgment: How expert nurses use intuition. *American Journal of Nursing, 87* (1), 23–31.

Calley, J.M., Dirksen, M., Engalla, M., & Hennrich, M.L. (1980). The Orem self-care nursing model. In J.P. Riehl & C. Roy (Eds.), *Conceptual models for nursing practice* (2nd ed.). New York: Appleton-Century-Crofts.

Callister, J. (1985). Lara's story. *UCSF Magazine, 8* (3), 40–45.

Coleman, L.J. (1980). Orem's self-care concept of nursing. In J.P. Riehl & C. Roy (Eds.), *Conceptual models for nursing practice* (2nd ed.). New York: Appleton-Century-Crofts.

Curtain, L. (1987). About nurses: Perceptions and misperceptions. *Nursing Management, 18* (1), 11–12.

Dickson, G.L., & Lee-Villasenor, H. (1982). Nursing theory and practice: A self-care approach. *Advances in Nursing Science, 5,* (1) 29–40.

Gilliss, C., Sparacino, P., Gortner, S., & Kenneth, H. (1985). Events leading to the treatment of coronary artery disease: Implications for nursing care. *Heart-Lung, 14* (4), 350–356.

Gortner, S., Gilliss, C., Moran, J., et al. (1985). Expected and realized benefits from coronary bypass surgery in relation to severity of illness. *Cardiovascular Nursing, 21* (3), 13–18.

Jacox, A. (1980). Strategies to promote nursing research. *Nursing Research, 29* (4), 213–217.

Johnson, J. (1972). Effects of structuring patients' expectations on their reactions to threatening events. *Nursing Research, 21* (6), 499–503.

Johnson, J., Fuller, S., Endress, M.P., & Rice, V. (1978). Altering patients' responses to surgery: An extension and replication. *Research in Nursing and Health, 1* (3), 111–121.

Johnson, S.H. (1985). Specialization with collaboration. *Dimensions of Critical Care Nursing, 4* (5), 259–260.

Joseph, L.S. (1980). Self-care and the nursing process. *Nursing Clinics of North America, 15* (1), 131–143.

King, D., Barnard, K., & Hoehn, R. (1981). Disseminating the results of nursing research. *Nursing Outlook, 29* (3), 164–169.

Lewinsohn, P.M., Sullivan, M.J., & Grosscup, S.J. (1982). Behavioral therapy: Clinical applications. In A.J. Rush (Ed.), *Short-term psychotherapies for depression.* New York: The Guilford Press.

Lewis, A., & Levy, J.S. (1982). *Psychiatric liaison nursing: The theory and clinical practice.* Reston, VA: Reston Publishing.

Luna-Raines, M. (1989). The confused response. In B. Riegel & D. Ehrenreich (Eds.), *Psychological aspects of critical care nursing*. Rockville, Maryland: Aspen Publishers.

McLean, P. (1982). Behavioral therapy: Theory and research. In A.J. Rush (Ed.), *Short-term psychotherapies for depression*. New York: The Guilford Press.

Minarik, P.A. (1984). The psychiatric liaison nurse's role with families in acute care. *Nursing Clinics of North America, 19* (1), 161–171.

Mullin, V.I. (1980). Implementing the self-care concept in the acute care setting. *Nursing Clinics of North America, 15* (1), 177–190.

Nelson, J.K.N., & Schilke, D.A. (1976). The evolution of psychiatric liaison nursing. *Perspectives in Psychiatric Care, 14*, 61.

Orem, D.E. (1985). *Nursing: Concepts of practice*, 3rd ed. New York: McGraw-Hill.

Poole, W. (1986). Clinical nurse specialists. *UCSF Magazine, 9* (3), 31–39.

The Science of Caring: Nursing at University of California, San Francisco. (1985). San Francisco: School of Nursing, University of California, San Francisco.

The Science of Caring: Nursing at University of California, San Francisco. (1986). San Francisco: School of Nursing, University of California, San Francisco.

Underwood, P.R. (1980). Facilitating self-care. In P.C. Pothier (Ed.), *Psychiatric nursing*. Boston: Little, Brown.

Weiss, S.J., & Davis, H.P. (1985). Validity and reliability of the collaborative practice scales. *Nursing Research, 34* (5), 299–305.

Wolanin, M.O., & Phillips, L.R.F. (1981). *Confusion: Prevention and care*. St. Louis: Mosby.

chapter thirteen

The Clinical Nurse Specialist in Private Collaborative Practice

Lora E. Burke

Collaborative or joint practice has been defined by the National Joint Practice Commission as "nurses and physicians collaborating as colleagues to provide patient care" (National Joint Practice Commission, 1977). Fagin and Lamberton (1981) noted that, through working together, health professionals are able to bring distinct yet different talents and abilities to the clinical setting, from which the recipient of their services will benefit. Some of the important characteristics of collaborative practice include both interdependent and cooperative decision making as well as the sharing of knowledge, goals, confidence, and mutual trust (Burchell, Thomas, & Smith, 1983).

Collaborative practice may take place in various settings. The setting described in this chapter is a private collaborative practice with a clinical nurse specialist and a cardiologist. This chapter also presents a case study of a patient cared for in such a practice. The interventions provided by the clinical nurse specialist are described with attention given to how these interventions differ from those of other caregivers. A patient representative of the practice was selected rather than one who presented as a catastrophic case with multiple needs. The methods of communication utilized with staff and patients by a clinical nurse specialist functioning independently are discussed. Patient outcomes are reviewed with discussion of how the clinical nurse specialist in particular made an impact on the case. How this role impacts on nursing practice on a particular unit and what research has to offer closes the chapter.

So that the reader may have a better understanding of the clinical nurse specialist delivering care in this unique setting, a brief description of the role and the practice will precede the case study presentation.

COLLABORATIVE PRACTICE ROLE

I am a clinical nurse specialist who is self-employed. I function as a consultant to the physician in the care of all patients in the collaborative practice. This includes hospitalized patients as well as those seen in the office. Activities that are performed regularly include making daily rounds on hospitalized patients, seeing new consultations in the hospital and in the office, assisting with procedures such as treadmill testing, and instructing and counseling patients and their families. When seeing a patient in consultation I obtain a complete history and perform a physical exam. I then present the patient to my associate in the presence of the patient, and he clarifies any questions he might have and confirms the physical findings. Once the course of action is determined, I explain this to the patient. Patients seen in consultation in the hospital are referred by another physician. In the office they are referred by a physician, another individual, or themselves.

Other patient-related activities I perform include telephone calls to patients in response to their questions or concerns, interpretation of test results, and counseling sessions with patients to assist them in dietary modification, coping with stress, weight reduction, and exercise. Home visits are made to selected patients. Because of the time involved, these are limited to patients for whom information significant to their management can be obtained by seeing the patient in the home setting. With the proliferation of home health agencies, it has become easier to make a referral and work with the nurse or therapist who can see the patient regularly.

Application for staff privileges was made to the hospital and approved before I was able to document interventions and write orders. This was a lengthy process that followed the recommendations of the Joint Practice Commission and the American Nurses' Association (ANA, 1978). It was strongly supported by nursing administration of the hospital as well as my associate.

The financial arrangements established by my associate and me allow me to be reimbursed on a fee-for-service and percentage of collectibles basis. My income is derived from a predetermined percentage of the collected receipts from the entire practice. Initially, this was based on only the parts of the practice in which I participate, such as hospital rounds, office follow-up visits, treadmill testing, and consultations. For the activities that I am able to perform independently, such as the educational and counseling sessions, I receive full reimbursement of fees from the practice. Because of a change in our inhouse computer and ability to track activities, we reduced the percentage and now base it on the collectibles of the entire practice.

To help meet the overhead expenses of office rent and staff salaries, I pay my associate a fixed amount every month. I pay for my own phone bill and personal equipment. Because I am self-employed, I must pay my own fringe benefits, such as health and disability insurance and monthly parking.

The majority of services provided by me are billed under my associate's name. Independent activities are billed under his title but clearly identified as a service provided by me. Laws do not exist as yet for me to bill independently (ANA, 1984). When billing third-party payers, it is important to describe the services provided and how they relate to the diagnosis (Campbell, 1982). An example would be the patient who has exogenous obesity, hyperlipidemia, and hypertension, who receives dietary counseling and teaching for the management of weight reduction and hypertension. This is a simple process that I learned from a billing consultant who has extensive experience.

Case Study

Mr. S was a 46-year-old, Hispanic, married male who was admitted to the coronary care unit (CCU) following 48 hours of chest pain associated with nausea and vomiting and diaphoresis. The chest pain subsided shortly after admission with no recurrence. There were minor ventricular arrhythmias the first 24 hours, which responded to a Lidocaine infusion, but no signs or symptoms of heart failure or pericarditis developed. The serial electro-cardiograms (ECG) showed unstable anteriolateral T waves for the first few days, which stabilized by the fifth day. The two-dimensional echocardiogram showed slight hypokinesia of the left lower ventricular septum. There was no pericardial effusion. Cardiac enzymes rose which confirmed an acute myocardial infarction.

Based on the above data, the nursing diagnoses in the acute period were:

1. Potential alteration in cardiac output
2. Anxiety, minimal
3. Potential activity intolerance
4. Knowledge deficit (regarding acute illness and follow-up care)
5. Potential self-concept disturbance in role performance

Mr. S was allowed to begin a progressive activity program within 48 hours, which consisted initially of sitting in the chair. Following transfer from the CCU to the telemetry unit, he was evaluated by physical therapy for continued progression of activity and by occupational therapy for an energy conservation program. The physical therapist and occupational therapist worked with nursing staff to begin his educational program regarding a heart attack. Mr. S progressed well without complications. On the seventh day a low-level treadmill evaluation was performed. He completed the submaximal exercise protocol without adverse symptoms. There were no arrhythmias or ECG changes during or following exercise. The following day he was discharged home with his only medications being a beta blocker, Timolol 10 mg twice a day, and Nitroglycerin as needed. Follow-up would occur in the office in 1 week.

Mr. S was referred by us to the outpatient cardiac rehabilitation program for monitored exercise sessions two times per week. The exercise prescription was based on the results of the submaximal treadmill done prior to discharge. This activity was supplemented by a progressive walking program at home.

Mr. S's social background showed that he was of Mexican descent. He was born and raised in California and had been married for 22 years. His wife, who was from Mexico, spoke limited English and did not work outside the home. They had two children, ages twelve and nine. Mr. S worked as a welder, a job he had held for several years. This involved lifting up to seventy-five pounds. He averaged 40 hours per week on the job. Mr. S and his family resided in a one-story house in Los Angeles, which they owned. They had a close family relationship and spent their leisure time doing family-oriented activities. He denied any significant amount of stress in his personal life.

His risk factors for coronary heart disease included a 25 year history of smoking one pack of cigarettes per day, which he had discontinued 1 year previously, and a serum cholesterol of 256. He was approximately 20 pounds overweight, had a sedentary life style, and identified stress in his work environment. There was no family history of heart disease or diabetes.

CLINICAL NURSE SPECIALIST INTERVENTION

Method of Patient Selection
As a clinical nurse specialist functioning in a private practice, criteria for case selection does not apply in the same manner as for a clinical nurse specialist in a staff position in an institution. All patients are usually seen by me on daily rounds. Their level of acuity usually does not influence their selection since I do not provide direct hands-on patient care.

Criteria for Patient Case Load
Criteria used when selecting patients for more extensive interventions focus on needs they or their family have that I can meet during the time spent at the hospital or through phone communication. Therefore, general criteria used are:

- Physical needs of the patient that I might assist nursing staff in meeting
- Emotional needs of the spouse or other family members that I am able to meet
- Educational needs of the patient and family
- Need for postdischarge follow-up that I may be able to assist in planning and coordinating

Criteria for Appropriateness of Type of Intervention
The amount of intervention delivered by a clinical nurse specialist in a private practice situation varies with the individual patient and the tim-

ing in the illness and recovery process. One patient may need a great deal of time while in the hospital and another may require frequent intervention following discharge.

Criteria used to determine the method or type of intervention are based on a needs assessment of the individual, done when seen on rounds or through discussion with staff. The primary subroles of the clinical nurse specialist in a private practice setting (educator/counselor and practitioner) are kept in mind when determining the services to be provided, as is the appropriateness of the level of need for clinical nurse specialist intervention.

In the case of Mr. S, the subroles of educator and counselor were utilized from the very beginning. The patient was seen by me for initial history and physical examination, which was then presented to my associate. Throughout this period I was able to assess Mr. S's responses to the situation. Upon completion of this process, the patient was provided an opportunity to ventilate his concerns and/or ask questions of us both. Time was also spent with Mrs. S. Additional time was spent by me with the couple in reexplaining the diagnosis and expected course of events. This method of intervention was repeated daily as part of rounds. Additional visits were made to the patient after rounds were completed, when I assessed a need for him to talk or have further information provided. His spouse was called and information was relayed to her on a regular basis. An interpreter was used when the information provided seemed to be fairly complicated and I could not be sure she understood it in English.

The educational program for a patient with an acute myocardial infarction (MI) is conducted by all members of the team: nursing, physical therapy, occupational therapy, dietary, and social services. Mr. S received a booklet on MIs two days after admission. I provided Mrs. S with a similar booklet in Spanish. My interventions were directed at meeting the specific needs of this couple, whatever they were that particular day. Since my time is flexible and the office is near by, I could arrange to spend longer periods of time with them some days or return when the wife could be present later.

Typically, a post-MI educational program follows an outline, and staff feel this must be reviewed fully prior to hospital discharge. Because I would be following the patient through office visits after discharge, there was no urgency to cover all material in a set time period. I focused on relaying information about whatever was on the patient's and spouse's mind that day. The spouse was given an opportunity to have a separate session with me, which we had once. This time was spent with me being a supportive listener while allowing Mrs. S to ventilate her concerns about the future, immediate and long-term, and discussing how she might best assist her husband.

While our patients receive instruction from each team member during their hospital stay, I see myself in the role of primary educator. I take responsibility for assuring that the patient and family have received and understood the information essential to know prior to discharge. In Mr. S's case, it was imperative that he know symptoms to be alert to, how to respond, how to use nitroglycerin, and what precautions to take. Also, patient understanding of activity allowances, dietary recommendations, and medications are very important; therefore, this specific information needs to be provided on more than one occasion. I covered this material in general terms early in the recovery course and repeated it several times, each time providing more specific guidelines. The MI booklet provided early in the hospitalization had general information on these topics. More specific printed information was provided on diet, medications, and activity as more was learned about Mr. S's prognosis.

While ample teaching or question-and-answer time is vital for the patient to have a good understanding of his illness and recovery process, it is also important that the patient understand the day-to-day activities, such as post-MI evaluation tests. An important intervention done by me as part of our rounds is preparing the patient for procedures he will undergo. Follow-up to this is interpreting the results of the tests to the patient and discussing the implications of these results for his prognosis. The spouse is provided with the same information.

The role of educator is the one I use most and is applied in all my usual functions. While it is a mode through which I am most effective in making changes, being able to provide counsel to the patient or family is helpful to them and rewarding to me. During any phase of an illness, the patient or family member may be in crisis. The clinical nurse specialist who serves as a primary care giver in an independent role can be well-acquainted with the individual and able to intervene in the crisis. Again, flexibility of my schedule allows me more control over my availability to the patient or relative; I, therefore, am able to meet the specific needs of a patient or family easily.

Mrs. S was very upset the day of her husband's admission. She could only think of him and the young children at home and was unable to take action in making arrangements. By allowing her to air her concerns, providing support, and assisting her in taking appropriate action, she was able to work through this crisis. She was also able to arrange additional support from her network of neighbors and friends. I was able to follow her on a regular basis during her husband's convalescence, mainly through regular telephone calls but also during joint and individual sessions.

Counselling is required during times other than a crisis. Assisting the patient and spouse to adjust to changes in lifestyle required by the illness is an ongoing process that continues well beyond discharge. Counseling may also be needed regarding resumption of sexual activity.

Both the patient and spouse may have fears they find difficult to verbalize. Many staff nurses do not feel comfortable discussing this topic and therefore never raise it, or do so but are unable to help the couple feel comfortable.

While intervening with Mr. and Mrs. S, I raised the topic early so they knew it would be discussed and felt free to ask questions. Initially, I counseled the patient alone so that I could assess his feelings and expectations as well as past habits and experiences. If there have been difficulties in the past or the patient has concerns about future sexual function, he may feel more comfortable expressing them without the spouse present. For the same reasons, I raised the topic with Mrs. S during a separate session. Prior to discharge, during a joint session, I reviewed the topic with them and facilitated their expression of concern to each other and provided information they could both hear.

The final in-hospital session took place the afternoon prior to discharge. I arranged for Mrs. S to come so that we could have a "wrap-up" session. Mr. S had a low-level treadmill evaluation that morning, so we had objective data on which to base activity progression. Time was spent answering many questions as well as conducting a general review of pertinent material. Treatment of chest pain and other symptoms and use of nitroglycerin and other medications were reviewed. A 5 × 7 medication card was provided at discharge for home use. At the first office visit, a wallet-sized card would be provided which would be updated regularly. The couple was also informed about the possibility of Mr. S experiencing a homecoming depression. They were given additional printed instructions and encouraged to call us at any time to ask questions or just talk. Arrangements were made for follow-up in the office 1 week later.

In reviewing the five nursing diagnoses made at the time of admission, the first one, potential alteration in cardiac output, never actualized. The second, anxiety, was anticipated and treated and never became a problem. Mr. S encountered no difficulty as he progressed in physical activities (diagnosis three), but the potential would be there for another 8 weeks. The fourth and fifth nursing diagnoses, knowledge deficit and potential self-concept disturbance in role performance, were being managed through the education and counseling which occurred in the hospital and were continued during follow-up.

A phone call to the couple was made during the week following discharge to check on Mr. S's progress and to see how they were coping. No major problems had occurred, and the time was used for general questioning and providing reassurance. One week after discharge, Mr. S was seen in the office for follow-up. He was seen weekly, initially, and gradually his visits were reduced to a less frequent schedule. Time was provided during his office visit for Mr. S, or his wife when she was able to accompany him, to ask questions or discuss in general how their adjustment was going. I usually initiated this by asking questions pertinent to various issues. My associate and I generally alternated seeing Mr. S. Even on the visits when I was not scheduled to see him, I would usually see him briefly to check on his progress and follow-up on the predischarge instructions.

An important area for clinical nurse specialist intervention with this patient population is modification of risk factors and lifestyle. There were four significant risk factors for progression of atherosclerosis and coronary heart disease that we needed to address with Mr. S. These were reviewed with him so priorities could be set and goals established. The sedentary lifestyle was already in the process of being modified by attending outpatient exercise sessions 2 to 3 times per week through the cardiac rehabilitation program. The stress in his work environment would not be an issue for at least 6 weeks but needed to be dealt with prior to his return. That left two risk factors, the cholesterol of 256 and being overweight. The elevated cholesterol was the most significant, since overall it is one of the most important risk factors. In a discussion with Mr. S, this was reviewed and he arrived at the decision to give priority to this area.

A nutritional counseling session was scheduled for both Mr. S and his wife, and he was given a set of forms on which to record his food intake for 5 days. This was to be completed and sent in prior to their appointment. An initial session was held in which his dietary habits were further assessed and the couple was instructed regarding cholesterol, the role it plays in the disease process, and where it is found in the diet. The couple seemed to have good comprehension of the material but were scheduled for two follow-up sessions so progress could be followed closely as well as further instructions given. Printed material including lists of fat and cholesterol content of foods and recipes were provided. They both had additional questions as they began to implement the diet.

In following the low-cholesterol, low-fat diet, Mr. S reduced his fat and caloric intake and began losing weight. This was further enhanced by the increased physical activity. At the 8-week post-heart attack stage, a symptom limited treadmill test was conducted. There were no ECG changes, arrhythmias, or symptoms during or following the evaluation. His exercise prescription was upgraded to allow a higher heart rate. He continued attending the exercise sessions and supplemented this with walking 30 to 45 minutes on the days he did not go to the rehabilitation sessions.

Mr. S was scheduled to return to work the tenth week postinfarction. Since his work involved lifting and carrying 50 to 75 pounds, we wanted to have him evaluated in a simulated situation. To do this, we had the therapist in cardiac rehabilitation monitor him while performing work loads equivalent to his job. There was an appropriate increase in heart rate and blood pressure without the occurrence of arrhythmias or angina.

A session with me was scheduled for Mr. S so we could review activity progression now that he would no longer be going to the exercise sessions and would be working full time. A major part of the time was devoted to talking about the stress in his work environment prior to his illness and how he planned to handle it. In doing so, I created specific situations and helped him work through how to best handle each one.

As Mr. S completed his recovery process and resumed his full schedule, his follow-up office visits were reduced to every three months. He continues to be followed in this manner and is usually seen by both my associate and me. If any problems requiring additional attention, such as increased serum cholesterol or weight gain, were to occur, I would schedule additional sessions with him so that I could assist him in modifying the situation. When his cholesterol level is checked, I call him to discuss the results, provide positive reinforcement, and make suggestions regarding diet.

From this account, the differences between the staff-nurse and clinical nurse specialist interventions are evident. The flexibility in schedules and the depth and breadth of the interventions in following the patient are not an option for a staff nurse. Being available to provide crisis intervention counseling in the evening, when there are no social workers and few hospital-employed clinical nurse specialists on duty, is somewhat unique to an independent clinical nurse specialist. The level of knowledge and expertise required to provide the services described are beyond the level of a baccalaureate-prepared nurse. The staff nurse also does not have the mobility to follow a patient from the coronary care unit to the convalescent units or the time to spend with the spouse once the mate has been moved from that unit.

The patient and spouse receive a fair amount of printed educational material in the hospital and office, plus other useful aids to help with medications and progress with exercise and weight. Except for the MI booklet that Mr. S received initially, all printed materials are either developed by the clinical nurse specialist or obtained by her from community or professional sources. No other patients in the hospital receive these materials.

Following the patient and spouse postdischarge and continuing specific interventions months later is an option most available to a privately employed clinical nurse specialist. A hospital-employed clinical nurse specialist could have provided most of these interventions, but in most circumstances would have had to turn over the postdischarge follow-up to a clinical nurse specialist in an outpatient setting, if that were available and the patient was going to that setting. In most settings, there is not a clinical nurse specialist available for outpatient follow-up.

Clinical Nurse Specialist/Health Team Communication

Communication is conducted through formal and informal methods. Using the written format is the most reliable means for reaching each member of the team. This consists of writing notes on the progress record, not the nurses' notes. Suggestions or approaches to care are recorded on the Kardex, as well as a brief medical and social history. A form was developed by the staff and myself for use with patients in the inpatient cardiac rehabilitation program. This form provides space for a brief cardiac history and assessment of knowledge level. An outline of the MI teaching content, with space for documentation of teaching done and evaluation of patient response, is included on the form. Utilization of this short form is a particularly good way to communicate specifically about this intervention with members of the rehabilitation team.

Verbal communication with the staff takes place during our daily rounds. When I return for meetings with the patient and spouse, I try to keep the staff informed of my interventions and their impact. A structured format for verbal communication takes place weekly in the cardiac rehabilitation rounds. The nursing staff presents the patients to the medical director and other team members. In this conference we discuss history, current illness, progress, problems and plans, and how the team could help the individual. Frequently individual communication between team members occurs following the conference. My associate and I had frequent discussions concerning Mr. S while making rounds during Mr. S's hospitalization or in the office prior to his follow-up visits. I dictated progress notes in the office, which were also read by my associate.

Clinical Nurse Specialist/Patient Communication

The principle method of communication with the patient is verbal one-to-one encounters. Small group discussions involving my associate, the patient, the spouse, and myself occur as part of rounds. As with Mrs. S, the spouse and I can also communicate through telephone calls. All verbal instructions are supplemented by printed material, which include diagrams as well as instructions with greater detail.

Joint evaluation of the patient's progress takes place during daily rounds and in the weekly cardiac rehabilitation conference attended by all the team members. Strategies to increase progress are discussed in this session.

IMPACT OF CLINICAL NURSE SPECIALIST INTERVENTION

Patient outcomes that are evaluated are patient's level of knowledge and understanding of the medical regimen and how the instructions are followed. This is not measured in a formal written test but through oral testing on follow-up visits. The patients are asked routinely what medicines they are taking and how. This uncovers any confusion or error and allows for immediate correction. An evaluation of the patient's general condition and progress in increasing activity are other ways to measure adherence.

In the case of Mr. S, another outcome important to evaluate was how he was doing in reaching his goal of reduced cholesterol and weight. Weight measurements were taken on every visit and did show progress, with a final weight loss being 18 pounds, two pounds short of the recommendations. Lipid profiles were checked every 3 months to determine his total cholesterol and high density lipoprotein (HDL). Through dietary changes and exercise, he was able to reduce his cholesterol to 198 and raise the HDL to 60, both in the target range of his goal and general recommendations.

One could argue that Mr. S would have achieved these goals and improvement in cardiovascular health without the intervention of the clinical nurse specialist. While the author does not have a controlled study to show the effect of no intervention, she does have significant experience in working with the cardiovascular patient population. Compliance has been studied extensively, and one of the factors that influences it is follow-up and reinforcement of the instructions (Burke, 1981). The attention of intervening in itself has a therapeutic effect. Scalzi and colleagues (1980) showed that provision of printed material had a positive effect on patient compliance. The material given to this patient often provoked questions later and served as a guideline for reference. The intervention of the clinical nurse specialist did increase the patient's and spouse's knowledge level, which seems to have affected his success in reaching the goals of risk factor reduction.

Method of Evaluation of Cost Effectiveness

Since an independent clinical nurse specialist is not salaried, cost effectiveness is viewed differently. The objectives I have in mind when intervening as I have described are improving care and reducing the risk of further events and readmissions. If this is accomplished, I know my time has been well spent.

Again, we have not been able to conduct a study to determine if our patients have a reduced length of stay or number of readmissions. That is clearly one of our goals and, because I am able to spend additional time with the patient and family and also coordinate our efforts with other team members, we may be able to accomplish our goals in a shorter period, or at least provide more comprehensive care in a given time period.

There is more communication with nursing staff regarding care of patients in our practice. Part of that is due to there being two nurses or a nurse and another team member exchanging information. Some team members and patients and families generally are more comfortable asking me, a nurse, for information and also feel I have more time to answer questions. My associate and I may invite a staff nurse to join us on our rounds. Increasing staff awareness of our concerns regarding a specific patient should have a positive effect on their nursing care.

ROLE OF THE CLINICAL NURSE SPECIALIST IN THE PRACTICE SETTING

I joined this practice in September 1982 though my associate invited me to join the practice earlier that year. He learned the value of a nurse in the practice when he had a graduate student conduct her clinical experience with him. Subsequently a nurse practitioner joined him in practice and was with him over 2 years before she died of an illness. I followed her and adopted the role.

One might ask why I pursued such a nontraditional role (Burke, 1983). For years, I had a dream of working with patients across the continuum of acute illness to regained health and, if possible, also in prevention. This position made that possible. It also provided the independence and creativity that I enjoy.

The development of role tasks came out of initial discussions as well as the precedents established by my predecessors. Since patient teaching and counseling is what I enjoy and do well, I assumed all related activities. Over time I developed more of these activities and am currently developing some group sessions for patients in the practice. As I became more familiar with the practice and patients, I assumed more activities, such as responsibility for patients' prothrombin time and Coumadin dosage in addition to follow-up of other lab test results. As the patients got to know me, they would call me with questions or to report problems. Since my associate has other responsibilities that I cannot share in (ECG, echo interpretation, etc. at the hospitals), my taking over these tasks reduces his hours.

With the exception of a very small minority, all the patients are seen by me. Alternating who sees the patient enables both of us to maintain good patient relationships. There is a small number of patients who will not accept being seen by a nurse, and therefore my associate always sees them. A few patients request that I always see them since they feel more comfortable with me.

I schedule only two follow-up patient appointments in an hour, compared to my associate who sees three. I spend the full 30 minutes with the patient, and possibly family, so that I can provide teaching and counseling. Patients have come to expect this attention and see me as having more time for listening and talking to them. I see this as one of the important differences between the physician and clinical nurse specialist. What I do with this time, and the rapport with the patient, are valuable contributions to the practice.

Where does support or resistance for this type of position come from? It is almost predictable. The main resistance, and there is not a great deal, comes from the medical community. This is not very apparent, but did become visible when my application for staff privileges was held up in the medical committee for 3 months. No resistance has been encountered from within nursing, and nursing administration has been most supportive. The staff in the office are very supportive and are probably my strongest promoters.

As one can imagine, it is difficult to conduct self-evaluation and peer review in such a setting. Peer review of our practice has been done once by a clinical nurse specialist who spent 2 full weeks with us. Graduate students who have clinical placement with us provide some feedback. My associate and I review our roles and tasks and the practice as a whole periodically. We do critique one another and make changes as needed to improve our individual roles as well as the joint practice. At the hospital where I have staff privileges, peer review has been conducted utilizing retrospective chart reviews.

As described in the beginning of this chapter, my position at the hospital where I see the majority of patients is that of an independent practitioner with staff privileges. The staff privileges allow me to do the activities described. As an independent practitioner, I carry no authority in terms of influencing staff. As a clinician who has established credibility with the staff, I serve as a role model who can influence care on a particular unit, and more so in individual cases. As described previously, during daily rounds I share the information relevant to the patient's case that could influence care.

In terms of affecting care on a particular unit, I was one of the leaders in organizing the patient education program on the post-CCU unit and developed the patient education recording form. Use of this form has improved the presentation of cases at the weekly rehabilitation conferences and also the communication between team members regarding interventions performed. I also shared with staff special patient education material I had available for loan to patients, so that I came to be known as a resource person, particularly in this area.

RESEARCH IN PRACTICE

Prior to my role as a clinical nurse specialist, I conducted research on patient education and compliance and anticipatory grief in spouses of the critically ill (Burke, 1978; Scalzi et al., 1980). The results of these studies, as well as the experience gained during the data collection, continue to make an impact on my nursing practice.

Thus far I have not conducted research as a clinical nurse specialist. There is certainly an interest in conducting studies in the future. One of the constraints of performing research in this type of arrangement is time and funding. As a self-employed consultant, there would be no financial provisions for coverage of time, supplies, and staff. It would be necessary to pursue external funding.

In addition to the previous reasons, time commitment is a factor. Because the practice can be quite time consuming, I hesitate to take on yet another project. In this setting there is no one else I can delegate to collect data. A graduate student who also has a commitment to the study would be a viable solution.

Unfortunately, I do not have a control group, and comparing it with another physician's practice is unacceptable. There would be innumerable variables confounding findings, and probably one could not obtain access to information on the patients in another practice. If the obstacles to doing research could be overcome, the first issue I would want to investigate is the effect of my presence on the patients in the practice. Do my interventions affect their compliance? Are there less hospital readmissions or planned admissions for a scheduled procedure? Is there reduced anxiety in the patient and family? Is there earlier discharge?

Gordon (1984) states that research into clinical practice will provide a critical evaluation of nursing practice and is essential for us to understand what is optimal nursing care and how we can provide it. Studies need to be done particularly on the role of the clinical nurse specialist. It is becoming important to look at different interpretations of the role in various settings, particularly at their effect on patient care and cost effectiveness. The clinical nurse specialist in the private practice setting could make significant impact on patient care. Many patients feel more comfortable with a non-physician provider and therefore would open up more about themselves and ask questions. As Felder (1983) pointed out, patients who have suffered a catastrophic, terminal, or chronic condition have different needs once they leave the inpatient setting and no longer need close medical supervision. The patient continues to need supportive care, education, and coordination of various services. These are services that can be delivered by the clinical nurse specialist in a very effective manner.

SUMMARY

In today's health care environment that increasingly necessitates successful collaborative relationships, I work as a self-employed clinical nurse specialist with the physician in our collaborative practice. As I described my involvement with Mr. and Mrs. S, I have differentiated the nursing role from the physician role. The advantages of collaborative practice are that it provides independence, creativity, and lets me provide quality nursing care across the health continuum. A disadvantage is lack of peer review. Clinical nurse specialists can succeed in private collaborative practice and make a difference in patient care delivery.

SPECIFIC QUESTIONS

1. Distinguish between patient teaching and counseling. Can all nurses do both?
2. Compare the benefits and risks for a clinical nurse specialist of self-employment, as described in this chapter, and employment by a department of nursing in an institution.
3. Identify the behaviors and strategies used by the author and her associate that enhanced their collaboration.
4. Based on the outcomes described in this chapter, how would you market yourself for a collaborative practice in your speciality?

REFERENCES

American Nurses' Association, Commission on Nursing Services. (1978). *Guidelines for appointment of nurses for individual practice privileges in health care organizations.* Kansas City, MO: American Nurses' Association.

American Nurses' Association, Council of Primary Health Care Practitioners and Joint Task Force on Third-party Reimbursement for Services of Nurses. (1984). *Obtaining third-party reimbursement: A nurse's guide to methods and strategies.* Kansas City, MO: American Nurses' Association.

Burchell, R.C., Thomas, D.A., & Smith, H.L. (1983). Some considerations for implementing collaborative practice. *American Journal of Medicine, 74* (9), 9–13.

Burke, L.E. (1978). Anticipatory grief in spouses of the critically ill. Master's thesis, University of California, Los Angeles, School of Nursing.

Burke, L.E. (1981). Learning and retention in the acute care setting. *Critical Care Quarterly, 4* (3), 67–73.

Burke, L.E. (1983). The clinical nurse specialist in collaborative practice. *Momentum* (ANA), *1* (2), 3–5.

Campbell, J.M. (1982). Practice management-reimbursement basics. *Pediatric Nursing, 8,* 424.

Fagin, C.M., & Lamberton, M.M. (1981). Nurse-physician collaboration: Evaluation of a nursing school-medical school joint practice. In L.H. Aiken (Ed.), *Health policy and nursing practice.* New York: McGraw-Hill.

Felder, L.A. (1983). Direct patient care and independent practice. In A.B. Hamric and J. Spross (Eds.), *The clinical nurse specialist in theory and practice.* Orlando, FL: Grune & Stratton.

Gordon, D.R. (1984). Research application: Identifying the use and misuse of formal models in nursing practice. In P. Benner (Ed.), *From novice to expert.* Menlo Park, CA: Addison-Wesley.

National Joint Practice Commission. (1977). *Statement on joint practice in primary care: Definitions and guidelines.* Chicago: National Joint Practice Commission.

Scalzi, C.C., Burke, L.E., & Greenland, S. (1980). Evaluation of an inpatient educational program for coronary patients and family. *Heart and Lung, 9* (5), 846–853.

part three

Views of the Future

chapter fourteen

Clinical Nurse Specialists and the Future of Nursing*

Margretta M. Styles

This book examines the clinical nurse specialist role as it was conceived and as it has developed—its intent, its components, and its effectiveness. It can readily be seen that clinical nurse specialists are at the cutting edge of nursing practice. The greater question must also be raised as to the place of the clinical nurse specialist movement within the evolution of all nursing. Specifically: Are clinical nurse specialists in the vanguard of the profession? Yes.

I believe that the future of all nursing is linked to the development of advanced nursing practice today. Advanced practitioners** are crucial to:

1. rational, systematic, relevant restructuring of the occupation
2. recruitment into nursing
3. the generation of knowledge for practice
4. the approach to key ethical issues in contemporary nursing, which are at the very heart of truly professional behavior

OCCUPATIONAL RESTRUCTURING

The structure of the occupation is many faceted and complex. For some decades now nursing has been in the process of reorganizing both vertically and horizontally. On the vertical axis we have been creating level after level, now ranging from the nurse's aide and the practical or vocational nurse to the associate-degree, diploma, baccalaureate, master's, and doctorally-prepared RNs. This has created so much confusion

---

*Adapted from an address on The Future of Advanced Practice presented at the Conference for Clinical Nurse Specialists and Nurse Practitioners, University of California, San Francisco, Department of Nursing and School of Nursing, February 11, 1988, San Francisco, California.

**As used throughout, the term "advanced practitioner" is intended to encompass clinical nurse specialists.

that we are now attempting to consolidate into two well-differentiated levels, the technical and the professional.

Within the evolutionary process, the clinical nurse specialist role has been created out of a need for greater knowledge and expertise and for more autonomous roles in nursing practice; the role has flourished because it successfully meets this need. Is a possible eventual outcome of the restructuring that the leading edge of today will represent the center of tomorrow? Is advanced nursing practice in 1988 the education and practice model for *all* nursing practice beyond the year 2000? Will *all* persons *entering* nursing in the next century be (1) postbaccalaureate prepared in primary and/or tertiary care, (2) practicing in a variety of settings, (3) fully accountable for care to their own patients, (4) serving as consultants to one another on special problems, and (5) engaged in improving nursing care through research? Will the term "advanced nursing practice" fade into the archives of nursing history only to mark the progress of this era?

In sum: In the future will there be only one NURSE and how will that nurse be prepared? Or will a hierarchical structure of nursing aides and technicians, nurses, and advanced practitioners persist and perhaps even further proliferate? The clinical nurse specialist role may hold the answer to the path chosen in nursing's current dilemma.

On the horizontal axis in the occupational restructuring, the subdivision of professional practice into specialties is occurring. Specialization is a phenomenon I have been studying for more than 4 years as an American Nurses' Foundation Distinguished Scholar. In analyzing more than 25 nursing specialties, I have found that the variability is staggering. Some specialties are well-established, with:

- Explicit statements on scope of practice, roles, curricula, and standards
- Graduate programs in the field
- Certification procedures
- Research support mechanisms
- Large vigorous specialty organizations for pulling all of this together and moving forward in a systematic, unified manner

Others specialties are newer, less well-defined, and are progressing tentatively. Moreover, ties to the profession as a whole are equally variable, with some specialties participating more actively than others in all-nursing organizations, such as the ANA, that serve as means for (1) setting standards and goals for all nursing and (2) enabling the total profession to take organized, concerted action.

We pride ourselves on diversity in nursing. What happens when diversity borders on anarchy, when random development and disorganization abound?

A synthesis of social systems theory tells us that if change—in this instance specialty differentiation—is to occur without disintegration of the total system (i.e., nursing) several conditions must exist. Three of those conditions are authority, homogeneity, and unity. Nursing specialties are developing with an absence or insufficiency of these essentials.

Until a single, central authority has been recognized for designating specialties and specialty standards, nursing is lacking in a source of authority for its specialties. Specialties are, in effect, self-declared and self-ordained. Thus they are susceptible to internal fluctuation and disorganization, and are especially vulnerable to outside forces competing for resources and power in the health care environment. Reimbursement and practice privileges are logically and historically linked to recognized specialties. In nursing, recognized by whom?

The absence of a single authority governing the development of specialties has led to extreme heterogeneity as to the specificity and caliber of standards of education and practice. Without a single authority there is very little hope for the development of greater standardization. The relative isolation and lack of parity of a specialty causes impotence within a fluctuating system of aggressive interests both internal and external to nursing.

Since specialization represents a division of practice within a profession, specialties, in the aggregate, should create a unity. They should all fit within the total range of services offered by the profession and be clearly complementary to and differentiated from one another. Just as there is currently no source for legitimization of specialties, there is no opportunity for this unity of purpose and fit to occur.

How can authority, homogeneity, and unity be provided for? Advanced nurse practitioners, throughout the specialties, must address this problem if nursing is to be empowered.

NURSE MANPOWER

There is clearly a mutual relationship between advanced practitioners and recruitment into nursing. On the one hand, the precipitous decline in entrants into nursing schools will diminish the recruitment pool for moving on to higher education and advanced practice. Therefore, to build and replenish the supply of advanced practitioners, recruits into nursing must be in sufficient numbers and of high caliber.

Advanced practice may serve as a magnet to draw the brightest and the best into nursing in a number of ways. Problems in the hospital environment related to economic incentives, advancement opportunities, status, and participation in decision-making create a negative image of nursing and inhibit recruitment. The American Hospital Association reports that 26.5 percent of hospitals utilize clinical nurse specialists with an average of four full-time and two part-time positions in those institutions (AHA, 1987). Clinical nurse specialists and nurse practitioners exert a very positive influence within the institutional environment and, I believe, as their numbers increase, will play a critical role in resolving the problems related to the practice setting.

Additionally, the current distribution and utilization of clinical nurse specialists and nurse practitioners indicates that they are broadening nursing practice with certain target populations. They are evolving new care delivery systems and nursing service models that create new roles, new markets, and new settings; this brings innovation and excitement to the field that will also draw recruits into nursing.

There is, however, another aspect to the magnetism of the advanced practitioner and this goes back to the question posed at the outset: Is the graduate-prepared advanced practitioner the prototype for the nurse of the future? Practice demands and professional evolution—the very survival of nursing in fact—may impel us in this direction. If not, we may be the only remaining profession prepared at the undergraduate level. Certainly this will undermine our claims to professional status and ultimately destroy our recruitment potential.

Those of us who are wrestling with the nurse recruitment problem nationally have long recognized that second-career college graduates represent a promising pool of recruits. To attract such persons to nursing, we must offer generic master's and doctoral programs. We must offer degrees that the post-baccalaureate status of this pool deserves and that all other professions provide for their graduates.

Thus, as magnets, nursing's master's and doctorally-prepared clinical nurse specialists and nurse practitioners may have two effects. They may draw others into the field through their influence upon the practice setting or they may draw all of professional nursing to their educational level through the model they set, or both.

RESEARCH

Research is another key element in the advanced practitioner's influence upon nursing's future. Clinical nurse specialists, by virtue of their advanced education at the master's or doctoral level and their supervision of clinical practice in a specialized area of nursing practice, are singularly qualified and responsible for promoting scientific inquiry and the dissemination of research-based knowledge.

By definition, the clinical specialist in nursing has a client-based practice and serves clients through direct intervention and supervision of other nurses in the practice setting—through the roles of educator, consultant, researcher or administrator (ANA, 1986). Though the number of doctorally prepared nurses principally involved in research for clinical practice has increased, in most clinical settings clinical nurse specialists are the only nurses well-prepared to contribute to research in their area of specialization by generating and refining research questions; interpreting research findings, and applying them to clinical practice; educating other nurses about research findings; collaborating in designing and conducting research; and communicating research findings through publication." (ANA, 1986, pp. 3-4).

The challenge for the future is to preserve, protect, and promote the clinical nurse specialists' research function in the midst of time constraints, attitudinal barriers, inadequate support services and other resources, personal knowledge and skill deficits, and other impediments. Given the nursing shortage, economic pressures, and the consequent reallocation of nursing resources in most clinical practice settings, they seldom have the luxury of time to devote solely to nursing research.

Nevertheless, advanced practitioners will need to set personal goals and be motivated to foster research generation and dissemination in *every* aspect of their multifaceted practice role and to fight for nursing research to be appropriately recognized in institutional priorities. To keep abreast of and add to the latest knowledge in the field will require both study and involvement with nurse researchers in projects, conferences, and publications focused on research for practice.

If advanced clinicians relinquish this responsibility, nursing practice will have no growing edge and will shrink to its narrowest, technical dimensions.

ETHICS

In addition to new knowledge, nursing's generative edge is also made up of our responses to various ethical dilemmas, the fourth area of challenge and opportunity for advanced practitioners.

Attention has been focused upon those ethical questions having to do with the rationing or withholding of treatments or new technology (e.g., distribution of transplant organs, use of experimental drugs, surrogate parenting, and heroic measures at both ends of the life continuum). The means to address such clinical dilemmas are being developed in government and in institutional procedures. We would assume that advanced practitioners are involved both in establishing those mechanisms, such as ethics committees, and in the decisions that are being made in individual cases.

There is, however, a neglected area of ethical dilemma, the administrative, supervisory or professional dilemma, arising out of cost containment efforts and the nursing shortage. Decisions to close units, thereby denying services to clients and income to the hospital, have always been difficult and are even more so under the current economic pressures when institutional survival is at stake. There have been more questions about the rights of nurses when faced with unsafe work assignments, for example, situations in which they feel inadequately prepared or in which there is inadequate staffing or support services. When forced to weigh institutional accountability and professional responsibility against patient abandonment, we are engaged in a no-win battle.

Clinical nurse specialists, who are called upon to counsel and supervise staff nurses facing such decisions, are, of course, doing more than providing advice to individuals. They are socializing the entire generation of professionals for whom they serve as supervisors and role models. How we deal with this growing category of ethical decisions (the administrative or professional dilemma) will indeed affect the future of nursing.

SUMMARY

Clinical nurse specialists are more than the generative edge of nursing practice. They are, as well, the vanguard of the profession. Clinical nurse specialists play a pivotal role in the restructuring of nursing, in recruitment into the field, in the development of the research base for practice, and in the approach to emerging ethical dilemmas of a clinical and administrative nature.

REFERENCES

American Hospital Association (1987). *Report of the hospital nursing personnel survey.* Chicago: American Hospital Association.

American Nurses' Association (1986). *The role of the clinical nurse specialist.* Kansas City, MO: American Nurses' Association.

chapter fifteen

Today—Assessment and Intuitions: Tomorrow—Projections

Diane M. Cooper

TODAY/TOMORROW

"Tomorrow begins today" Kelly (1987) reminded us. In the same editorial she went on to raise the reader's awareness of the fact that "tomorrow, in fact, reaches back to the past, to the series of events and conditions that formed the foundation for today" (p. 59). Few of us would argue with either statement. Truisms like those cited by Kelly engender head nodding and an inner feeling of contentment at the rightness of their meaning. The other side of these succinct statements, however, is that often truisms point out facts of which we need reminding in order to complete undone tasks. Phrases such as "a stitch in time saves nine" and "opportunity knocks but once" challenge us to action. Similarly, the notion that "tomorrow begins today" prods and forces the reader to reflect on the reality that what occurs today, what is done or not done today, affects and predicts something about tomorrow. This is true for families as well as for nations, for individuals as well as for professions.

Nursing is one profession increasingly aware of the effect of the past on its present. Articles have appeared documenting the impact of history on various aspects of and trends in nursing (Baer, 1987; Buhler-Wilkerson, 1987; Church, 1987; O'Brien, 1987; Reverby, 1987; Rogge, 1987). At the same time, nurse authors focus on nursing's tomorrow—its future. Not long ago, an entire issue of *Nursing Outlook* (1987, 35) was devoted to capturing noted nurse leaders' predictions about the future of the nursing profession in the year 2020. Although the visions of the contributors differed somewhat, the majority of their opinions and suggestions regarding nursing's future emanated from the dictum that, in fact, "tomorrow is now."

TRENDS AND ACCOMPLISHMENTS

It would be inconsistent with the adage quoted by Kelly to move too quickly in this chapter to making predictions for the clinical nurse specialist's future without pausing to recount some of the significant occurrences of the past that are affecting nursing today. For in taking time to highlight a few of today's achievements in nursing, we are apt to be better informed about tomorrow's possibilities as well as its problems. And, although clinical nurse specialists have not been involved directly in each of the accomplishments presented here, all of them in some way impact on individuals functioning in that role.

One of the positive trends evidenced by the appearance of this text, the numerous articles generated for the journal *Clinical Nurse Specialist*, the writings in the now classic book *The Clinical Nurse Specialist in Theory and Practice* (Hamric & Spross, 1983), and in the many articles written by and about clinical nurse specialists for other journals as well, is that clinical nurse specialists are communicating formally with one another with increasing frequency. In assessing the evolution of this communication, one observes that it appears to be less random than in the past; it is more focused. Indeed, in general, the topics currently addressed by clinical nurse specialists reveal their sense of urgency in responding to issues critical to them, whether role issues or assessment and reactions to trends in health care. A positive outcome of this expansion in writing about the role of the clinical nurse specialist is the increased likelihood of the development of a body of knowledge concerning the "is-ness," the "what-ness," the creative and futuristic possibilities of this pivotal role within professional nursing. Additionally, through these writings, other members of the profession, including clinical nurse specialists, are made aware of the significance of clinical nurse specialists' accomplishments.

More particularly, one observes increased sharing of methods of role evaluation specific to the role of the clinical nurse specialist. This area, long one of interest and concern to many clinical nurse specialists, is increasingly evident in the literature (Baker, 1987; Brown & Wilson, 1987; Fenton, 1985; Holt, 1987; Steele & Fenton, 1988). Welch-McCaffrey stands out as one of the earliest clinical nurse specialists to systematically log the number and types of activities she carried out with patients (Welch-McCaffrey & D'Agostino, 1984). Several other authors (Cooper, Minarik & Sparacino) within this book describe the methods by which they also attempted to document their effectiveness, and their impact on patient care. This demonstration of documentation will assist greatly in helping other clinical nurse specialists to objectively quantify the significant impact they make on patient care. Once logged, these data can serve as powerful tools in support of the role.

Yet another milestone in nursing was reached when the findings of Dr. Dorothy Brooten and her colleagues at the University of Pennsylvania School of Nursing, were reported in the Fall 1986 issue of the *New England Journal of Medicine* (Brooten et al., 1986). This study documented the fact that low-birth-weight infants who had continuing access to clinical nurse specialists left the hospital two weeks earlier than infants in a control group. Not only did these infants do equally as well as those who remained in the hospital, but hospital charges were approximately $18,500 per child less.

These and other examples of data collection by and about clinical nurse specialists add support to a statement about nursing's future made by Geraldine Felton (1987), professor and dean, at the University of Iowa and president-elect of the American Academy of Nursing:

> Without question the history of nursing's growth and the development of authority over nursing practice must be principally the history of graduate education and university-based research and scholarship that nurture an astonishing advance and diffusion of knowledge in nursing. (p. 126)

Nurses witnessed an additional major achievement in April 1986 when, as a result of the passage of the Health Research Extension Act of 1985, a National Center for Nursing Research was established at the National Institutes of Health. Armed with a budget of $23.3 million for fiscal year 1988, its director, Ada Sue Hinshaw, PhD, FAAN, forecast a goal of funding 320 research trainees by the year 1991 (Nursing research, 1988). Not only does the establishment of this center bode well for nurses prepared at the graduate level, but, more significantly, it ensures acceleration in building a body of knowledge and a theoretical base for nursing.

Yet again, the June 1988 issue of *The American Nurse* announced the publication of a new ANA document entitled "Nursing Case Management" (Case management, 1988). The publication "describes a health care delivery process whose goals are to provide quality health care, decrease fragmentation, enhance the client's quality of life, and contain costs" (p. 5). The individuals proposed to be addressed through the case management approach range from the frail chronically disabled to those experiencing acute exacerbations of serious illnesses. Seven models of the case management approach are already in existence. This creative approach to nursing care has high potential for increasing the public's awareness of the skills of the advanced nurse practitioner in providing health care. Because the case management approach finds its basis in promoting *health* care, the nurse has been appropriately identified to interact and plan with the patient. Certainly many "eyes" will be observing the effectiveness of such a health care delivery plan.

Even though the majority of nursing's achievements, and those of clinical nurse specialists in particular, have been positive, nursing can little afford to rest on its laurels. In response to the nursing shortage, in 1988 the AMA Board of Trustees adopted a plan to create a new category of health care worker "to give bedside care to patients" (AMA shortage, 1988; Salahuddin, 1988). These individuals, to be called Registered Care Technologists, would undertake between 9 and 18 months of training at community or technical colleges before assuming positions and be regulated by physician licensing boards. Although James E. Davis, MD, AMA president, justified the creation of this class of workers by stating that "organized nursing is . . . going all out for graduate nurses to get more 'supernurses', but we all know that the real need is at the bedside" (Salahuddin, 1988, p. 16), Margretta Styles, then president of the American Nurses' Association, summarized organized nursing's view when she stated, "This new breed of health care worker will only create more confusion as well as accountability and liability problems, without addressing the real need, which is for more support systems for nurses" (AMA shortage, 1988, p. 1).

Nurses, and clinical nurse specialists in particular, cannot rest on their laurels. Instead, the American Academy of Nursing urges all nurses to be busy about considering their "preferred future," "not a future that may happen because of lack of foresight or failure of strategy" but evolving out of a vision of "what is desirable, what is highly valued, and above all, is most worthwhile to society" (Aydelotte, 1987, p. 114).

PREFERRED FUTURE

In predicting the future in the decade after the turn of the century, Aydelotte (1987) proposed, among other things, that hospitals as we know them will change; they will "consist of multiple intensive care units offering highly specialized scientific and technological services . . . patients will remain in them for short periods" (p. 117). She forecast increased emphasis and value being placed on health promotion. As a result of this trend, Aydelotte predicted programs will be developed for those interested in focusing on maintaining health. Additionally, economic constraints will continue to affect the care that health care professionals are able to provide; consequently change will have to occur in methods of health care delivery to ensure that quality is maintained. Finally, Aydelotte proposed that health care will be divided into four major branches: health promotion, chronic disease management, trauma and severe illness, and care of the frail elderly and dying (p. 118). Several of Aydelotte's predictions come as no surprise, as trends in the direction suggested have already begun. Each of the predictions, however, impacts on the future of nursing, most particularly on where and how advanced practitioners of nursing will practice.

In a further attempt to ferret out what nursing's preferred future might look like, a group of nurse leaders convened (Sullivan et al., 1987). The first phase of the study in which the leaders participated involved forty nurse experts generating twenty forecast statements potentially reflective of nursing's "intentional" future. Phase two of the study involved a different set of thirty-five nurses, among them seven clinical nurse specialists, rating the forecast statements generated previously for "probability and desirability of occurrence" (Sullivan et al., 1987, p. 233). Three major themes evolved from the twenty forecast statements regarding nursing's future, those being concern for: "shifting nursing's level of autonomy in society and health care, strengthening of patients' rights in health care, and increasing the interrelationship of high technology with humanistic caring by nurses" (p. 234).

Interestingly, the nurse leaders involved in formulating the forecast statements for the study cited above predicted that the changes in nursing over the next twelve years, or the period between now and the year 2000, would be "barely noticeable." On the other hand, they predicted "significant accomplishments in nursing," by the year 2020. Perhaps leaders in nursing need to be more aggressive in encouraging the members of the profession, advanced practitioners in particular, to move their accomplishments over the next 12 years into "noticeable" reality. Nursing can ill afford to quietly address problems while the profession is widely discussed in the public arena (Ringold, 1988; Will, 1988).

A "Future's Quiz" prepared by the nurse leaders involved in the study and subsequently assessed by the thirty-five nurses invited to test it is both thought-provoking and revealing. Each clinical nurse specialist should take the time to score the quiz and judge the results privately. It is difficult not to be catapulted into the future when asked to decide whether or not you believe that, in the future, nurses will "enforce state-prescribed economic sanctions when clients do not comply with health care regimens" or that some nurses will work in an environment where "robots take over many technical nursing tasks and procedures in hospital settings" (Sullivan et al., 1987, p. 234).

Aydelotte and the American Academy of Nursing are not alone in urging that nurses take the time to predict and begin planning their "preferred" future. Those outside of nursing also urge forward thinking by professionals involved in health care. One author goes so far as to suggest that creative thinking or intuition "be nurtured" (Kaiser, 1987, p. 15).

INTUITION

Leland Kaiser, a health care consultant and associate professor at the University of Colorado's Graduate School of Business Administration, wrote an article containing food for thought. The article, "The Intuitive Manager and Innovation" (Kaiser, 1987), urges leaders within health care to seek out experiences that exercise intuition. Reminding us that "intuition is beyond thinking" and that in fact "thinking tends to block it" (p. 16), Kaiser went on to say that in order to address the problems of today and in the 1990's, we need to develop our intuition much as individuals interested in analyzing both their conscious and unconscious thoughts push themselves to remember their dreams. Intuition, Kaiser reminded the reader, is paying attention to one's hunches, seizing flashes of insight, and opening one's mind to the possibility of solutions to problems that in a more analytical mode would never be given consideration.

Throughout the article on intuition and innovation, the reader is urged by Kaiser to develop the intuitive aspect of the mind precisely because, if developed, the individual will be more likely to possess the capacity for dreaming new realities, of catapulting reality onto new plateaus, and of going to "places" never thought possible. Aware of the fact that analysis (i.e., thinking), "is often too slow a tool" to use when rapid changes are needed, he pointed out that humans should take delight in the fact that they have another mode of reflection available to them, a way in which answers, even whole new visions of reality, can evolve expeditiously.

Certainly Kaiser is not alone in encouraging visionary thinking in addressing current issues in health care. Numerous recognized leaders speak to the need for "visionaries" in health care. Responding to an interviewer's question, Goldsmith, author of *Can Hospitals Survive: The New Competitive Health Care Market*, goes so far as to say that only leaders with vision "will be here in 5 years" (Goman, 1988, p. 14).

In spite of the urging for visionaries evidenced in the literature, members of the health care professions, nurses included, are faced with two factors that may constrain their potential for intuition. First, traditionally, nurses have not been encouraged to be risk-takers or to exercise the intuitive aspect of their minds. Perhaps because of the emphasis on science, analytical thinking, and varying degrees of "fitting into the mold," intuition has not been a highly developed nor valued attribute among most nurses. Secondly, nurses, not unlike other members of society, believe that "what is," or that which appears to be occurring in any present situation, is a greater reality than "what could be." Because of this latter fact, nurses often turn to solutions to problems that "work in the short term" but "may not be right in the long term" (Kaiser, 1987, p. 17). In such situations, slight modifications in the status quo are perceived as significant changes, only to be followed by the realization that little if anything has actually changed.

Intuitor's Projections
In an often-quoted article addressing the future of health care up until the year 2028, Kaiser (1986) divided the next 40 years into three distinct periods. These periods, termed "Futures," each involving different

time frames, can be described succinctly. The initial period, lasting from 1986–1991, is referred to as "the white water period." During this time frame, the "name of the game is organizational survival. . . . There will be winning hospitals and losing hospitals" (Kaiser, 1986, p. 12). The second future, lasting from 1991–2007, "belongs to the winners of the shakeout period" (Kaiser, 1986, p. 13). This second future will be marked by technological and organizational growth. The third and last future "will take medical care to the outer limits of present imagination" (Kaiser, 1986, p. 14).

During this latter period, lasting 20 years, such developments as the prolongation of the life span and organ regeneration will occur. Obviously, the fashioner of these three time frames is an intuitive thinker, yet he clearly pointed out that "the challenge is surviving long enough to get there" (Kaiser, 1986, p. 13).

In order to survive even the "white water period" of the future lasting until 1991, much change will need to occur. As Goertzen (1987) reminded us, "Visions are easier said than done" (p. 121). Nurses, not normally intuitive thinkers, of necessity will need to nurture, to exercise their "wide angle vision." Nurses will choose to make the visions they identify become a reality or they will continue to propose safe solutions to problems that work in the short run. Either way, the future will continue to challenge nursing.

FUTURE REALITIES

To some, the notions suggested in the "Futures Quiz" as well as other predictions about the future seem impossible, to others improbable, and to the majority, better if not thought about too long or taken too seriously. And yet, thinking about the future of nursing is a task each of us has been called to undertake. It is, as Aydelotte (1987) stated, the only way we can make "strategic decisions" (p. 114). Whether or not nurses, clinical nurse specialists among them, choose to grapple with the future, they have already been taken there by recent trends in economics, burgeoning health care needs, changing populations, increased longevity of the population, and decreased enrollment in nursing schools. Cognizant of these multiple changes, nursing can no longer afford to be "other-controlled, other directed . . . neither autonomous nor independent," as Schlotfeldt (1987, p. 226) warned us. And so nursing, as it has done on numerous occasions before, faces a difficult future. Yet nurses can be consoled by Barnum's (1987) observation, "nursing is at its best when things really get tough" (p. 221). Furthermore, Barnum wrote that if it were true that nursing excelled during times of tribulations, then "we're about to come into our own because it's hard to envision a more challenging era" than the one that lies ahead (p. 221).

Acknowledging the impact of multiple factors on health care and the need for creativity in proposing solutions, the remainder of this chapter will look to the clinical nurse specialist's future and propose some possibilities. The projections will respond to the question, How might the clinical nurse specialist look in the years to come? It is believed by some that if human beings can imagine a reality, it has increased likelihood of coming into being. These forecasts are projected with that hope.

In order to get from "what is" to "what can be," clinical nurse specialists of the future will be more experienced in intuitive thinking. In the past, conferences held specifically for clinical nurse specialist participants often involved a series of noted speakers, most often from traditional settings, describing various facets of the role as *they* performed them. In the near future, cognizant of the fact that intuitive thinkers may appear "in the most unlikely places" (Kaiser, 1987, p. 15), clinical nurse specialist conferences will focus on capturing the participants' intuition. Imagine a conference where clinical nurse specialists submit in writing their visions of the best possible future for individuals functioning in that role. Once the attendees convened, these visions of the future could be shared and then strategies devised about how clinical nurse specialists might make such visions work in reality.

"Intuition is not a respecter of persons or necessarily a companion of high status individuals" (Kaiser, 1987, p. 15). Because of this fact, both novice and experienced clinical nurse specialists in the scenario described above and in other discussions will propose "futures" that will move nursing specialization forward immensely. Faculty, too, will encourage expansion of graduate students' reflective abilities, so that speculating about the future of the role becomes more natural. Clinical nurse specialists of the future will be prepared to address issues within the larger context of health care in addition to the physiological and psychological needs of their patients. These clinical nurse specialists will have a greater awareness of the health care world, including knowledge of marketing, fiscal issues, and of the multiple options available to them in meeting the needs of consumers. Because of their knowledge and expertise, clinical nurse specialists will propose new solutions to problems in a proactive way. They will not wait to react.

"By the early 1990s," stated Jeffrey Bauer, senior research associate with the University of Colorado Graduate School of Business in Denver, "consumers will be paying more than 50 percent of their health care costs" (Goman, 1988, p. 9). This same consumer, he added, "is just now realizing how many choices he or she really has" (Goman, 1988, p. 9). Capitalizing on this fact, in the future whenever clinical nurse specialists convene, consumer input will be sought.

As a consequence of the increased emphasis on health versus illness care and the demand for quality, clinical nurse specialists will devise new ways of meeting patients' needs. Consumer input regarding the "fit" of the services rendered by specialists will be ongoing. As always, the patient in whatever setting will be the clinical nurse specialist's focus of attention, but now that focus will be expanded. Advanced practitioners, realizing the significance of marketing strategies, will pay heed to the sound advice of Bauer, who pointed out that "marketing is not just telling the customer what you have to offer. It is first finding out what the customer wants and then providing that" (Goman, 1988, p. 9).

A forward-thinking example of the inclusion of the consumer's point of view was manifested in the program prepared by a group in 1987 when, at their annual clinical nurse specialist conference, they included the benefits manager for a large chain of supermarkets. This individual spoke of the cost of insuring the thousands of employees working for that corporation. Several times during his address he prodded the clinical nurse specialists in the audience to approach his and like companies if they felt they could demonstrate ways in which health care could be provided more efficiently and effectively. Currently we see trends in the direction of meeting the nonhospitalized members of society's health care needs through the case management approach. Case management will take hold because the members of society will value the emphasis on *health* maintenance, teaching, and personalized care (high touch care) provided by nurses. Although some clinical nurse specialists will always practice in tertiary care centers, increasingly, clinical nurse specialists will move to ambulatory and home care settings where their skills will focus on the care of the aged, persons with AIDS (acquired immune deficiency syndrome), and the terminally ill. Clinical nurse specialists also will increase their functioning in collaborative and private practice. Because many patients will choose to have their own nurse, as well as their own doctor, individuals will become clearer about the strengths of each professional group.

Recording data about the effect of their interventions and on outcomes will be commonplace among clinical nurse specialists. Computers will assist in data retrieval and analysis. These data will act as a basis for evaluation of the individual clinical nurse specialist's level of expertise. Over time, comparison of these results between individuals and groups will reveal the behaviors distinctive of levels of expertise. Clinical nurse specialists at the highest end of the continuum will be acknowledged widely by both the profession and society.

The text *The Clinical Nurse Specialist in Theory and Practice* (Hamric & Spross, 1983) ended with future projections. Among the forecasts was the plea that clinical nurse specialists and nurse practitioners prepared at the graduate level join forces, that they merge their titles and be known as "Advanced Registered Nurse Practitioners" (ARNPs) (p. 292). This overdue feat will come to pass. Although to some individuals within nursing the demarcations between the roles are so separate that they should never be merged, the future demands otherwise. In particularly poignant words where this subject is concerned, Bauer exhorted, "The most successful people in future health care will be those who are creative and open to different ways of doing things. . . . Inflexible people with rigidly held views are going to be overwhelmed by those who can adapt to new ideas and directions . . . 'the one right way' doesn't exist anymore" (Goman, 1988, p. 9).

This writer reflects on the positive experience of working with master's-prepared nurse practitioners, nurse midwives, and nurse anesthetists in the early 1980s in creating a statement regarding advanced practice for the California Nurses' Association (CNA, 1984). Although, no doubt, each member of the group began the task with a certain amount of anxiety and trepidation, each relaxed, sighed deeply, and delighted in the common language we shared where speciality practice and patient care were concerned.

In the future, clinical nurse specialists will value the opportunities to work together with other master's-prepared clinicians, of moving with the patient between settings, and of becoming a more vital force in health care by virtue of the fact that the once separate groups are "woven together." If clinical nurse specialists combining their expertise can improve patient care immeasurably (see Chapter 12), imagine what might happen to health care and the profession of nursing if ARNPs got together? The future has been described as the "age of specialization and cooperation between specialists" (Goman, 1988, p. 10). Nowhere will that be more evident than among ARNPs.

Once unified, the talent within the ARNP group will march forcibly against their common enemy and in pursuit of a "golden opportunity" (Styles, 1987, p. 229). Issues such as poverty, human despair, inequitable health care, discrimination against women and minorities, ignorance and repression will be dealt with from a nursing perspective (Styles, 1987, p. 229). ARNPs are reminded of "the possibility of extinction" (Styles, 1987, p. 229), of the need of groups in nursing to acknowledge their differences in order for survival to be insured (Fagin, 1988 Personal communication), of the destructiveness of "horizontal violence" (Stevens, 1988), or the degrading of members of the profession in any way. Already fortified with some of the tools of "competition in modern society" (Styles, 1987, p. 229), ARNPs will add others, among them "knowledge and expertise of a higher and higher order; public sanction through licensing and economic policies . . . and power in institutional and governmental political processes" (Styles, 1987, p. 229). ARNPs will have developed a strong political voice.

Certainly the creation of the Registered Care Technologists was an attempt on the part of physicians to deal with the nursing shortage. The future will prove this stopgap approach to have been an ineffective response given that leaders in health care predict that hospitals will see one highly skilled nurse supervising the operation of the cybernated patient care unit with a "remaining staff" required to have higher-level cognitive skills (Kaiser, 1986, p. 16). If, as projected, computers and robots will replace 50 percent of the current employees working in hospitals, those who do survive will be the best, the brightest, and the most caring. Who is better prepared to meet the hospital patients' needs of the future than the ARNP, presently referred to as the clinical nurse specialist?

Numerous authors envision medical centers where teams of physicians and nurses recognized for their skill in working with extremely complex procedures unite. These teams, having worked together over time and collected data, will be sought out by consumers precisely for their level of expertise and the procedures they can perform. ARNPs will be pivotal in overseeing and monitoring the patient's progress and providing high touch throughout the patient's procedure and during the transition into the community. Because it has long been known that "poor care is expensive" and that the "right diagnosis delivered promptly, the correct procedures, and a practitioner who doesn't make mistakes have always made good economic sense" (Goman, 1988, p. 10), ARNPs will be sought out to supervise, deliver, consult on, and problem-solve patient care in the future. In select situations ARNPs, presently termed nurse practitioners, will replace physicians because of their ability to deliver cost-effective quality care. Just as our peer ARNPs, presently called nurse midwives, have demonstrated their competency and unique approach to the birthing experience for many pregnant individuals, so will other ARNPs demonstrate their skill in settings yet to be imagined.

ARNPs will be leaders in addressing the ethics of the issues cited above, as well as the ethics of "cost containment," who will receive care and who will not, who will receive a renovated organ and who will not, when, where, and how individuals choose to die, and whether or not nurses can refuse to provide care when an individual requires it.

CRISIS OR OPPORTUNITY

ARNPs face a future of uncertainty. Bauer stated in regard to health care, "much of what the future holds is totally unpredictable. This is a period when virtually anything can happen" (Goman, 1988, p. 9). Abundene stated, "It will take a concerted effort . . . to help doctors let go of power, to assist nurses to trust their knowledge and growing authority (Goman, 1988, p. 8). Definitely for some, the years immediately ahead represent a time of crisis. Goman (1988) wisely reminded us, "In Chinese, the ideogram for crisis combines two characters: one is the symbol for danger, the other for opportunity" (p. 8). Nurses have met crisis before and conquered it. If doubtful, read George Will's editorial for

May 23, 1988 (Will, 1988), entitled "The Dignity of Nursing," then follow it by reading June's editorial responses. This writer chooses to admire again the depth of the eastern mentality when it sees both danger and opportunity in crisis.

Clinical nurse specialists can be counted among those nurses who bring more clinical savvy, more creativity in practice, and more risk-taking to role implementation than almost any other group of nurses. Many have demonstrated these talents repeatedly. Watch out for what they will do in the next two decades!

SUMMARY

The preface of this book called for increased efforts in describing the "is-ness" of the role of the clinical nurse specialist. Each of the chapters that followed, especially the chapters in Part II, meticulously recorded the world and work of the clinical nurse specialist. As the book comes to a close and one assesses the contemporary health care scene, new horizons appear. Everything becomes possible for the clinical nurse specialist; the role is, as some have described, the most flexible, malleable nursing role, "difficult to pinpoint." The logging of what it is clinical nurse specialists do and what it is they accomplish will continue to be important, but for new reasons: it will speak to the worth of ARNPs, and it will reduce the likelihood of the extinction of nursing due to decreased numbers. For in joining with our peers prepared at the master's and doctoral level, we will demonstrate to society the value of advanced preparation and finely honed clinical skills. As educated, articulate professionals, ARNPs will speak to a new generation and, because of that generation's ability to identify the ARNP's worth, nursing will again attract the best and brightest students. Nursing will emerge strong and fully professional. Seventy thousand master's-prepared clinicians united cannot but help to bring nursing into a remarkable future. "A hospital cannot move into a future it cannot imagine" said Kaiser (1986, p. 18) and neither can ARNPs. The editors and contributors to this book give its readers a mandate: exercise your intuition!

REFERENCES

AMA shortage plan stirs controversy. (1988). *The Pennsylvania Nurse, 43*(7), 1.

Aydelotte, M. (1987). Nursing's preferred future. *Nursing Outlook, 35,* 114–120.

Baer, E. (1987). "A cooperative venture" in pursuit of professional status: A research journal for nursing. *Nursing Research, 36,* 18–25.

Baker, P. (1987). Model activities for clinical nurse specialists' role development. *Clinical Nurse Specialist, 1,* 119.

Barnum, B. (1987). Nursing: Now, then, and maybe again. *Nursing Outlook, 35,* 219–221.

Brooten, D., Kumer, S., & Brown, L.P., et al., (1986). A randomized clinical trial of early hospital discharge and home follow-up of very-low-birth-weight infants. *New England Journal of Medicine, 315* (15), 934–939.

Brown, M., & Wilson, C. (1987). Time management and the clinical nurse specialist. *Clinical Nurse Specialist, 1,* 32–38.

Buhler-Wilkerson, K. (1987). Left carrying the bag: Experiments in visiting nursing, 1877-1909. *Nursing Research, 36,* 42–47.

California Nurses' Association. (1984). *Position statement on specialization in nursing practice.* San Francisco: California Nurses' Association.

Case management, career plan described. (1988). *The American Nurse, 20*(6) 5.

Church, O. (1987). From custody to community in psychiatric nursing. *Nursing Research, 36,* 48–55.

Felton, G. (1987). Obstacles to nursing's preferred future. *Nursing Outlook, 35,* 126–128.

Fenton, M. (1985). Identifying competencies of clinical nurse specialists. *Journal of Nursing Administration, 15,* 31–37.

Goertzen, I. (1987). Making nursing's vision a reality. *Nursing Outlook, 35,* 121–123.

Goman, C. (1988). Forecast '88: Ten leading healthcare experts discuss the future. *Healthcare Forum, 31,* (1) 8–17.

Hamric, A., & Spross, J. (1983). *The clinical nurse specialist in theory and practice.* Orlando, FL: Grune & Stratton.

Holt, F. (1987). Executive practice role. Editorial. *Clinical Nurse Specialist, 1,* 116–118.

Kaiser, L. (1986). Anticipating your high-tech tomorrow. *Healthcare Forum, 29*(6) 12–20.

Kaiser, L. (1987). The intuitive manager and innovation. *Healthcare Forum, 30*(6) 15–17.

Kelly, L. (1987). To touch tomorrow. *Nursing Outlook, 35*(2) 59.

Nursing research on fast track at national center. (1988). *The American Nurse, 20*(6) 27.

O'Brien, P. (1987). "All a woman's life can bring": The domestic roots of nursing in Philadelphia 1830–1855. *Nursing Research, 36,* 12–17.

Reverby, S. (1987). A caring dilemma: Womanhood and nursing in historical perspective. *Nursing Research, 36*(1), 5–11.

Ringold, E. (1988). Nursing in crisis. *McCall's, CXV* (2), 54–65.

Rogge, M. (1987). Nursing and politics: A forgotten legacy. *Nursing Research, 36*(1), 26–30.

Salahuddin, M. (1988). AMA seeks new nursing job category. *The Pennsylvania Nurses, 43*(7), 16, 3.

Schlotfeldt, R. (1987). Reflection on nursing, 1987. *Nursing Outlook, 35*(5), 226–228.

Steele, S., & Fenton, M. (1988). Expert practice of clinical nurse specialists. *Clinical Nurse Specialist, 2,* 45–51.

Stevens, S. (1988). Mutual support: A remedy for the autoimmune factor in nursing. Presentation at conference, Molding the Future: The clinical nurse specialist. Columbia, SC: Richland Memorial Hospital.

Styles, M. (1987). The tarnished opportunity. *Nursing Outlook, 35,* 229.

Sullivan, T., Lee, J., & Warnick, M., et al.,(1987). Nursing 2020: A study of nursing's future. *Nursing Outlook, 35,* 233–235.

Welch-McCaffrey, D., & D'Agostino, J. (1984). Documenting role effectiveness. Presented at conference on Progress, Promise, and Controversy. Good Samaritan Medical Center, Scottsdale, Arizona.

Will, G. (1988). The dignity of nursing. *Newsweek, CXI* (21), 80.

Bibliography

AMA shortage plan stirs controversy. (1988). *The Pennsylvania Nurse, 43* (7), 1, 15.

American Academy of Nursing. (1983). *Magnet hospitals: Attraction and retention of professional nurses.* Kansas City, MO: American Nurses' Association.

American Association of Critical Care Nurses. (1987). *AACN position statement: The critical care clinical nurse specialist: Role definition.* Newport Beach, CA: American Association of Critical Care Nurses.

American Hospital Association. (1987). *Report of the hospital nursing personnel survey.* Chicago: American Hospital Association.

American Nurses' Association. (1980). *Nursing: A social policy statement.* Kansas City, MO: American Nurses' Association.

American Nurses' Association. (1986). *Clinical nurse specialists: Distribution and utilization.* Kansas City, MO: American Nurses' Association.

American Nurses' Association. (1986). *The role of the clinical nurse specialist.* Kansas City, MO: American Nurses' Association.

American Nurses' Association, Commission on Nursing Services. (1978). *Guidelines for appointment of nurses for individual practice privileges in health care organizations.* Kansas City, MO: American Nurses' Association.

American Nurses' Association, Council of Primary Health Care Practitioners and Joint Task Force on Third-party Reimbursement for Services of Nurses. (1984). *Obtaining third-party reimbursement: A nurse's guide to methods and strategies.* Kansas City, MO: American Nurses' Association.

American Nurses' Association. (1988). *Nursing Case Management.* Kansas City, MO: American Nurses' Association.

Anderson, T., & Siden, A. (1982). A clinical study of the Guillain-Barre syndrome. *Acta Neurologica Scandinavica, 66,* 316–327.

Andreoli, K.G. (1986). Specialization and the graduate curriculum: Where does it fit? In *Patterns in specialization: Challenge to the curriculum.* New York: National League for Nursing.

Aradine, C. (1980). Home care for young children with long-term tracheostomies. *Maternal Child Nursing, 5* (2), 121–125.

Aradine, C., & Deynes, M.J. (1972). Activities and pressures of clinical nurse specialists. *Nursing Research, 21* (5), 411–418.

Armacost, B. (1973). On becoming a nurse-manager of psychiatry. In J. Riehl & J. McVay (Eds.), *The clinical nurse specialist: Interpretations.* New York: Appleton-Century-Crofts.

Aydelotte, M. (1987). Nursing's preferred future. *Nursing Outlook, 35,* 114–120.

Ayers, R., Padilla, G.V., Baker, V.E., & Crary, W.G. (1971). *The clinical nurse specialist: An experiment in role effectiveness and role development.* Duarte, CA: City of Hope National Medical Center.

Backshieder, J. (1971). The clinical nursing specialist as a practitioner. *Nursing Forum, 10* (4), 359–377.

Baer, E. (1987). "A cooperative venture" in pursuit of professional status: A research journal for nursing. *Nursing Research, 36,* 18–25.

Baker, C., & Kramer, M. (1970). To define or not to define: The role of the clinical specialist. *Nursing Forum, 9* (1), 41–55.

Baker, P.O. (1987). Model activities for clinical nurse specialist role development. *Clinical Nurse Specialist, 1* (3), 119–123.

Baker, V.E (1973). Retrospective explorations in role development. In J. Riehl & J. McVay (Eds.), *The clinical nurse specialist: Interpretations.* New York: Appleton-Century-Crofts.

Bang, A., Morse, J., & Campion, E. (1984). Transition of VA acute care hospital into acute and long-term care. In T. Wetle & J. Rowe (Eds.), *Older veterans: Linking VA and community resources.* Cambridge, MA: Harvard University Press, pp. 69–88.

Barnard, K.E. (1980). Knowledge for practice: Directions for the future. *Nursing Research, 29* (4), 208–212.

Barnes, J.C., & Smith, W.L. (1978). The VATER association. *Radiology, 126,* 445–450.

Barnum, B. (1987). Nursing: Now, then, and maybe again. *Nursing Outlook, 35,* 219–221.

Barrett, J. (1971). Administrative factors in development of new nursing practice roles. *Journal of Nursing Administration, 1* (4), 25–29.

Barrett, J. (1972). The nurse specialist practitioner: A study. *Nursing Outlook, 20* (8), 524–527.

Barron, A.M. (1983). The CNS as consultant. In A. Hamric & J. Spross (Eds.), *The clinical nurse specialist in theory and practice.* Orlando, FL: Grune & Stratton.

Beare, P. (1988). The ABCs of external consultation. *Clinical Nurse Specialist, 2,* 35–38.

Beck, A. (1976). *Cognitive therapy and the emotional disorders.* New York: New American Library.

Beeber, L. & Scicchitani, B. (1980). Should the clinical nurse specialist be free of administrative responsibility? *Perspectives in Psychiatric Care, 18* (6), 250–269.

Beecroft, P., & Papenhausen, J. (1985). CNS survey. Unpublished research.

Beecroft, P., & Papenhausen, J. (1987). Editorial opinion. *Clinical Nurse Specialist, 1,* 53.

Beecroft, P., & Papenhausen, J. (1988). Editorial opinion. *Clinical Nurse Specialist, 2,* 1–2.

Benner, P. (1984). *From novice to expert.* Menlo Park, CA: Addison-Wesley.

Benner, P. (1985). The oncology clinical nurse specialist: An expert coach. *Oncology Nursing Forum, 12* (2), 40–44.

Benner, P., & Tanner, C. (1987). Clinical judgment: How expert nurses use intuition. *American Journal of Nursing, 87* (1), 23–31.

Blake, P. (1977). The clinical specialist as nurse consultant. *Journal of Nursing Administration, 7* (10), 33–36.

Blount, M., Burges, S., Crigler, L., et al. (1981). Extending the influence of the clinical nurse specialist. *Nursing Administration Quarterly, 6* (1), 53–63.

Boucher, R. (1972). *Similarities and differences in the perception of the role of the clinical specialist,* Vol. I. Kansas City, MO: American Nurses' Association.

Brigman, C., Dickey, C., & Zegeer, L.J. (1983). The agitated-aggressive patient. *American Journal of Nursing, 83* (10), 1408–1412.

Brodish, M.S., Chamings, P.A., & Tranbarger, R.E. (1987). Fostering a research focus for the clinical nurse specialist. *Clinical Nurse Specialist, 1* (3), 99–104.

Brooten, D., Kumer, S., & Brown, L.P., et al. (1986). A randomized clinical trial of early hospital discharge and home follow-up of very-low-birth-weight infants. *New England Journal of Medicine, 315* (15), 934–939.

Brown, E.L. (1948). *Nursing for the future.* New York: Russell Sage Foundation.

Brown, M. & Wilson, C. (1987). Time management and the clinical nurse specialist. *Clinical Nurse Specialist, 1* (1), 32–38.

Brown, S.S. (1983). Administrative support. In A. Hamric & J. Spross (Eds.), *The clinical nurse specialist in theory and practice.* Orlando, FL: Grune & Stratton.

Bruce, S. (1972). *Valuation of functions of the role of the clinical nursing specialist,* Vol. II. Kansas City, MO: American Nurses' Association.

Buhler-Wilkerson, K. (1987). Left carrying the bag: Experiments in visiting nursing, 1877–1909. *Nursing Research, 36,* 42–47.

Burchell, R.C., Thomas, D.A., & Smith, H.L. (1983). Some considerations for implementing collaborative practice. *American Journal of Medicine, 74* (9), 9–13.

Burke, L.E. (1978). Anticipatory grief in spouses of the critically ill. Master's thesis, University of California, Los Angeles, School of Nursing.

Burke, L.E. (1981). Learning and retention in the acute care setting. *Critical Care Quarterly, 4* (3), 67–73.

Burke, L.E. (1983). The clinical nurse specialist in collaborative practice. *Momentum, 1* (2), 3–5.

Butts, P. (1974). The clinical specialist vs. the clinical supervisor. *Supervisor Nurse, 5* (4), 38–44.

Cahill, I. (1973). The development of maternity nursing as a specialty. In J. Riehl & J. McVay (Eds.), *The clinical nurse specialist: Interpretations.* New York: Appleton-Century-Crofts.

California Nurses' Association. (1984). *Position statement on specialization in nursing practice.* San Francisco: California Nurses' Association.

Calkin, J.D. (1984). A model for advanced nursing practice. *Journal of Nursing Administration, 14* (1), 24–30.

Calley, J.M., Dirksen, M., Engalla, M., & Hennrich, M.L. (1980). The Orem self-care nursing model. In J.P. Riehl & C. Roy (Eds.), *Conceptual models for nursing practice,* (2nd ed.). New York: Appleton-Century-Crofts.

Callister, J. (1985). Lara's story. *UCSF Magazine, 8* (3), 40–45.

Campbell, J.M. (1982). Practice management-reimbursement basics. *Pediatric Nursing, 8,* 424.

Caplan, G. (1970). *The theory and practice of mental health consultation.* New York: Basic Books.

Case management, career plan described. (1988). *The American Nurse, 20* (6) 5.

Castronovo, F. (1975). The effective use of the clinical specialist. *Supervisor Nurse, 6* (5), 48–56.

Chambers, J., Dangel, R., & Germon, K., et al. (1987). Clinical nurse specialist collaboration: Development of a generic job description and standards of performance. *Clinical Nurse Specialist, 1,* 124–127.

Chang, M. (1984). The effect of diaphragmatic and pursed lip breathing on oral temperature. *Proceedings of Octoberquest '84: Nursing Research Conference.*

Chang, M. (1985). Temperature changes with breathing effort. *American Journal of Nursing, 85* (7), 775.

Christman, L. (1965). The influence of specialization on the nursing profession. *Nursing Science, 3* (6), 446–453.

Christman, L. (1987). The future of the nursing profession. *Nursing Administration Quarterly, 11*, 1–8.

Church, O. (1987). From custody to community in psychiatric nursing. *Nursing Research, 36*, 48–55.

Cipriano, P.F. (1986). Certification: Self-regulation for specialty practice. In *Patterns in specialization: Challenge to the curriculum.* New York: National League for Nursing.

Colavecchio, R., Tescher, B., & Scalzi, C. (1974). A clinical ladder for nursing practice. *The Journal of Nursing Administration, 4*, 54–58.

Colavecchio, R., Tescher, B., & Scalzi, C. (1975). A clinical ladder for nursing practice . . . University of California Health Care Facilities. *Nursing Digest, 3*, 5–9.

Coleman, L.J. (1980). Orem's self-care concept of nursing. In J.P. Riehl & C. Roy (Eds.), *Conceptual models for nursing practice* (2nd ed.). New York: Appleton-Century-Crofts.

Colerick, E.J., Mason, P.B., & Proulx, J.R. (1980). Evaluation of the clinical nurse specialist role: Development and implementation of a dual purpose framework. *Nursing Leadership, 3* (3), 26–34.

Cooper, D.M. (1983). A refined expert: The clinical nurse specialist after five years. *Momentum, 1* (3), 1–2.

Cooper, D.M. (1989). *Steroids, vitamin A, and soft tissue healing: What does it say for practice?* (Manuscript in process).

Coutant, N. (1982). Rage: Implied neurological correlates. *Journal of Neurosurgical Nursing, 14* (1), 28–33.

Crabtree, M. (1979). Effective utilization of clinical specialists within the organizational structure of hospital nursing service. *Nursing Administration Quarterly, 4* (1): 1–11.

Crawford-Gamble, T. (1986). An application of Levine's conceptual model. *Perioperative Nursing Quarterly, 2*, 63–70.

Cronenwett, L. (1986). The research role of the clinical nurse specialist. *Journal of Nursing Administration, 16* (4), 10–11.

Cronenwett, L. (1986). Research contributions of clinical nurse specialists. *Journal of Nursing Administration, 16* (6), 6–7.

Curtain, L. (1987). About nurses: Perceptions and misperceptions. *Nursing Management, 18* (1), 11–12.

Curtin, L. (1984). Wound management: Care and cost—an overview. *Nursing Management, 15*, 34–37.

Davidson, K.R., Donovan, K.B., & Gilman, C.S., et al. (1978). A descriptive study of the attitudes of psychiatrists toward the new role of the nurse therapist. *Journal of Psychiatric Nursing and Mental Health Services, 16* (11), 24–28.

Davis, D.S., Greig, A.E., Burkholder, J., & Keating, T. (1984). Evaluating advanced practice nurses. *Nursing Management, 15* (3), 44–47.

del Bueno, D.J., & Price, M.S. (1987). Interviewing for a CNS position? Ask the right questions. *Clinical Nurse Specialist, 1* (4), 179–184.

DeWitt, K. (1900). Specialties in nursing. *American Journal of Nursing, 1* (1), 14–17.

Dickson, G.L., & Lee-Villasenor, H. (1982). Nursing theory and practice: A self-care approach. *Advances in Nursing Science, 5,* 29–40.

Diers, D. (1985). Preparation of practitioners, clinical specialists, and clinicians. *Journal of Professional Nursing, 1* (1), 41–47.

Dirschel, K. (1976). The conception, gestation, and delivery of the clinical nursing specialist. In R. Rotkovich (Ed.), *Quality patient care and the role of the clinical nursing specialist.* New York: Wiley.

Disch, J. (1978). The clinical specialist in a large peer group. *Journal of Nursing Administration, 8* (12), 17–20.

Donoghue, M. & Spross, J.A. (1984). The future of the oncology clinical nurse specialist. *Oncology Nursing Forum, 11* (1), 74–78.

Edlund, B.J., & Hodges, L.C. (1983). Preparing and using the clinical nurse specialist. *Nursing Clinics of North America, 18* (3), 499–507.

Edlund, B.J., Hodges, L.C., & Poteet, G.W. (1987). Consultation: Doing it and doing it well. *Clinical Nurse Specialist, 1,* 86–90.

Edwards, J. (1971). Clinical specialists are not effective—why? *Supervisor Nurse, 2* (8), 38–41, 45, 47, 51.

Ehrlich, H., & Hunt, T.K. (1968). Effect of cortisone and vitamin A on wound healing. *Annals of Surgery, 167,* 324–328.

Everson, S. (1981). Integration of the role of clinical specialist. *The Journal of Continuing Education in Nursing, 12* (2), 16–19.

Fagin, C. (1967). The clinical specialist as supervisor. *Nursing Outlook, 15* (1), 34–36.

Fagin, C.M., & Lamberton, M.M. (1981). Nurse–physician collaboration: Evaluation of a nursing school–medical school joint practice. In L.H. Aiken (Ed.), *Health policy and nursing practice.* New York: McGraw-Hill.

Fanslow, C. (1976). Rehabilitation nursing. In R. Rockovitch (Ed.), *Quality patient care and the role of the clinical nursing specialist.* New York: Wiley.

Fawcett, J. (1984a). *Analysis and evaluation of conceptual models of nursing.* Philadelphia: F.A. Davis.

Fawcett, J. (1984b). The metaparadigm of nursing: Current status and future refinement. *Image. Journal of Nursing Scholarship, 16,* 84–87.

Feild, L. (1983). Current trends in education and implications for the future. In A.B. Hamric, and J. Spross (Eds.), *The clinical nurse specialist in theory and practice.* Orlando, FL: Grune & Stratton.

Felder, L.A. (1983). Direct patient care and independent practice. In A.B. Hamric and J. Spross (Eds.), *The clinical nurse specialist in theory and practice.* New York: Grune & Stratton.

Felton, G. (1987). Obstacles to nursing's preferred future. *Nursing Outlook, 35,* 126–128.

Fenton, M.V. (1985). Identifying competencies of clinical nurse specialists. *Journal of Nursing Administration, 15,* 31–37.

ヮguson, V. (1983). Foreward. In *Magnet hospitals: Attraction and retention of professional nurses.* Kansas City, MO: American Nurses' Association.

Fife, B., & Lemler, S. (1983). The psychiatric nurse specialist: A valuable asset in the general hospital. *Journal of Nursing Administration, 13* (4), 14–17.

Fralic, M.F. (1988). Nursing's precious resource: The clinical nurse specialist. *Journal of Nursing Administration, 18* (2), 5–6.

Freeman, B., Carwell, G., & McCraw, J. (1981). The quantitative study of the use of dextranomer in the management of infected wounds. *Surgery, Gynecology, & Obstetrics, 153*, 81–86.

Gallant, B., & McLane, A. (1979). Outcome criteria: A process for validation at the ûnit level. *Journal of Nursing Administration, 9* (1), 14–21.

Gallessich, J. (1983). *The profession and practice of consultation.* San Francisco: Jossey-Bass.

Georgopoulos, B., & Christman, L. (1970). The clinical nurse specialist: A role model. *American Journal of Nursing, 70* (5), 1030–1039.

Georgopoulos, B., & Jackson, M. (1970). Nursing kardex behavior in an experimental study of patient units with and without clinical nurse specialists. *Nursing Research, 19* (3), 196–218.

Georgopoulos, B., & Sana, J. (1971). Clinical nursing specialization and intershift report behaviour. *American Journal of Nursing, 71* (3), 538–545.

Gilliss, C., Sparacino, P., Gortner, S., & Kenneth, H. (1985). Events leading to the treatment of coronary artery disease: Implications for nursing care. *Heart-Lung, 14* (4), 350–356.

Girouard, S. (1978). The role of the clinical specialist as change agent: An experiment in preoperative teaching. *International Journal of Nursing Studies, 15* (2), 57–65.

Girouard, S. (1983). Theory-based practice: Functions, obstacles and solutions. In A.B. Hamric and J. Spross (Eds.), *The clinical nurse specialist in theory and practice.* Orlando, FL: Grune & Stratton.

Gleason, J., & Flynn, K. (1987). The surgical clinical nurse specialist as consultant in a tertiary care setting. *Clinical Nurse Specialist, 1*, 129–132.

Goertzen, I. (1987). Making nursing's vision a reality. *Nursing Outlook, 35*, 121–123.

Goman, C. (1988). Forecast '88: Ten leading healthcare experts discuss the future. *Healthcare Forum, 31* (1), 8–17.

Gordon, D.R. (1984). Research application: Identifying the use and misuse of formal models in nursing practice. In P. Benner (Ed.), *From novice to expert.* Menlo Park, CA: Addison-Wesley.

Gortner, S., Gilliss, C., Moran, J., et al. (1985). Expected and realized benefits from coronary bypass surgery in relation to severity of illness. *Cardiovascular Nursing, 21* (3), 13–18.

Gracey, D.R., McMichan, J.C., Divertie, M.B., & Howard, F.M. (1982). Respiratory failure in Guillain-Barre syndrome: A six-year experience. *Mayo Clinic Proceedings, 57*, 742–746.

Gresham, M. (1983) Joint appointments. In A. Hamric & J. Spross (Eds.), *The clinical nurse specialist in theory and practice.* Orlando, FL: Grune & Stratton.

Gross, N., Mason, W., & McEachern, A. (1958). *Explorations in role analysis.* New York: Wiley.

Hamric, A. (1983). Role development and role function. In A. Hamric & J. Spross (Eds.), *The clinical nurse specialist in theory and practice.* (pp. 187–206). Orlando, FL: Grune & Stratton.

Hamric, A., & Spross, J. (1983) *The clinical nurse specialist in theory and practice.* Orlando, FL: Grune & Stratton.

Hardy, M. (1983). Role differentiation with specialization and its effects on quality patient care. In N. Chaska (Ed.), *The nursing profession: A time to speak.* New York: McGraw-Hill.

Henderson, V. (1981). Implementing the clinical nurse specialist role: A success story. *Nursing Management, 12*, (11), 55–58.

Hendrix, M., & La Godna, G. (1982). Consultation: A political process aimed at change. In J. Lancaster & W. Lancaster (Eds.), *The nurse as a change agent.* St. Louis: Mosby.

Hirsch, J., Sparacino, P., & Doyle, M.B., et al. (1987). On the scene: Section II— University of California, San Francisco. *Nursing Administration Quarterly, 11*, 47–61.

Hodges, L.C., Poteet, G.W., & Edlund, B.J. (1985). Teaching clinical nurse specialist to lead . . . and to succeed. *Nursing and Health Care, 6* (4), 193– 196.

Hodgman, E.C. (1983). The CNS as researcher. In A.B. Hamric & J. Spross (Eds.), *The clinical nurse specialist in theory and practice.* Orlando, FL: Grune & Stratton.

Hoeffer, B., & Murphy, S. (1984). Specialization in nursing practice. In *Issues in professional nursing practice.* Kansas City, MO: American Nurses' Association, pp. 1–10.

Holt, F.M. (1984). A theoretical model for clinical specialist practice. *Nursing and Health Care, 5*, (8), 445–449.

Holt, F.M. (1987). Executive practice role. Editorial. *Clinical Nurse Specialist, 1* (3), 116–118.

Howell, L.J. (1980). *Preschool children after open heart surgery: Parental childrearing practices.* Master's thesis, University of California, San Francisco.

Hunt, T.K. (1976). Control of wound healing with cortisone and vitamin A. In J.J. Longacre (Ed.), *The ultrastructure of collagen.* Springfield, IL: Thomas.

Hunt, T.K., Ehrlich, H.P., Garcia, J., & Dunphy, J.E. (1969). Effect of vitamin A on reversing the inhibitory effect of cortisone on healing of open wounds in animals and man. *Annals of Surgery, 170*, 633–641.

Jackson, B. (1973). Hospital administrators need to know about clinical specialists. *Supervisor Nurse, 4* (9), 29–34.

Jacobsson, S., Rothman, U., Arturson, G., et al. (1976). A new principle for the cleansing of infected wounds. *Scandinavian Journal of Plastic and Reconstructive Surgery, 10*, 65–72.

Jacox, A. (1974). Nursing research and the clinician. *Nursing Outlook, 22* (6), 382–385.

Jacox, A. (1980). Strategies to promote nursing research. *Nursing Research, 29* (4), 213–217.

James, W. (1958). *Talks to teachers.* New York: W.W. Norton and Company.

Johnson, D., Wilcox, J., & Moidel, H. (1967). The clinical nurse specialist as a practitioner. *American Journal of Nursing, 67* (11), 2298–2303.

Johnson, J. (1972). Effects of structuring patients' expectations on their reactions to threatening events. *Nursing Research, 21* (6), 499–503.

Johnson, J.E., Fuller, S.S., Endress, M.P., & Rice, V.H. (1978). Altering patients' responses to surgery: An extension and replication. *Research in Nursing and Health, 1* (3), 111–121.

Johnson, S.H. (1985). Specialization with collaboration. *Dimensions of Critical Care Nursing, 4* (5), 259–260.

Joseph, L.S. (1980). Self-care and the nursing process. *Nursing Clinics of North America, 15* (1), 131–143.

Kaiser, L. (1986). Anticipating your high-tech tomorrow. *Healthcare Forum, 29* (6), 12–18.

Kaiser, L. (1987). The intuitive manager and innovation. *Healthcare Forum, 30* (6), 15–17.

Kelly, L. (1987). To touch tomorrow. *Nursing Outlook, 35* (2), 59.

Kennedy, L., Neidlinger, S., & Scroggins, K. (1987). Effective comprehensive discharge planning for hospitalized elderly. *The Gerontologist, 27,* 577–580.

King, D., Barnard, K.E., & Hoehn, R. (1981). Disseminating the results of nursing research. *Nursing Outlook, 29* (2), 164–169.

Kohnke, M. (1978). *Case for consultation in nursing: Designs for professional practice.* New York: Wiley.

Kubler-Ross, E. (1969). *On death and dying.* New York: Macmillan.

Kwong, M., Manning, M.P., & Koetters, T.L. (1982). The role of the oncology clinical nurse specialist: Three personal views. *Cancer Nursing, 5* (6), 427–434.

Lange, F. (1979). The multi-faceted role of the nurse consultant. *Journal of Nursing Education, 8,* 30–34.

Laureau, S.C. (1985). The nurse as clinical consultant. *Topics in Clinical Nursing, 2,* 79–84.

Lawrence, P.R. (1969). How to deal with resistance to change. *Harvard Business Review, 47* (1), 4–6.

Lee, A.R. (1977). Creating a mental health consultation package for community agencies. *Hospital and Community Psychiatry, 28* (10), 745–748.

Levine, M. (1967). The four conservation principles of nursing. *Nursing Forum, 6,* 45–59.

Levine, M. (1969). *Introduction to clinical nursing.* Philadelphia: F.A. Davis.

Levine, M. (1969). The pursuit of wholeness. *American Journal of Nursing, 69,* 93–98.

Levine, M. (1971). Holistic nursing. *Nursing Clinics of North America, 6,* 253–264.

Levine, M. (1978). *Introduction to clinical nursing* (2nd ed.). Philadelphia: F.A. Davis.

Lewin, K. (1947, June). Frontiers in group dynamics: Concept, method and reality in social science, social equilibria and social change. *Human Relations, 1,* 5–41.

Lewinsohn, P.M., Sullivan, M.J., & Grosscup, S.J. (1982). Behavioral therapy: Clinical applications. In A.J. Rush (Ed.), *Short-term psychotherapies for depression.* New York: The Guilford Press.

Lewis, A. & Levy, J.S. (1982). *Psychiatric liaison nursing: The theory and clinical practice.* Reston, VA: Reston Publishing.

Lewis, E.P. (1970). *The clinical nurse specialist.* New York: American Journal of Nursing, Educational Services Division.

Linde, B., & Janz, N. (1979). Effect of a teaching program on knowledge and compliance of cardiac patients. *Nursing Research, 28* (5), 282–286.

Littell, S. (1981). The clinical nurse specialist in a private medical practice. *Nursing Administration Quarterly, 6* (1), 77–85.

Little, D. & Carnevali, D. (1967). Nurse specialist effect on tuberculosis. *Nursing Research, 16* (4), 321–326.

Luna-Raines, M. (1989). The confused response. In B. Riegel & D. Ehrenreich (Eds.) *Psychological Aspects of critical care nursing.* Rockville, Maryland: Aspen Publishers.

MacPhail, J. (1971). Reasonable expectations for the nurse clinician. *Journal of Nursing Administration, 1* (5), 16–18.

Malone, B.L. (1986). Evaluation of the clinical nurse specialist. *American Journal of Nursing, 86* (12), 1375–1377.

Mather, J. (1984). An overview of the Veterans Administration and its services for older veterans. In T. Wetle & J. Rowe (Eds.), *Older veterans: Linking VA and community resources.* Cambridge: Harvard University Press, pp. 35–48.

Mayo, A.A. (1944). Advanced courses in clinical nursing. *American Journal of Nursing, 44* (6), 579–585.

McCorkle, R. & Young, K. (1978). Development of a symptom distress rating scale. *Cancer Nursing, 1* (5), 373–378.

McCormick, R. & Parkevich, T. (1979). *Patient and family education: Tools, techniques and theory.* New York: Wiley.

McGann, M. (1975). The clinical specialist: From hospital, to clinic, to community. *Journal of Nursing Administration, 5* (3), 33–37.

McGee, R.F., Powell, M.L., Broadwell, D.C., & Clark, J.C. (1987). A delphi survey of oncology clinical nurse specialist competencies. *Oncology Nursing Forum, 14* (2), 29–34.

McLean, P. (1982). Behavioral therapy: Theory and research. In A.J. Rush (Ed.), *Short-term psychotherapies for depression.* New York: The Guilford Press.

Mensh, I. (1979). Acute, reversible, psychotic reactions in geriatric patients. In O.J. Kaplan (Ed.), *Psychopathology of aging.* New York: Academic Press.

Minarik, P.A. (1984). The psychiatric liaison nurse's role with families in acute care. *Nursing Clinics of North America, 19* (1), 161–171.

Montemuro, M.A. (1987). The evolution of the clinical nurse specialist: Response to the challenge of professional nursing practice. *Clinical Nurse Specialist, 1,* 106–110.

Morath, J. (1983). Putting leaders, consultants and teachers on the line. *Nursing Management, 14,* (1), 50–52.

Morath, J.M. (1988). The clinical nurse specialist: Evaluation issues. *Nursing Management, 19* (3), 72–80.

Moritz, D.A. (1978). Understanding anger. *American Journal of Nursing, 78* (1), 81–83.

Mullin, V.I. (1980). Implementing the self-care concept in the acute care setting. *Nursing Clinics of North America, 15* (1), 177–190.

Mumford, E., Schlesinger, H.J., Glass, G.V., et al. (1984). A new look at evidence about reduced cost of medical utilization following mental health treatment. *American Journal of Psychiatry, 141* (10), 1145–1158.

Munro, B.H. (1987). The research role of the clinical nurse specialist. *Clinical Nurse Specialist, 1* (1), 7.

Murphy, J. (1971). If p (additional nursing care), then q (quality of patient welfare)? In M. Batey (Ed.), *Communicating nursing research.* Boulder, CO: Western Interstate Commission for Higher Education.

National Joint Practice Commission. (1977). *Statement on joint practice in primary care: Definitions and guidelines.* Chicago: National Joint Practice Commission.

National League for Nursing. (1958). *The educational preparation of the clinical nurse specialist in psychiatric nursing.* New York: National League for Nursing.

National League for Nursing. (1969). *A review of the preparation and roles of the clinical nurse specialist: Extending the boundaries of nursing education.* New York: National League for Nursing.

Neidlinger, S., Kennedy, L., & Scroggins, K. (1987). Effective and cost efficient discharge planning for hospitalized elders. *Nursing Economics, 5* (5), 225–230.

Nelson, J.K.N., & Schilke, D.A. (1976). The evolution of psychiatric liaison nursing. *Perspectives in Psychiatric Care, 14,* 61.

Nichols, E., Barstow, R., & Cooper, D. (1983). Relationship between the incidence of phlebitis and frequency of changing IV tubing and percutaneous site. *Nursing Research, 32* (4). 247–252.

Niessner, P. (1979). The clinical specialist's contribution to quality nursing care. *Nursing Leadership, 2* (1), 21–30.

Noll, M. (1987). Internal consultation as a framework for clinical nurse specialist practice. *Clinical Nurse Specialist, 1,* 46–50.

Novaco, R.W. (1976). The functions and regulation of the arousal of anger. *American Journal of Psychiatry, 133* (10), 1124–1128.

Nursing research on fast track at national center. (1988) *The American Nurse, 20* (6) 27.

O'Brien, P. (1987). "All a woman's life can bring": The domestic roots of nursing in Philadelphia 1830–1855. *Nursing Research, 36,* 12–17.

O'Connor, P. (1984). Resumes: Opening the door. *Nursing Economics, 2,* 428–431.

Oda, D. (1977). Specialized role development: A three-phase process. *Nursing Outlook, 25* (6), 374–377.

Oda, D.S. (1985). Community health nursing in innovative school health roles and programs. In S.E. Archer and R.P. Fleshman (Eds.), *Community health nursing.* Monterey, CA: Wadsworth Health Sciences.

Oda, D, Sparacino, P., & Boyd, P. (1988). Role advancement for the experienced clinical nurse specialist. *Clinical Nurse Specialist, 2* (4), 167–171.

Odello, E. (1973). The clinical specialist in a line position. *Supervisor Nurse, 4* (9), 36–41.

Oncology Nursing Society. (1987). The scope of advanced oncology nursing practice. *ONS News, 2* (2), 1.

Oncology Nursing Society and ANA. (1987). *Standards for oncology nursing practice.* Kansas City, MO: Oncology Nursing Society and ANA.

Oredsson, S., Gottrup, F., Beckmann, A., & Hohn, D. (1983). Activation of chemotactic factors in serum and wound fluid by dextranomer. *Surgery, 94,* 453–457.

Orem, D.E. (1985). *Nursing: Concepts of practice* (3rd ed.). New York: McGraw-Hill.

Padilla, G. & Padilla, G. (1979). Nursing roles to improve patient care. *Nursing Digest, 6* (4), 1–13.

Panicucci, C. (1983). Functional assessment of the older adult in the acute care setting. *The Nursing Clinics of North America, 18* (2), 355–363.

Parkis, E. (1974). The management role of the clinical specialist. (Part 1). *Supervisor Nurse, 5* (9), 44–51.

Parkis, E. (1974). The management role of the clinical specialist. (Part 2). *Supervisor Nurse, 5* (10), 24–35.

Paulen, A. (1985). Practice issues for the oncology clinical nurse specialist. *Oncology Nursing Forum, 12* (2), 37–39.

Peplau, H. (1952). *Interpersonal relations in nursing.* New York: G.P. Putnam's.

Peplau, H. (1965). Specialization in professional nursing. *Nursing Science, 3* (4), 268–287.

Pfeiffer, E. (1977). Psychopathology and social pathology. In J. Birren and K.W. Schaie (Eds.), *Handbook of the psychology of aging.* New York: Van Nostrand Reinhold.

Pollock, S.E. (1987). Clinical nursing research: The needed link for unifying professional nursing. *Clinical Nurse Specialist, 1* (1), 8–12.

Poole, W. (1986). Clinical nurse specialists. *UCSF Magazine, 9* (3), 31–39.

Poteet, G.W. (1987). Consultation. *Clinical Nurse Specialist, 1* (2), 85.

Pozen, M.W., Stechmiller, J.A., Harris, W., et al. (1977). A nurse rehabilitator's impact on patients with myocardial infarction. *Medical Care, 15* (10), 830–837.

Prydum, M. (1983). Guillain-Barre syndrome: Disease process. *Journal of Neurosurgical Nursing, 15* (1), 27–32.

Raskind, M., Alvarez, C., & Pietrzyk, M., et al. (1976). Helping the elderly psychiatric patient in crisis. *Geriatrics, 31,* 51–56.

Redman, B.K. (1980). *Process of patient teaching in nursing.* St. Louis: Mosby.

Reiter, F. (1966). The nurse clinician. *American Journal of Nursing, 66* (2), 274–280.

Reverby, S. (1987). A caring dilemma: Womanhood and nursing in historical perspective. *Nursing Research, 36* (1). 5–11.

Rew, L. (1988). AFFIRM the role of the clinical specialist in private practice. *Clinical Nurse Specialist, 2* (1). 39–43.

Ringold, E. (1988). Nursing in crisis. *McCall's, CXV* (2), 54–65.

Roberts, L.R. (1987). Clinical nurse specialist: Line or staff using Lewin's field theory to resolve the issue. *Clinical Nurse Specialist, 1* (1), 39–44.

Robichaud, A.M., & Hamric, A.B. (1986). Time documentation of clinical nurse specialist activities. *Journal of Nursing Administration, 16* (1), 31–36.

Rodgers, J.A. (1973). Theoretical considerations in the process of change. *Nursing Forum, 12* (2), 160–174.

Rogge, M. (1987). Nursing and politics: A forgotten legacy. *Nursing Research, 36* (1). 26–30.

Ropper, A.H. & Shahant, B.T. (1984). Pain in Guillain-Barre syndrome. *Archives of Neurology, 41,* 511–514.

Ruben, R.J., Newton, L., Jornsay, D., et al. (1982). Home care of the pediatric patient with a tracheotomy. *Annals of Otology, Rhinology, and Laryngology, 91* (6), Part 1: 633–640.

Salahuddin, M. (1988). AMA seeks new nursing job category. *The Pennsylvania Nurse, 43* (7), 16, 3.

Sarbin, T., & Allen, V. (1968). Role theory. In G. Lindzey and E. Aronson (Eds.), *Handbook of social psychology.* Menlo Park, CA: Addison-Wesley.

Scalzi, C.C., Burke, L.E., & Greenland, S. (1980). Evaluation of an inpatient educational program for coronary patients and family. *Heart and Lung, 9* (5), 846–853.

Schlotfeldt, R. (1987). Reflection on nursing, 1987. *Nursing Outlook, 35* (5). 226–228.

SDVAMC. (1984). *Functions and responsibilities of the clinical nurse specialist.* San Diego: San Diego Veterans Administration Medical Center Nursing Service.

Shaefer, J. (1973). The satisfied clinician: Administrative support makes the difference. *Journal of Nursing Administration, 3* (4), 17–20.

Siehl, S. (1982). The clinical nurse specialist in oncology. *Nursing Clinics of North America, 17* (4), 753–761.

Sills, G.M. (1983). The role and function of the clinical nurse specialist. In N.L. Chaska (Ed.), *The nursing profession: A time to speak.* New York: McGraw-Hill.

Simms, L. (1965). The clinical nursing specialist: An experiment. *Nursing Outlook, 13* (8), 26–28.

Sisson, R. (1987). Co-workers' perceptions of the clinical nurse specialist role. *Clinical Nurse Specialist, 1,* 13–17.

Smith, M. (1974). Perceptions of head nurses, clinical nurse specialists, nursing educators, and nursing office personnel regarding performance of selected nursing activities. *Nursing Research, 23* (6), 505–511.

Sneed, N.V. (1987). Collaboration as a means to achieving the clinical nurse specialist research role expectations. *Clinical Nurse Specialist, 1* (1), 70–74.

Sovie, M. (1984). The economics of magnetism. *Nursing Economics, 2* (2): 85–92.

Sparacino, P.S.A., & Durand, B.A. (1986). Editorial on specialization in advanced nursing practice. *Momentum, 4* (2), 1–4.

Spross, J., & Hamric, A.B. (1983). A model for future clinical specialist practice. In A.B. Hamric & J. Spross (Eds.), *The clinical nurse specialist in theory and practice.* (pp. 291–306) Orlando, FL: Grune & Stratton.

Starck, P. (1983). Factors influencing the role of the oncology clinical nurse specialist. *Oncology Nursing Forum, 10* (4), 54–58.

Steele, S. & Fenton, M. (1988). Expert practice of clinical nurse specialists. *Clinical Nurse Specialist, 2* (1), 45–51.

Stevens, B. (1976). Accountability of the clinical specialist: An administrator's viewpoint. *Journal of Nursing Administration, 6* (2), 30–32.

Styles, M. (1987). The tarnished opportunity. *Nursing Outlook, 35,* 229.

Styles, M.M. (1987). Nursing today and a vision for the future. *Nursing Economics, 5,* 103–117.

Suedfeld, P. (1969). Introduction and historical background. In J.P. Zubeck (Ed.), *Sensory deprivation: 15 years of research.* New York: Appleton-Century-Crofts.

Sullivan, T.J., Lee, J.L., & Warnick, M.L., et al. (1987). Nursing 2020: A study of nursing's future. *Nursing Outlook, 35* (5), 233–235.

Tarsitano, B.J., Brophy, E.B., & Snyder, D.J. (1986). A demystification of the clinical nurse specialist role: Perceptions of clinical nurse specialists and nurse administrators. *Journal of Nursing Education, 25,* (1) 4–9.

The Science of Caring: Nursing at University of California, San Francisco. (1985). San Francisco: School of Nursing, University of California, San Francisco.

The Science of Caring: Nursing at University of California, San Francisco. (1986). San Francisco: School of Nursing, University of California, San Francisco.

Thornton, R. & Nardi, P.M. (1975). The dynamics of role acquisition. *American Journal of Sociology, 80* (4), 870–885.

Topham, D.L. (1987). Role theory in relation to role of the clinical nurse specialist. *Clinical Nurse Specialist, 1* (2), 81–84.

Tucker, J.A., & Silberman, H.D. (1972). Tracheotomy in pediatrics. *Annals of Otology, Rhinology, and Laryngology, 81,* 818–824.

Turner, R.H. (1978). The role and the person. *American Journal of Sociology, 84* (1), 1–23.

Underwood, P.R. (1980). Facilitating self-care. In P.C. Pothier (Ed.), *Psychiatric nursing*. Boston: Little, Brown.

University of California, San Francisco. (1983). *Philosophy: Department of Nursing*. San Francisco: University of California, San Francisco.

University of California, San Francisco Medical Center. (1986). Clinical nurse specialists: Role markers for the clinical nurse specialist. (Unpublished) Presented by M. Inturrisi & D. Oda, *CNS role development and evaluation*, at UCSF Conference, "Create the Future Now," February 12–13, 1987, San Francisco, CA.

Veterans Administration. (1984). *A summary of veterans administration benefits*. VA Pamphlet 27-82-2. Department of Veterans Benefits.

Walker, D. (1983). Administrative utilization of the CNS. In A. Hamric & J. Spross (Eds.), *The clinical nurse specialist in theory and practice*. Orlando, FL: Grune & Stratton.

Walker, M. (1986). How nursing service administrators view clinical nurse specialists. *Nursing Management, 17* (3), 52–54.

Weiss, S.J., & Davis, H.P. (1985). Validity and reliability of the collaborative practice scales. *Nursing Research, 34* (5), 299–305.

Welch-McCaffrey, D. (1985). Rationale, development and evaluation of a chemotherapy certification course for nurses. *Cancer Nursing, 8* (5), 255–262.

Welch-McCaffrey, D. (1986). Role performance issues for oncology clinical nurse specialists. *Cancer Nursing, 9* (6), 287–294.

Welch-McCaffrey, D. (1987). 2001: An oncology nurse odyssey. *Innovations in Oncology Nursing, 3* (4), 1, 12.

Welch-McCaffrey, D., & Dodge, J. (1988). Acute confusional states in elderly cancer patients. *Seminars in Oncology Nursing 4*, 208–216.

Werner, J.S., Bumann, R.M., & O'Brien, J.A. (1988). Clinical nurse specialization: An annotated bibliography. *Clinical Nurse Specialist, 2* (1): 14–15.

Wetmore, R.F., Handler, S.D., & Potsic, W.P. (1982). Pediatric tracheostomy experience during the past decade. *Annals of Otology, Rhinology, and Laryngology, 91* (6) Part 1: 628–632.

Will, G. (1988). The dignity of nursing. *Newsweek, CXI*: no 21 p. 80.

Wolanin, M.O., & Phillips, L.R.F. (1981). *Confusion: Prevention and care*. St. Louis: Mosby.

Woodrow, M., & Bell, J. (1971). Clinical specialization: Conflict between reality and theory. *Journal of Nursing Administration, 1* (6), 23–28.

Wyers, M.E.A., Grove, S.K., & Pastorino, C. (1985). Clinical nurse specialist: In search of the right role. *Nursing and Health Care, 6* (4), 203–207.

Yasko, J. (1985). The predicted effect of recent health care trends on the role of the oncology clinical nurse specialist. *Oncology Nursing Forum, 12* (2), 58–61.

Index